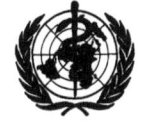 

WORLD HEALTH ORGANIZATION

INTERNATIONAL AGENCY FOR RESEARCH ON CANCER

IARC MONOGRAPHS
ON THE
EVALUATION OF THE CARCINOGENIC RISK OF CHEMICALS TO HUMANS

Some Pharmaceutical Drugs

VOLUME 24

This publication represents the views and expert opinions
of an IARC Working Group on the
Evaluation of the Carcinogenic Risk of Chemicals to Humans
which met in Lyon,
19-26 February 1980

Septembre 1980

INTERNATIONAL AGENCY FOR RESEARCH ON CANCER

IARC MONOGRAPHS

In 1971, the International Agency for Research on Cancer (IARC) initiated a programme on the evaluation of the carcinogenic risk of chemicals to humans involving the production of critically evaluated monographs on individual chemicals.

The objective of the programme is to elaborate and publish in the form of monographs critical reviews of data on carcinogenicity for groups of chemicals to which humans are known to be exposed, to evaluate those data in terms of human risk with the help of international working groups of experts in chemical carcinogenesis and related fields, and to indicate where additional research efforts are needed.

International Agency for Research on Cancer 1980

ISBN 92 832 1224 X

PRINTED IN SWITZERLAND

CONTENTS

LIST OF PARTICIPANTS 5

NOTE TO THE READER 9

PREAMBLE 11
    Background 11
    Objective and Scope 11
    Selection of Chemicals for Monographs 12
    Working Procedures 12
    Data for Evaluations 13
    The Working Group 13
    General Principles for Evaluating the Carcinogenic Risk of Chemicals ... 14
    Explanatory Notes on the Monograph Contents 20

GENERAL REMARKS ON THE SUBSTANCES CONSIDERED 33

THE MONOGRAPHS
    Clofibrate 39
    Dapsone 59
    Dihydroxymethylfuratrizine 77
    Hydralazine and hydralazine hydrochloride 85
    Methoxsalen 101
    Nafenopin 125
    Phenacetin 135
    Phenazopyridine and phenazopyridine hydrochloride 163
    Phenelzine and phenelzine sulphate 175
    Phenoxybenzamine and phenoxybenzamine hydrochloride 185
    Proflavine, proflavine dihydrochloride, proflavine hemisulphate and proflavine
        monohydrochloride 195
    Reserpine 211
    Rifampicin 243
    Spironolactone 259

Sulfafurazole (Sulphisoxazole) 275
Sulfamethoxazole 285

GENERAL CONSIDERATIONS ON *N*-NITROSATABLE DRUGS 297

SUPPLEMENTARY CORRIGENDA TO VOLUMES 1-23 315

CUMULATIVE INDEX TO MONOGRAPHS 317

IARC WORKING GROUP ON THE EVALUATION OF THE CARCINOGENIC RISK OF CHEMICALS TO HUMANS:

SOME PHARMACEUTICAL DRUGS

Lyon, 19-26 February 1980

Members[1]

R. Althouse, University of Oxford, Clinical Medical School, John Radcliffe Hospital, Oxford, UK

B.K. Armstrong, NHRMRC Research Unit in Epidemiology and Preventive Medicine, The University of Western Australia, Department of Medicine, Medical School Building, The Queen Elizabeth II Medical Centre, Nedlands, Western Australia 6009, Australia *(Vice-chairman; Co-rapporteur section 3.3)*

G. Della Porta, Director, Division of Experimental Oncology A, Istituto Nazionale per lo Studio et la Cura dei Tumori, Via G. Venezian 1, 20133 Milan, Italy

G.D. Friedman, Department of Medical Methods Research, Kaiser-Permanente Medical Care Program, 3700 Broadway, Oakland CA 94611, USA

C.A. Johnson, Secretary and Scientific Director, British Pharmacopoeia Commission, Market Towers, 1 Nine Elms Lane, London S.E., UK

A. Jori, Istituto di Ricerche Farmacologiche 'Mario Negri', Via Eritrea 62, 20157 Milan, Italy

R. Preussmann, Institut für Toxikologie und Chemotherapie, Deutsches Krebsforschungszentrum, Im Neuenheimer Feld 280, 6900 Heidelberg 1, Federal Republic of Germany *(Chairman; Co-rapporteur section 3.1)*

---

[1] Unable to attend: N.P. Napalkov, Director, Petrov Research Institute of Oncology, Leningradskaya Street 68, Pesochny-2, Leningrad 188646, USSR

J.K. Reddy, Northwestern University, Department of Pathology, The Medical School, Ward Memorial Building, 303 E. Chicago Avenue, Chicago IL 60611, USA

J.P. Seiler, Eidgenössische Forschungsanstalt für Obst-, Wein und Gartenbau, CH 8820 Wädenswil, Switzerland *(Co-rapporteur section 3.2)*

S. Shapiro, Co-director, Drug Epidemiology Unit, Boston University Medical Center, 777 Concord Avenue, Cambridge MA 02138, USA

T.H. Shepard, Department of Pediatrics, University of Washington, Seattle WA 98105, USA

B. Teichmann, Akademie der Wissenschaften der DDR, Zentralinstitut für Krebsforschung, Lindenberger Weg 80, 1115 Berlin-Buch, German Democratic Republic

B. Toth, The Eppley Institute for Research in Cancer, The University of Nebraska Medical Center, 42nd and Dewey Avenue, Omaha NE 68105, USA

N.M. Woolhouse, University of Ghana Medical School, Department of Biochemistry, P.O. Box 4236, Accra, Ghana *(Co-rapporteur section 3.2)*

Representatives from the National Cancer Institute

T. Cameron and D. Tidwell, National Cancer Institute, Division of Cancer Cause & Prevention, Landow Building, Rm 3C39, Bethesda MD 20014, USA

Representative from SRI International

J. Johansson, SRI International, 333 Ravenswood Avenue, Menlo Park CA 94025, USA *(Rapporteur sections 2.1 & 2.2)*

Representative from the Pharmaceutical Manufacturers' Association

J.M. Price, Vice-President Medical Affairs, Norwich-Eaton Pharmaceuticals, 17 Eaton Avenue, PO Box 191, Norwich NY 13815, USA

Representative from the World Health Organization

J.-F. Bertaux, Medical Officer, Pharmaceuticals, World Health Organization, 1211 Geneva 27, Switzerland

Representative from the Commission of the European Communities

M.-T. van der Venne, Commission of the European Communities, Health and Safety Directorate, Bâtiment Jean Monnet, Plateau du Kirchberg, Luxembourg, Grand Duchy of Luxembourg

Representative from the World Federation of Association of Clinical Toxicology Centres and Poison Control Centres

C. Vigneau, World Federation of Association of Clinical Toxicology Centres and Poison Control Centres, IARC

Secretariat

    C. Agthe, Director's Office, IARC, Lyon

    H. Bartsch, Division of Chemical and Biological Carcinogenesis *(Co-rapporteur section 3.2)*

    J.R.P. Cabral, Division of Chemical and Biological Carcinogenesis

    B. Dodet, Division of Chemical and Biological Carcinogenesis

    M. Friesen, Division of Chemical and Biological Carcinogenesis

    A. Geser, Division of Human Cancer and Field Programmes

    L. Griciute[1], Division of Chemical and Biological Carcinogenesis

    V. Khudoley, Division of Chemical and Biological Carcinogenesis

    A. Likhachev, Division of Chemical and Biological Carcinogenesis

    D. Mietton, Division of Chemical and Biological Carcinogenesis *(Library assistant)*

    R. Montesano, Division of Chemical and Biological Carcinogenesis *(Co-rapporteur section 3.1)*

    H. Ohshima, Division of Chemical and Biological Carcinogenesis

    C. Partensky, Division of Chemical and Biological Carcinogenesis *(Technical editor)*

    I. Peterschmitt, Division of Chemical and Biological Carcinogenesis, WHO, Geneva *(Bibliographic researcher)*

    R. Saracci, Division of Human Cancer and Field Programmes *(Co-rapporteur section 3.3)*

    L. Simonato, Division of Human Cancer and Field Programmes

    L. Tomatis, Director, Division of Chemical and Biological Carcinogenesis *(Head of the Programme)*

---

[1] Present address: The Oncological Institute of the Lithuanian SSR, 2 Polocko Street, 232007 Vilnius, Lithuanian SSR

E. Ward, Chârost, France *(Editor)*

J.D. Wilbourn, Division of Chemical and Biological Carcinogenesis *(Secretary)*

Secretarial assistance

A. Beevers
M.-J. Ghess
S. Reynaud
J. Smith

NOTE TO THE READER

The term 'carcinogenic risk' in the IARC Monograph series is taken to mean the probability that exposure to the chemical will lead to cancer in humans.

Inclusion of a chemical in the monographs does not imply that it is a carcinogen, only that published data have been examined. Equally, the fact that a chemical has not yet been evaluated in a monograph does not mean that it is not carcinogenic.

Anyone who is aware of published data that may alter the evaluation of the carcinogenic risk of a chemical for humans is encouraged to make this information available to the Division of Chemical and Biological Carcinogenesis, International Agency for Research on Cancer, Lyon, France, in order that the chemical may be considered for re-evaluation by a future Working Group.

Although every effort is made to prepare the monographs as accurately as possible, mistakes may occur. Readers are requested to communicate any errors to the Division of Chemical and Biological Carcinogenesis, so that corrections can be reported in future volumes.

IARC MONOGRAPH PROGRAMME ON THE EVALUATION OF THE CARCINOGENIC RISK OF CHEMICALS TO HUMANS

PREAMBLE

BACKGROUND

In 1971, the International Agency for Research on Cancer (IARC) initiated a programme on the evaluation of the carcinogenic risk of chemicals to humans with the object of producing monographs on individual chemicals[1]. The criteria established at that time to evaluate carcinogenic risk to humans were adopted by all the working groups whose deliberations resulted in the first 16 volumes of the *IARC Monograph* series. In October 1977, a joint IARC/WHO *ad hoc* Working Group met to re-evaluate these guiding criteria; this preamble reflects the results of their deliberations(1) and those of a subsequent IARC *ad hoc* Working Group which met in April 1978(2).

OBJECTIVE AND SCOPE

The objective of the programme is to elaborate and publish in the form of monographs critical reviews of data on carcinogenicity for groups of chemicals to which humans are known to be exposed, to evaluate those data in terms of human risk with the help of international working groups of experts in chemical carcinogenesis and related fields, and to indicate where additional research efforts are needed.

The monographs summarize the evidence for the carcinogenicity of individual chemicals and other relevant information. The critical analyses of the data are intended to assist national and international authorities in formulating decisions concerning preventive measures. No recommendations are given concerning legislation, since this depends on risk-benefit evaluations, which seem best made by individual governments and/or other international agencies. In this connection, WHO recommendations on food additives(3), drugs(4), pesticides and contaminants(5) and occupational carcinogens(6) are particularly informative.

---

[1] Since 1972, the programme has undergone considerable expansion, primarily with the scientific collaboration and financial support of the US National Cancer Institute, Bethesda, MD.

The *IARC Monographs* are recognized as an authoritative source of information on the carcinogenicity of environmental chemicals. The first users' survey, made in 1976, indicates that the monographs are consulted routinely by various agencies in 24 countries.

Since the programme began in 1971, 24 volumes have been published(7) in the *IARC Monograph* series, and 531 separate chemical substances have been evaluated (see also cumulative index to the monographs, p. 317). Each volume is printed in 4000 copies and distributed *via* the WHO publications service (see inside covers for a listing of IARC publications and back outside cover for distribution and sales services).

SELECTION OF CHEMICALS FOR MONOGRAPHS

The chemicals (natural and synthetic, including those which occur as mixtures and in manufacturing processes) are selected for evaluation on the basis of two main criteria: (a) there is evidence of human exposure, and (b) there is some experimental evidence of carcinogenicity and/or there is some evidence or suspicion of a risk to humans. In certain instances, chemical analogues were also considered. The scientific literature is surveyed for published data relevant to the monograph programme. In addition, the IARC *Survey of Chemicals Being Tested for Carcinogenicity*(8) often indicates those chemicals that are to be scheduled for future meetings.

Inclusion of a chemical in a volume does not imply that it is carcinogenic, only that the published data have been examined. The evaluations must be consulted to ascertain the conclusions of the Working Group. Equally, the fact that a chemical has not appeared in a monograph does not mean that it is without carcinogenic hazard.

As new data on chemicals for which monographs have already been prepared and new principles for evaluating carcinogenic risk receive acceptance, re-evaluations will be made at subsequent meetings, and revised monographs will be published as necessary.

WORKING PROCEDURES

Approximately one year in advance of a meeting of a working group, a list of the substances to be considered is prepared by IARC staff in consultation with other experts. Subsequently, all relevant biological data are collected by IARC; in addition to the published literature, US Public Health Service Publication No. 149(9) has been particularly valuable and has been used in conjunction with other recognized sources of information on chemical carcinogenesis and systems such as CANCERLINE, MEDLINE and TOXLINE. The major collection of data and the preparation of first drafts for the sections on chemical and physical properties, on production, use, occurrence and on analysis are carried out by SRI International, Stanford, CA, USA under a separate contract with the US National Cancer Institute. Most of the data so obtained on production, use and occurrence refer to the

PREAMBLE

United States and Japan; SRI International and IARC supplement this information with that from other sources in Europe. Bibliographical sources for data on mutagenicity and teratogenicity are the Environmental Mutagen Information Center and the Environmental Teratology Information Center, both located at the Oak Ridge National Laboratory, TN, USA.

Six to nine months before the meeting, reprints of articles containing relevant biological data are sent to an expert(s), or are used by the IARC staff, for the preparation of first draft monographs. These drafts are edited by IARC staff and are sent prior to the meeting to all participants of the Working Group for their comments. The Working Group then meets in Lyon for seven to eight days to discuss and finalize the texts of the monographs and to formulate the evaluations. After the meeting, the master copy of each monograph is verified by consulting the original literature, then edited and prepared for reproduction. The monographs are usually published within six months after the Working Group meeting.

DATA FOR EVALUATIONS

With regard to biological data, only reports that have been published or accepted for publication are reviewed by the working groups, although a few exceptions have been made. The monographs do not cite all of the literature on a particular chemical: only those data considered by the Working Group to be relevant to the evaluation of the carcinogenic risk of the chemical to humans are included.

Anyone who is aware of data that have been published or are in press which are relevant to the evaluations of the carcinogenic risk to humans of chemicals for which monographs have appeared is urged to make them available to the Division of Chemical and Biological Carcinogenesis, International Agency for Research on Cancer, Lyon, France.

THE WORKING GROUP

The tasks of the Working Group are five-fold: (a) to ascertain that all data have been collected; (b) to select the data relevant for the evaluation; (c) to ensure that the summaries of the data enable the reader to follow the reasoning of the committee; (d) to judge the significance of the results of experimental and epidemiological studies; and (e) to make an evaluation of the carcinogenic risk of the chemical.

Working Group participants who contributed to the consideration and evaluation of chemicals within a particular volume are listed, with their addresses, at the beginning of each publication (see p. 5). Each member serves as an individual scientist and not as a representative of any organization or government. In addition, observers are often invited from national and international agencies, organizations and industries.

GENERAL PRINCIPLES FOR EVALUATING THE CARCINOGENIC RISK OF CHEMICALS

The widely accepted meaning of the term 'chemical carcinogenesis', and that used in these monographs, is the induction by chemicals of neoplasms that are not usually observed, the earlier induction by chemicals of neoplasms that are usually observed, and/or the induction by chemicals of more neoplasms than are usually found - although fundamentally different mechanisms may be involved in these three situations. Etymologically, the term 'carcinogenesis' means the induction of cancer, that is, of malignant neoplasms; however, the commonly accepted meaning is the induction of various types of neoplasms or of a combination of malignant and benign tumours. In the monographs, the words 'tumour' and 'neoplasm' are used interchangeably. (In scientific literature the terms 'tumourigen', 'oncogen' and 'blastomogen' have all been used synonymously with 'carcinogen', although occasionally 'tumourigen' has been used specifically to denote a substance that induces benign tumours.)

Experimental Evidence

Qualitative aspects

Both the interpretation and evaluation of a particular study as well as the overall assessment of the carcinogenic activity of a chemical involve several qualitatively important considerations, including: (a) the experimental parameters under which the chemical was tested, including route of administration and exposure, species, strain, sex, age, etc.; (b) the consistency with which the chemical has been shown to be carcinogenic, e.g., in how many species and at which target organ(s); (c) the spectrum of neoplastic response, from benign neoplasia to multiple malignant tumours; (d) the stage of tumour formation in which a chemical may be involved: some chemicals act as complete carcinogens and have initiating and promoting activity, while others are promoters only; and (e) the possible role of modifying factors.

There are problems not only of differential survival but of differential toxicity, which may be manifested by unequal growth and weight gain in treated and control animals. These complexities should also be considered in the interpretation of data, or, better, in the experimental design.

Many chemicals induce both benign and malignant tumours; few instances are recorded in which only benign neoplasms are induced by chemicals that have been studied extensively. Benign tumours may represent a stage in the evolution of a malignant neoplasm or they may be 'end-points' that do not readily undergo transition to malignancy. If a substance is found to induce only benign tumours in experimental animals, the chemical should be suspected of being a carcinogen and requires further investigation.

Hormonal carcinogenesis

Hormonal carcinogenesis presents certain distinctive features: the chemicals involved occur both endogenously and exogenously; in many instances, long exposure is required; tumours occur in the target tissue in association with a stimulation of non-neoplastic growth, but in some cases, hormones promote the proliferation of tumour cells in a target organ. Hormones that occur in excessive amounts, hormone-mimetic agents and agents that cause hyperactivity or imbalance in the endocrine system may require evaluative methods comparable with those used to identify chemical carcinogens; particular emphasis must be laid on quantitative aspects and duration of exposure. Some chemical carcinogens have significant side effects on the endocrine system, which may also result in hormonal carcinogenesis. Synthetic hormones and anti-hormones can be expected to possess other pharmacological and toxicological actions in addition to those on the endocrine system, and in this respect they must be treated like any other chemical with regard to intrinsic carcinogenic potential.

Quantitative aspects

Dose-response studies are important in the evaluation of carcinogenesis: the confidence with which a carcinogenic effect can be established is strengthened by the observation of an increasing incidence of neoplasms with increasing exposure.

The assessment of carcinogenicity in animals is frequently complicated by recognized differences among the test animals (species, strain, sex, age), route(s) of administration and in dose/duration of exposure; often, target organs at which a cancer occurs and its histological type may vary with these parameters. Nevertheless, indices of carcinogenic potency in particular experimental systems [for instance, the dose-rate required under continuous exposure to halve the probability of the animals remaining tumourless[10]] have been formulated in the hope that, at least among categories of fairly similar agents, such indices may be of some predictive value in other systems, including humans.

Chemical carcinogens differ widely in the dose required to produce a given level of tumour induction, although many of them share common biological properties, which include metabolism to reactive [electrophilic[11-13]] intermediates capable of interacting with DNA. The reason for this variation in dose-response is not understood, but it may be due either to differences within a common metabolic process or to the operation of qualitatively distinct mechanisms.

Statistical analysis of animal studies

Tumours which would have arisen had an animal lived longer may not be observed because of the death of the animal from unrelated causes, and this possibility must be allowed for. Various analytical techniques have been developed which use the assumption of independence of competing risks to allow for the effects of intercurrent mortality on the final numbers of tumour-bearing animals in particular treatment groups.

For externally visible tumours and for neoplasms that cause death, methods such as Kaplan-Meier (i.e., 'life-table', 'product-limit', or 'actuarial') estimates(10), with associated significance tests(14,15), are recommended.

For internal neoplasms which are discovered 'incidentally'(14) at autopsy but which did not cause the death of the host, different estimates(16) and significance tests(14,15) may be necessary for the unbiased study of the numbers of tumour-bearing animals.

All of these methods(10,14-16) can be used to analyse the numbers of animals bearing particular tumour types, but they do not distinguish between animals with one or many such tumours. In experiments which end at a particular fixed time, with the simultaneous sacrifice of many animals, analysis of the total numbers of internal neoplasms per animal found at autopsy at the end of the experiment is straightforward. However, there are no adequate statistical methods for analysing the numbers of particular neoplasms that kill an animal.

Evidence of Carcinogenicity in Humans

Evidence of carcinogenicity in humans can be derived from three types of study, the first two of which usually provide only suggestive evidence: (1) reports concerning individual cancer patients (case reports), including a history of exposure to the supposed carcinogenic agent; (2) descriptive epidemiological studies in which the incidence of cancer in human populations is found to vary (spatially or temporally) with exposure to the agent; and (3) analytical epidemiological studies (e.g., case-control or cohort studies) in which individual exposure to the agent is found to be associated with an increased risk of cancer.

An analytical study that shows a positive association between an agent and a cancer may be interpreted as implying causality to a greater or lesser extent, if the following criteria are met. (a) There is no identifiable positive bias. [By 'positive bias' is meant the operation of factors in study design or execution which lead erroneously to a more strongly positive association between an agent and disease than in fact exists. Examples of positive bias include, in case-control studies, better documentation of exposure to the agent for cases than for controls, and, in cohort studies, the use of better means of detecting cancer in individuals exposed to the agent than in individuals not exposed.] (b) The possibility of positive confounding has been considered. [By 'positive confounding' is meant a situation in which the relationship between an agent and a disease is rendered more strongly positive than it truly is as a result of an association between that agent and another agent which either causes or prevents the disease. An example of positive confounding is the association between coffee consumption and lung cancer, which results from their joint association with cigarette smoking.]   (c) The association is unlikely to be due to chance alone. (d) The association is strong. (e) There is a dose-response relationship.

In some instances, a single epidemiological study may be strongly indicative of a cause-effect relationship; however, the most convincing evidence of causality comes when several independent studies done under different circumstances result in 'positive' findings.

Analytical epidemiological studies that show no association between an agent and a cancer ('negative' studies) should be interpreted according to criteria analogous to those listed above: (a) there is no identifiable negative bias; (b) the possibility of negative confounding has been considered; and (c) the possible effects of misclassification of exposure or outcome have been weighed.

In addition, it must be recognized that in any study there are confidence limits around the estimate of association or relative risk. In a study regarded as 'negative', the upper confidence limit may indicate a relative risk substantially greater than unity; in that case, the study excludes only relative risks that are above this upper limit. This usually means that a 'negative' study must be large to be convincing. Confidence in a 'negative' result is increased when several independent studies carried out under different circumstances are in agreement.

Finally, a 'negative' study may be considered to be relevant only to dose levels within or below the range of those observed in the study and is pertinent only if sufficient time has elapsed since first human exposure to the agent. Experience with human cancers of known etiology suggests that the period from first exposure to a chemical carcinogen to development of clinically observed cancer is usually measured in decades and may be in excess of 30 years.

Experimental Data Relevant to the Evaluation of Carcinogenic Risk to Humans

No adequate criteria are presently available to interpret experimental carcinogenicity data directly in terms of carcinogenic potential for humans. Nonetheless, utilizing data collected from appropriate tests in animals, positive extrapolations to possible human risk can be approximated.

Information compiled from the first 24 volumes of the *IARC Monographs*(17-19) shows that of the 37 chemicals, groups of chemicals or manufacturing processes now generally accepted to cause or probably to cause cancer in humans, all but possibly two (arsenic and benzene) of those which have been tested appropriately produce cancer in at least one animal species. For several of the chemicals that are carcinogenic for humans (aflatoxins, 4-aminobiphenyl, diethylstilboestrol, melphalan, mustard gas and vinyl chloride), evidence of carcinogenicity in experimental animals preceded evidence obtained from epidemiological studies or case reports.

In general, the evidence that a chemical produces tumours in experimental animals is of two degrees: (a) *sufficient evidence* of carcinogenicity is provided by the production of malignant tumours; and (b) *limited evidence* of carcinogenicity reflects qualitative and/or quantitative limitations of the experimental results.

For many of the chemicals evaluated in the first 24 volumes of the *IARC Monographs* for which there is *sufficient evidence* of carcinogenicity in animals, data relating to carcinogenicity for humans are either insufficient or nonexistent. In the absence of adequate data on humans, it is reasonable, for practical purposes, to regard such chemicals as if they presented a carcinogenic risk to humans.

Sufficient evidence of carcinogenicity is provided by experimental studies that show an increased incidence of malignant tumours: (i) in multiple species or strains, and/or (ii) in multiple experiments (routes and/or doses), and/or (iii) to an unusual degree (with regard to incidence, site, type and/or precocity of onset). Additional evidence may be provided by data concerning dose-response, mutagenicity or structure.

In the present state of knowledge, it would be difficult to define a predictable relationship between the dose (mg/kg bw/day) of a particular chemical required to produce cancer in test animals and the dose which would produce a similar incidence of cancer in humans. The available data suggest, however, that such a relationship may exist(20,21), at least for certain classes of carcinogenic chemicals. Data that provide *sufficient evidence* of carcinogenicity in test animals may therefore be used in an approximate quantitative evaluation of the human risk at some given exposure level, provided that the nature of the chemical concerned and the physiological, pharmacological and toxicological differences between the test animals and humans are taken into account. However, no acceptable methods are currently available for quantifying the possible errors in such a procedure, whether it is used to generalize between species or to extrapolate from high to low doses. The methodology for such quantitative extrapolation to humans requires further development.

Evidence for the carcinogenicity of some chemicals in experimental animals may be *limited* for two reasons. Firstly, experimental data may be restricted to such a point that it is not possible to determine a causal relationship between administration of a chemical and the development of a particular lesion in the animals. Secondly, there are certain neoplasms, including lung tumours and hepatomas in mice, which have been considered of lesser significance than neoplasms occurring at other sites for the purpose of evaluating the carcinogenicity of chemicals. Such tumours occur spontaneously in high incidence in these animals, and their malignancy is often difficult to establish. An evaluation of the significance of these tumours following administration of a chemical is the responsibility of particular Working Groups preparing individual monographs, and it has not been possible to set down rigid guidelines; the relevance of these tumours must be determined by considerations which include experimental design and completeness of reporting.

Some chemicals for which there is *limited evidence* of carcinogenicity in animals have also been studied in humans with, in general, inconclusive results. While such chemicals may indeed be carcinogenic to humans, more experimental and epidemiological investigation is required.

Hence *'sufficient evidence'* of carcinogenicity and *'limited evidence'* of carcinogenicity do not indicate categories of chemicals: the inherent definitions of those terms indicate varying degrees of experimental evidence, which may change if and when new data on the chemicals become available. The main drawback to any rigid classification of chemicals with regard to their carcinogenic capacity is the as yet incomplete knowledge of the mechanism(s) of carcinogenesis.

In recent years, several short-term tests for the detection of potential carcinogens have been developed. When only inadequate experimental data are available, positive results in validated short-term tests (see p. 23) are an indication that the compound is a potential carcinogen and that it should be tested in animals for an assessment of its carcinogenicity. Negative results from short-term tests cannot be considered sufficient evidence to rule out carcinogenicity. Whether short-term tests will eventually be as reliable as long-term tests in predicting carcinogenicity in humans will depend on further demonstrations of consistency with long-term experiments and with data from humans.

EXPLANATORY NOTES ON THE MONOGRAPH CONTENTS

Chemical and Physical Data (Section 1)

The Chemical Abstracts Service Registry Number, the latest Chemical Abstracts Primary Name (9th Collective Index)(22) and the IUPAC Systematic Name(23) are recorded in section 1. Other synonyms and trade names are given, but no comprehensive list is provided. Further, some of the trade names are those of mixtures in which the compound being evaluated is only one of the ingredients.

The structural and molecular formulae, molecular weight and chemical and physical properties are given. The properties listed refer to the pure substance, unless otherwise specified, and include, in particular, data that might be relevant to carcinogenicity (e.g., lipid solubility) and those that concern identification. In this volume, ultra-violet spectrometric data are expressed in a new symbol devised by the International Union of Spectroscopists, A (1%, 1 cm), i.e., absorbance of a 1% solution examined as a 1-cm layer.

A separate description of the composition of technical products includes available information on impurities and formulated products.

Production, Use, Occurrence and Analysis (Section 2)

The purpose of section 2 is to provide indications of the extent of past and present human exposure to this chemical.

Synthesis

Since cancer is a delayed toxic effect, the dates of first synthesis and of first commercial production of the chemical are provided. In addition, methods of synthesis used in past and present commercial production are described. This information allows a reasonable estimate to be made of the date before which no human exposure could have occurred.

Production

Since Europe, Japan and the United States are reasonably representative industrialized areas of the world, most data on production, foreign trade and uses are obtained from those countries. It should not, however, be inferred that those nations are the sole or even the major sources or users of any individual chemical.

Production and foreign trade data are obtained from both governmental and trade publications by chemical economists in the three geographical areas. In some cases, separate production data on organic chemicals manufactured in the United States are not available because their publication could disclose confidential information. In such cases, an indication of the minimum quantity produced can be inferred from the number of companies reporting commercial production. Each company is required to report on individual chemicals if the sales value or the weight of the annual production exceeds a specified minimum level. These levels vary for chemicals classified for different uses, e.g., medicinals and plastics; in fact, the minimal annual sales value is between $1000 and $50,000 and the minimal annual weight of production is between 450 and 22, 700 kg. Data on production in some European countries are obtained by means of general questionnaires sent to companies thought to produce the compounds being evaluated. Information from the completed questionnaires is compiled by country, and the resulting estimates of production are included in the individual monographs.

Use

Information on uses is meant to serve as a guide only and is not complete. It is usually obtained from published data but is often complemented by direct contact with manufacturers of the chemical. In the case of drugs, mention of their therapeutic uses does not necessarily represent current practice nor does it imply judgement as to their clinical efficacy.

Statements concerning regulations and standards (e.g., pesticide registrations, maximum levels permitted in foods, occupational standards and allowable limits) in specific countries are mentioned as examples only. They may not reflect the most recent situation, since such legislation is in a constant state of change; nor should it be taken to imply that other countries do not have similar regulations.

Occurrence

Information on the occurrence of a chemical in the environment is obtained from published data including that derived from the monitoring and surveillance of levels of the chemical in occupational environments, air, water, soil, foods and tissues of animals and humans. When available, data on the generation, persistence and bioaccumulation of a chemical are also included.

Analysis

The purpose of the section on analysis is to give the reader an indication, rather than a complete review, of methods cited in the literature. No attempt is made to evaluate critically or to recommend any of the methods.

Biological Data Relevant to the Evaluation of Carcinogenic Risk to Humans (Section 3)

In general, the data recorded in section 3 are summarized as given by the author; however, comments made by the Working Group on certain shortcomings of reporting, of statistical analysis or of experimental design are given in square brackets. The nature and extent of impurities/contaminants in the chemicals being tested are given when available.

Carcinogenicity studies in animals

The monographs are not intended to cover all reported studies. Some studies are purposely omitted (a) because they are inadequate, as judged from previously described criteria(24-27) (e.g., too short a duration, too few animals, poor survival); (b) because they only confirm findings that have already been fully described; or (c) because they are judged irrelevant for the purpose of the evaluation. In certain cases, however, such studies are mentioned briefly, particularly when the information is considered to be a useful supplement to other reports or when it is the only data available. Their inclusion does not, however, imply acceptance of the adequacy of their experimental design and/or of the analysis and interpretation of their results.

Mention is made of all routes of administration by which the compound has been adequately tested and of all species in which relevant tests have been done(5, 26). In most cases, animal strains are given. [General characteristics of mouse strains have been reviewed (28).] Quantitative data are given to indicate the order of magnitude of the effective carcinogenic doses. In general, the doses and schedules are indicated as they appear in the paper; sometimes units have been converted for easier comparison. Experiments in which the compound was administered in conjunction with known carcinogens and experiments on factors that modify the carcinogenic effect are also reported. Experiments on the carcinogenicity of known metabolites, chemical precursors, analogues and derivatives are also included.

Other relevant biological data

Lethality data are given when available, and other data on toxicity are included when considered relevant. The metabolic data are restricted to studies that show the metabolic fate of the chemical in animals and humans, and comparisons of data from animals and humans are made when possible. Information is also given on absorption, distribution, excretion and placental transfer.

Prenatal toxicity

Data on effects on reproduction, teratogenicity, feto- and embryotoxicity from studies in experimental animals and from observations in humans are also included. There appears to be no causal relationship between teratogenicity (29) and carcinogenicity, but chemicals often have both properties. Evidence of prenatal toxicity suggests transplacental transfer, which is a prerequisite for transplacental carcinogenesis.

Indirect tests (mutagenicity and other short-term tests)

Data from indirect tests are also included. Since most of these tests have the advantage of taking less time and being less expensive than mammalian carcinogenicity studies, they are generally known as 'short-term' tests. They comprise assay procedures which rely on the induction of biological and biochemical effects in *in vivo* and/or *in vitro* systems. The endpoint of the majority of these tests is the production not of neoplasms in animals but of changes at the molecular, cellular or multicellular level: these include the induction of DNA damage and repair, mutagenesis in bacteria and other organisms, transformation of mammalian cells in culture, and other systems.

The short-term tests are proposed for use (a) in predicting potential carcinogenicity in the absence of carcinogenicity data in animals, (b) as a contribution in deciding which chemicals should be tested in animals, (c) in identifying active fractions of complex mixtures containing carcinogens, (d) for recognizing active metabolites of known carcinogens in human and/or animal body fluids and (e) to help elucidate mechanisms of carcinogenesis.

Although the theory that cancer is induced as a result of somatic mutation suggests that agents which damage DNA *in vivo* may be carcinogens, the precise relevance of short-term tests to the mechanism by which cancer is induced is not known. Predictions of potential carcinogenicity are currently based on correlations between responses in short-term tests and data from animal carcinogenicity and/or human epidemiological studies. This approach is limited because the number of chemicals known to be carcinogenic in humans is insufficient to provide a basis for validation, and most validation studies involve chemicals that have been evaluated for carcinogenicity only in animals. The selection of chemicals is in turn limited to those classes for which data on carcinogenicity are available. The results of validation studies could be strongly influenced by such selection of chemicals and by the proportion of carcinogens in the series of chemicals tested; this should be kept in mind when evaluating the predictivity of a particular test. The usefulness of any test is reflected by its ability to classify carcinogens and noncarcinogens, using the animal data as a standard; however, animal tests may not always provide a perfect standard. The attainable level of correlation between short-term tests and animal bioassays is still under investigation.

Since many chemicals require metabolism to an active form, tests that do not take this into account may fail to detect certain potential carcinogens. The metabolic activation systems used in short-term tests (e.g., the cell-free systems used in bacterial tests) are meant to approximate the metabolic capacity of the whole organism. Each test has its advantages and limitations; thus, more confidence can be placed in the conclusions when negative or positive results for a chemical are confirmed in several such test systems. Deficiencies in metabolic competence may lead to misclassification of chemicals, which means that not all tests are suitable for assessing the potential carcinogenicity of all classes of compounds.

The present state of knowledge does not permit the selection of a specific test(s) as the most appropriate for identifying potential carcinogenicity. Before the results of a particular test can be considered to be fully acceptable for predicting potential carcinogenicity, certain criteria should be met: (a) the test should have been validated with respect to known animal carcinogens and found to have a high capacity for discriminating between carcinogens and noncarcinogens, and (b), when possible, a structurally related carcinogen(s) and noncarcinogen(s) should have been tested simultaneously with the chemical in question. The results should have been reproduced in different laboratories, and a prediction of carcinogenicity should have been confirmed in additional test systems. Confidence in positive results is increased if a mechanism of action can be deduced and if appropriate dose-response data are available. For optimum usefulness, data on purity must be given.

The short-term tests in current use that have been the most extensively validated are the *Salmonella typhimurium* plate-incorporation assay(30-34), the X-linked recessive lethal test in *Drosophila melanogaster*(35), unscheduled DNA synthesis(36) and *in vitro* transformation(34,37). Each is compatible with current concepts of the possible mechanism(s) of carcinogenesis.

An adequate assessment of the genetic activity of a chemical depends on data from a wide range of test systems. The monographs include, therefore, data not only from those already mentioned, but also on the induction of point mutations in other systems(38-43), on structural(44) and numerical chromosome aberrations, including dominant lethal effects (45), on mitotic recombination in fungi(38) and on sister chromatid exchanges(46-48).

The existence of a correlation between quantitative aspects of mutagenic and carcinogenic activity has been suggested (5,45-51), but it is not sufficiently well established to allow general use.

Further information about mutagenicity and other short-term tests is given in references 46-54.

Case reports and epidemiological studies

Observations in humans are summarized in this section.

Summary of Data Reported and Evaluation (Section 4)

Section 4 summarizes the relevant data from animals and humans and gives the critical views of the Working Group on those data.

Experimental data

Data relevant to the evaluation of the carcinogenicity of the chemical in animals are summarized in this section. The animal species mentioned are those in which the carcinogenicity of the substance was clearly demonstrated. Tumour sites are also indicated. If the substance has produced tumours after prenatal exposure or in single-dose experiments, this is indicated. Dose-response data are given when available.

Results from validated mutagenicity and other short-term tests and from tests for prenatal toxicity are reported if the Working Group considered the data to be relevant.

Human data

Human exposure to the chemical is summarized on the basis of data on production, use and occurrence. Case reports and epidemiological studies that are considered to be pertinent to an assessment of human carcinogenicity are described. Other biological data which are considered to be relevant are also mentioned.

Evaluation

This section comprises the overall evaluation by the Working Group of the carcinogenic risk of the chemical to humans. All of the data in the monograph, and particularly the summarized information on experimental and human data, are considered in order to make this evaluation.

References

1. IARC (1977) IARC Monograph Programme on the Evaluation of the Carcinogenic Risk of Chemicals to Humans. Preamble. *IARC intern. tech. Rep. No. 77/002*

2. IARC (1978) Chemicals with *sufficient evidence* of carcinogenicity in experimental animals - *IARC Monographs* volumes 1-17. *IARC intern. tech. Rep. No. 78/003*

3. WHO (1961) Fifth Report of the Joint FAO/WHO Expert Committee on Food Additives. Evaluation of carcinogenic hazard of food additives. *WHO tech. Rep. Ser., No. 220*, pp. 5, 18, 19

4. WHO (1969) Report of a WHO Scientific Group. Principles for the testing and evaluation of drugs for carcinogenicity. *WHO tech. Rep. Ser., No. 426*, pp. 19, 21, 22

5. WHO (1974) Report of a WHO Scientific Group. Assessment of the carcinogenicity and mutagenicity of chemicals. *WHO tech. Rep. Ser.*, No. 546

6. WHO (1964) Report of a WHO Expert Committee. Prevention of cancer. *WHO tech. Rep. Ser., No. 276*, pp. 29, 30

7. IARC (1972-1980) *IARC Monographs on the Evaluation of the Carcinogenic Risk of Chemicals to Humans*, Volumes 1-24, Lyon, France

   Volume 1 (1972) Some Inorganic Substances, Chlorinated Hydrocarbons, Aromatic Amines, *N*-Nitroso Compounds and Natural Products (19 monographs), 184 pages

   Volume 2 (1973) Some Inorganic and Organometallic Compounds (7 monographs), 181 pages

   Volume 3 (1973) Certain Polycyclic Aromatic Hydrocarbons and Heterocyclic Compounds (17 monographs), 271 pages

   Volume 4 (1974) Some Aromatic Amines, Hydrazine and Related Substances, *N*-Nitroso Compounds and Miscellaneous Alkylating Agents (28 monographs), 286 pages

   Volume 5 (1974) Some Organochlorine Pesticides (12 monographs), 241 pages

   Volume 6 (1974) Sex Hormones (15 monographs), 243 pages

Volume 7 (1974) Some Anti-thyroid and Related Substances, Nitrofurans and Industrial Chemicals (23 monographs), 326 pages

Volume 8 (1975) Some Aromatic Azo Compounds (32 monographs), 357 pages

Volume 9 (1975) Some Aziridines, *N*-, *S*- and *O*-Mustards and Selenium (24 monographs), 268 pages

Volume 10 (1976) Some Naturally Occurring Substances (32 monographs), 353 pages

Volume 11 (1976) Cadmium, Nickel, Some Epoxides, Miscellaneous Industrial Chemicals and General Considerations on Volatile Anaesthetics (24 monographs), 306 pages

Volume 12 (1976) Some Carbamates, Thiocarbamates and Carbazides (24 monographs), 282 pages

Volume 13 (1977) Some Miscellaneous Pharmaceutical Substances (17 monographs), 255 pages

Volume 14 (1977) Asbestos (1 monograph), 106 pages

Volume 15 (1977) Some Fumigants, the Herbicides 2,4-D and 2,4,5-T, Chlorinated Dibenzodioxins and Miscellaneous Industrial Chemicals (18 monographs), 354 pages

Volume 16 (1978) Some Aromatic Amines and Related Nitro Compounds - Hair Dyes, Colouring Agents, and Miscellaneous Industrial Chemicals (32 monographs), 400 pages

Volume 17 (1978) Some *N*-Nitroso Compounds (17 monographs), 365 pages

Volume 18 (1978) Polychlorinated Biphenyls and Polybrominated Biphenyls (2 monographs), 140 pages

Volume 19 (1979) Some Monomers, Plastics and Synthetic Elastomers, and Acrolein (17 monographs), 513 pages

Volume 20 (1979) Some Halogenated Hydrocarbons (25 monographs), 609 pages

Volume 21 (1979) Sex Hormones (II) (22 monographs), 583 pages

Volume 22 (1980) Some Non-Nutritive Sweetening Agents (2 monographs), 208 pages

Volume 23 (1980) Some Metals and Metallic Compounds (4 monographs), 438 pages

Volume 24 (1980) Some Pharmaceutical Drugs (16 monographs), 337 pages

8. IARC (1973-1979) *Information Bulletin on the Survey of Chemicals Being Tested for Carcinogenicity*, Numbers 1-8, Lyon, France

   Number 1 (1973) 52 pages
   Number 2 (1973) 77 pages
   Number 3 (1974) 67 pages
   Number 4 (1974) 97 pages
   Number 5 (1975) 88 pages
   Number 6 (1976) 360 pages
   Number 7 (1978) 460 pages
   Number 8 (1979) 604 pages

9. PHS 149 (1951-1976) Public Health Service Publication No. 149, *Survey of Compounds which have been Tested for Carcinogenic Activity*, Washington DC, US Government Printing Office

   1951   Hartwell, J.L., 2nd ed., Literature up to 1947 on 1329 compounds, 583 pages

   1957   Shubik, P. & Hartwell, J.L., Supplement 1, Literature for the years 1948-1953 on 981 compounds, 388 pages

   1969   Shubik, P. & Hartwell, J.L., edited by Peters, J.A., Supplement 2, Literature for the years 1954-1960 on 1048 compounds, 655 pages

   1971   National Cancer Institute, Literature for the years 1968-1969 on 882 compounds, 653 pages

   1973   National Cancer Institute, Literature for the years 1961-1967 on 1632 compounds, 2343 pages

   1974   National Cancer Institute, Literature for the years 1970-1971 on 750 compounds, 1667 pages

   1976   National Cancer Institute, Literature for the years 1972-1973 on 966 compounds, 1638 pages

10. Pike, M.C. & Roe, F.J.C. (1963) An actuarial method of analysis of an experiment in two-stage carcinogenesis. *Br. J. Cancer, 17*, 605-610

11. Miller, E.C. & Miller, J.A. (1966) Mechanisms of chemical carcinogenesis: nature of proximate carcinogens and interactions with macromolecules. *Pharmacol. Rev., 18*, 805-838

12. Miller, J.A. (1970) Carcinogenesis by chemicals: an overview - G.H.A. Clowes Memorial Lecture. *Cancer Res., 30*, 559-576

13. Miller, J.A. & Miller, E.C. (1976) *The metabolic activation of chemical carcinogens to reactive electrophiles.* In: Yuhas, J.M., Tennant, R.W. & Reagon, J.D., eds, *Biology of Radiation Carcinogenesis,* New York, Raven Press

14. Peto, R. (1974) Guidelines on the analysis of tumours rates and death rates in experimental animals. *Br. J. Cancer, 29*, 101-105

15. Peto, R. (1975) Letter to the editor. *Br. J. Cancer, 31*, 697-699

16. Hoel, D.G. & Walburg, H.E., Jr (1972) Statistical analysis of survival experiments. *J. natl Cancer Inst., 49*, 361-372

17. IARC Working Group (1980) An evaluation of chemicals and industrial processes associated with cancer in humans based on human and animal data : *IARC Monographs* Volumes 1 to 20. *Cancer Res., 40,* 1-12

18. IARC (1979) *IARC Monographs on the Evaluation of the Carcinogenic Risk of Chemicals to Humans,* Supplement 1, *Chemicals and Industrial Processes Associated with Cancer in Humans,* Lyon, France

19. IARC (1979) *Annual Report 1979*, Lyon, International Agency for Research on Cancer, pp. 89-99

20. Rall, D.P. (1977) *Species differences in carcinogenesis testing.* In: Hiatt, H.H., Watson, J.D. & Winsten, J.A., eds, *Origins of Human Cancer*, Book C, Cold Spring Harbor, NY, Cold Spring Harbor Laboratory, pp. 1383-1390

21. National Academy of Sciences (NAS) (1975) *Contemporary Pest Control Practices and Prospects: the Report of the Executive Committee*, Washington DC

22. Chemical Abstracts Services (1978) *Chemical Abstracts Ninth Collective Index (9CI), 1972-1976*, Vols 76-85, Columbus, Ohio

23. International Union of Pure & Applied Chemistry (1965) *Nomenclature of Organic Chemistry*, Section C, London, Butterworths

24. WHO (1958) Second Report of the Joint FAO/WHO Expert Committee on Food Additives. Procedures for the testing of intentional food additives to establish their safety and use. *WHO tech. Rep. Ser., No. 144*

25. WHO (1967) Scientific Group. Procedures for investigating intentional and unintentional food additives. *WHO tech. Rep. Ser., No. 348*

26. Berenblum, I., ed. (1969) Carcinogenicity testing. *UICC tech. Rep. Ser., 2*

27. Sontag, J.M., Page, N.P. & Saffiotti, U. (1976) Guidelines for carcinogen bioassay in small rodents. *Natl Cancer Inst. Carcinog. tech. Rep. Ser., No. 1*

28. Committee on Standardized Genetic Nomenclature for Mice (1972) Standardized nomenclature for inbred strains of mice. Fifth listing. *Cancer Res., 32*, 1609-1646

29. Wilson, J.G. & Fraser, F.C. (1977) *Handbook of Teratology*, New York, Plenum Press

30. Ames, B.N., Durston, W.E., Yamasaki, E. & Lee, F.D. (1973) Carcinogens are mutagens: a simple test system combining liver homogenates for activation and bacteria for detection. *Proc. natl Acad. Sci. USA, 70*, 2281-2285

31. McCann, J., Choi, E., Yamasaki, E. & Ames, B.N. (1975) Detection of carcinogens as mutagens in the *Salmonella*/microsome test: assay of 300 chemicals. *Proc. natl Acad. Sci. USA, 72*, 5135-5139

32. McCann, J. & Ames, B.N. (1976) Detection of carcinogens as mutagens in the *Salmonella*/microsome test: assay of 300 chemicals: discussion. *Proc. natl Acad. Sci. USA, 73*, 950-954

33. Sugimura, T., Sato, S., Nagao, M., Yahagi, T., Matsushima, T., Seino, Y., Takeuchi, M. & Kawachi, T. (1977) *Overlapping of carcinogens and mutagens*. In: Magee, P.N., Takayama, S., Sugimura, T. & Matsushima, T., eds, *Fundamentals in Cancer Prevention*, Baltimore, University Park Press, pp. 191-215

34. Purchase, I.F.M., Longstaff, E., Ashby, J., Styles, J.A., Anderson, D., Lefevre, P.A. & Westwood, F.R. (1976) Evaluation of six short term tests for detecting organic chemical carcinogens and recommendations for their use. *Nature, 264,* 624-627

35. Vogel, E. & Sobels, F.H. (1976) *The function of* Drosophila *in genetic toxicology testing.* In: Hollaender, A., ed., *Chemical Mutagens: Principles and Methods for Their Detection,* Vol. 4, New York, Plenum Press, pp. 93-142

36. San, R.H.C. & Stich, H.F. (1975) DNA repair synthesis of cultured human cells as a rapid bioassay for chemical carcinogens. *Int. J. Cancer, 16,* 284-291

37. Pienta, R.J., Poiley, J.A. & Lebherz, W.B. (1977) Morphological transformation of early passage golden Syrian hamster embryo cells derived from cryopreserved primary cultures as a reliable *in vitro* bioassay for identifying diverse carcinogens. *Int. J. Cancer, 19,* 642-655

38. Zimmermann, F.K. (1975) Procedures used in the induction of mitotic recombination and mutation in the yeast *Saccharomyces cerevisiae*. *Mutat. Res., 31,* 71-86

39. Ong, T.-M. & de Serres, F.J. (1972) Mutagenicity of chemical carcinogens in *Neurospora crassa*. *Cancer Res., 32,* 1890-1893

40. Huberman, E. & Sachs, L. (1976) Mutability of different genetic loci in mammalian cells by metabolically activated carcinogenic polycyclic hydrocarbons. *Proc. natl Acad. Sci. USA, 73,* 188-192

41. Krahn, D.F. & Heidelburger, C. (1977) Liver homogenate-mediated mutagenesis in Chinese hamster V79 cells by polycyclic aromatic hydrocarbons and aflatoxins. *Mutat. Res., 46,* 27-44

42. Kuroki, T., Drevon, C. & Montesano, R. (1977) Microsome-mediated mutagenesis in V79 Chinese hamster cells by various nitrosamines. *Cancer Res., 37,* 1044-1050

43. Searle, A.G. (1975) The specific locus test in the mouse. *Mutat. Res., 31,* 277-290

44. Evans, H.J. & O'Riordan, M.L. (1975) Human peripheral blood lymphocytes for the analysis of chromosome aberrations in mutagen tests. *Mutat. Res., 31,* 135-148

45. Epstein, S.S., Arnold, E., Andrea, J., Bass, W. & Bishop, Y. (1972) Detection of chemical mutagens by the dominant lethal assay in the mouse. *Toxicol. appl. Pharmacol., 23,* 288-325

46. Perry, P. & Evans, H.J. (1975) Cytological detection of mutagen-carcinogen exposure by sister chromatid exchanges. *Nature, 258*, 121-125

47. Stetka, D.G. & Wolff, S. (1976) Sister chromatid exchanges as an assay for genetic damage induced by mutagen-carcinogens. I. *In vivo* test for compounds requiring metabolic activation. *Mutat. Res., 41*, 333-342

48. Bartsch, H. & Grover, P.L. (1976) *Chemical carcinogenesis and mutagenesis.* In: Symington, T. & Carter, R.L., eds, *Scientific Foundations of Oncology*, Vol. IX, *Chemical Carcinogenesis,* London, Heinemann Medical Books Ltd, pp. 334-342

49. Hollaender, A., ed. (1971a,b, 1973, 1976) *Chemical Mutagens: Principles and Methods for Their Detection,* Vols 1-4, New York, Plenum Press

50. Montesano, R. & Tomatis, L., eds (1974) *Chemical Carcinogenesis Essays (IARC Scientific Publications No. 10),* Lyon, International Agency for Research on Cancer

51. Ramel, C., ed. (1973) Evaluation of genetic risk of environmental chemicals: report of a symposium held at Skokloster, Sweden, 1972. *Ambio Spec. Rep., No. 3*

52. Stoltz, D.R., Poirier, L.A., Irving, C.C., Stich, H.F., Weisburger, J.H. & Grice, H.C. (1974) Evaluation of short-term tests for carcinogenicity. *Toxicol. appl. Pharmacol., 29*, 157-180

53. Montesano, R., Bartsch, H. & Tomatis, L., eds (1976) *Screening Tests in Chemical Carcinogenesis (IARC Scientific Publications No. 12),* Lyon, International Agency for Research on Cancer

54. Committee 17 (1976) Environmental mutagenic hazards. *Science, 187*, 503-514

GENERAL REMARKS ON THE SUBSTANCES CONSIDERED

This twenty-fourth volume of *IARC Monographs* covers a number of miscellaneous pharmaceutical drugs. Certain other drugs have been considered in previous volumes of monographs in this series (IARC, 1973, 1974a,b,c, 1975, 1976a,b, 1977, 1979). Since new data had become available on several of these - phenacetin, phenoxybenzamine and reserpine - the monographs on these substances were updated.

Many pharmaceutical drugs contain amine groups, which, in principle, can be converted to *N*-nitroso compounds by reaction *in vitro* with nitrite under conditions similar to those prevailing in the human stomach. Monographs on such drugs were not prepared; however, a short section briefly describes the chemistry of *N*-nitrosation processes and lists references to studies of carcinogenicity and mutagenicity in which the drugs were tested in combination with nitrite or in which the *N*-nitrosation products themselves were administered. Some of the drugs can react *in vivo* with nitrite to form *N*-nitrosamines, several of which were evaluated by a previous Working Group (IARC, 1978).

The Working Group felt that full consideration of the problem of *N*-nitrosation and its relevance to the human situation should be deferred to a future meeting, since many classes of compounds, including drugs, pesticides and other industrial chemicals, can undergo such reactions; further evidence is needed to assess the extent of nitrosation processes in humans *in vivo*.

Regulatory requirements that include assay, identification and limit tests for impurities in pharmaceutical-grade drugs or pharmaceutical products are given in various national and international pharmacopoeias, such as the *British Pharmacopoeia, The US Pharmacopeia,* the *WHO International Pharmacopoeia* and the *European Pharmacopoeia;* and such information is given for a number of drugs considered in this volume. No attempt was made to give such requirements in detail in the sections on analysis; however, simple and effective methods for testing the purity of both pure and formulated drugs are outlined. In certain cases, however, it should be noted that the content of active ingredient stated may be somewhat misleading when considered in isolation; thus, the range given takes into account not only variations in the content of the substance itself but also possible variations in the methods of analysis.

When evaluating drug-cancer relationships in humans, the Working Group stressed that the following points should be considered:

(1) The disease for which the drug is given may predispose to cancer.

(2) The prescribing of a drug may increase the possibility of diagnosis of the cancer

without increasing its true incidence; this assumes that in some cases the cancer may go undiagnosed unless the drug is prescribed or some similar event occurs.

(3) When drugs are used in combination, it is virtually impossible, on the basis of epidemiological data, to incriminate a particular component of the combination.

When evaluating experiments carried out to investigate the carcinogenicity of drugs in experimental animals, the Working Group noted that:

(1) Drugs are often tested at doses higher than the therapeutic dose.

(2) The purity and chemical form of the compound being tested are not always given.

(3) In tests of photoactive compounds, the protocol used was not adequate to evaluate the carcinogenicity of the compound alone.

Most of the drugs considered are used currently; some are being phased out; others may be phased out in future; and others may be considered for future use or for uses different from their present ones. Some details of present use patterns are provided for all compounds, since these may be particularly important for epidemiological studies.

Evaluations of carcinogenic risk were made purely on the basis of the available scientific data, taking into account both the experimental and human results. Any risk/benefit evaluations leading to legislative decisions are the prerogative of others.

References

IARC (1973) *IARC Monographs on the Evaluation of the Carcinogenic Risk of Chemicals to Humans,* Volume 2, *Some Inorganic and Organometallic Compounds,* pp. 53-57

IARC (1974a) *IARC Monographs on the Evaluation of the Carcinogenic Risk of Chemicals to Humans,* Volume 4, *Some Aromatic Amines, Hydrazine and Related Substances, N-Nitroso Compounds and Miscellaneous Alkylating Agents*

IARC (1974b) *IARC Monographs on the Evaluation of the Carcinogenic Risk of Chemicals to Humans,* Volume 6, *Sex Hormones*

IARC (1974c) *IARC Monographs on the Evaluation of the Carcinogenic Risk of Chemicals to Humans,* Volume 7, *Some Anti-thyroid and Related Substances, Nitrofurans and Industrial Chemicals,* pp. 53-65, 67-76, 85-94, 143-146, 147-150, 161-169, 171-180, 181-184, 185-193

IARC (1975) *IARC Monographs on the Evaluation of the Carcinogenic Risk of Chemicals to Humans,* Volume 9, *Some Aziridines, N-, S-, & O-Mustards and Selenium,* pp. 67-73, 85-94, 95-105, 125-134, 135-136, 157-166, 167-180, 209-216, 235-241

IARC (1976a) *IARC Monographs on the Evaluation of the Carcinogenic Risk of Chemicals to Humans,* Volume 11, *Cadmium, Nickel, Some Epoxides, Miscellaneous Industrial Chemicals and General Considerations on Volatile Anaesthetics,* pp. 285-293

IARC (1976b) *IARC Monographs on the Evaluation of the Carcinogenic Risk of Chemicals to Humans,* Volume 12, *Some Carbamates, Thiocarbamates and Carbazides,* pp. 85-95, 177-181

IARC (1977) *IARC Monographs on the Evaluation of the Carcinogenic Risk of Chemicals to Humans,* Volume 13, *Some Miscellaneous Pharmaceutical Substances*

IARC (1978) *IARC Monographs on the Evaluation of the Carcinogenic Risk of Chemicals to Humans,* Volume 17, *Some N-Nitroso Compounds*

IARC (1979) *IARC Monographs on the Evaluation of the Carcinogenic Risk of Chemicals to Humans,* Volume 21, *Sex Hormones (II)*

THE MONOGRAPHS

CLOFIBRATE

1. Chemical and Physical Data

1.1 Synonyms and trade names

Chem. Abstr. Services Reg. No.: 637-07-0

Chem. Abstr. Name: Propanoic acid, 2-(4-chlorophenoxy)-2-methyl, ethyl ester

IUPAC Systematic Name: Ethyl 2-(4-chlorophenoxy)-2-methylpropionate

Synonyms: 2-(4-Chlorophenoxy)-2-methylpropanoic acid ethyl ester; 2-(*para*-chlorophenoxy)-2-methylpropionic acid ethyl ester; ethyl chlorophenoxyisobutyrate; ethyl *para*-chlorophenoxyisobutyrate; ethyl 2-(*para*-chlorophenoxy)isobutyrate; ethyl α-(4-chlorophenoxy)-isobutyrate; ethyl α-(*para*-chlorophenoxy)isobutyrate; ethyl 2-(4-chlorophenoxy)-2-methylpropionate; ethyl 2-(*para*-chlorophenoxy)-2-methylpropionate; ethyl-α-(4-chlorophenoxy)-α-methylpropionate; ethyl-α-(*para*-chlorophenoxy)-α-methylpropionate; ethyl clofibrate

Trade names: Amotril; Amotril S; Angiokapsul; Anparton; Antilipid; Antilipide; Apolan; Arterioflexin; Artes; Ateculon; Ateriosan; Aterosol; Athebrate; Atheromide; Atheropront; Athranid-Wirkstoff; Atrolen; Atromid; Atromida; Atromidin; Atromid-S; Atrovis; AY 61123; Azionyl; Bioscleran; Bresit; Cartagyl; Cinnarizin; Citiflus; Claripex; Clobrat; Clobren-5F; Clobren-SF; Clofar; Clofibram; Clofibrat; Clofinit; Clofipront; CPIB; Deliva; Dura Clofibrat; Elpi; EPIB; Fibralem; Gerastop; Hyclorate; ICI 28257; Klofiran; Levatrom; Lipamid; Lipavil; Lipavlon; Lipide 500; Lipidsenker; Lipofacton; Lipomid; Liponorm; Liporeduct; Liporil; Liposid; Liprin; Liprinal; Lobetrin; Miscleron; Negalip; Neo-Atromid; Normalip; Normat; Normet; Oxan 600; Persantinat; Recolip; Regardin; Regelan; Regelan N; Robigram; Scrobin; Serofinex; Serotinex; Skerolip; Skleromex; Skleromexe; Sklero-Tablinen; Sklero-Tabuls; Ticlobran; Vincamin compositum; Xyduril; Yoclo

1.2 Structural and molecular formulae and molecular weight

$$Cl-\langle\bigcirc\rangle-O-\underset{CH_3}{\overset{CH_3}{\underset{|}{\overset{|}{C}}}}-COOC_2H_5$$

$C_{12}H_{15}ClO_3$ Mol. wt: 242.7

1.3 Chemical and physical properties of the pure substance

From Wade (1977) or Windholz (1976) unless otherwise specified

(a) *Description:* Clear, almost colourless oily liquid
(b) *Boiling-point:* 148-150°C at 2.7 kPa (20 mm Hg)
(c) *Density:* d^{20} 1.138-1.144
(d) *Refractive index:* $n_{19.5-20.5}^D$ = 1.500-1.505 (British Pharmacopoeia Commission, 1973)
(e) *Spectroscopy data:* λ_{max} (dehydrated ethanol): 226 nm, A(1%, 1 cm) = 910; 280 nm, A(1%, 1 cm) = 87; 288 nm, A(1%, 1 cm) = 62 (British Pharmacopoeia Commission, 1973). Infrared spectral data have been tabulated (US Pharmacopeial Convention, Inc., 1975).
(f) *Solubility:* Practically insoluble in water; readily miscible with ethanol, acetone, chloroform and diethyl ether
(g) *Stability:* Sensitive to oxidation and light; easily hydrolysed

1.4 Technical products and impurities

Various national and international pharmacopoeias give specifications for the purity of clofibrate in pharmaceutical products. For example, clofibrate is available in the US as a USP grade containing 97.0-0-103.0% active ingredient calculated on the anhydrous basis; it should not contain more than 0.2% water or more than 0.003% *para*-chlorophenol. In the *British Pharmacopoeia,* stringent methods are described to ensure that clofibrate does not contain free phenolic materials and related volatile substances (British Pharmacopoeia Commission, 1973). A number of specifically identified, related impurities have been reported in commercially available samples of clofibrate such as 4-bromo- and 2,4-dichloro-derivatives (Johansson & Ryhage, 1976).

CLOFIBRATE

It is available in the US in 500 mg doses as capsules containing 90.0-110.0% of the stated amount of clofibrate (US Pharmacopoeial Convention Inc., 1975); 500 mg doses as capsules are also available in the UK (British Pharmacopoeia Commission, 1973). In Japan, clofibrate is available in 125, 250 and 500 mg doses as capsules.

2. Production, Use, Occurrence and Analysis

2.1 Production and use

(a) Production

Clofibric acid was first synthesized in 1947, but the ethyl ester, clofibrate, was not mentioned until 1961 (Windholz, 1976). The effect of clofibrates on reducing plasma lipids was discovered by Thorp & Waring (1962).

One reported method of producing clofibrate involves use of *para*-chlorophenol, chloroform and acetone as starting materials, to give clofibric acid, which is subsequently esterified with ethanol. It is not known, however, whether this is the only method used for commercial production.

No evidence was found that clofibrate has ever been produced in commercial quantities in the US. Imports through the principal US customs districts amounted to 475.8 thousand kg in 1977 (US International Trade Commission, 1978) and to 196.4 thousand kg in 1978 (US International Trade Commission, 1979).

There are about 10 producers of clofibrate in western Europe, with an annual production of 50,000-100,000 kg. It is believed to be produced by one company each in Austria, the Federal Republic of Germany, Scandinavia, Switzerland and the UK; by two companies in Spain; and by three companies in Italy. Production in eastern Europe is about 50,000-100,000 kg/yr; only small quantities are exported.

Clofibrate is produced by two companies in Japan, which had a combined annual production of about 65 thousand kg in 1975-1978.

(b) Use

Clofibrate is used to lower plasma lipid levels. It appears to cause mobilization of cholesterol from tissues, and xanthomatous deposits often regress; it also causes inhibition of cholesterol synthesis and increased excretion of neutral sterols. The drug is usually used orally in a dose of 2 g per day taken in 2-4 portions (Goodman & Gilman, 1975).

Following the report of a WHO-sponsored cooperative study of the use of clofibrate in the primary prevention of ischaemic heart disease (Committee of Principal Investigators, 1978), it was withdrawn in the Federal Republic of Germany and in Norway in early 1979. In a number of other countries, including France, Italy, Sweden, Switzerland, the UK and the US (where the drug is available only on prescription), practitioners have been advised to reserve its use for patients with high plasma lipid concentrations that are refractory to dietary measures and to consider carefullly the risks and benefits of the treatment. It was reintroduced in the Federal Republic of Germany in August 1979 (WHO, 1979).

The US Food and Drug Administration (1979) has recommended that, due to the possible risk of malignancy and definitely increased risk of cholelithiasis in humans, clofibrate is presently indicated only in limited circumstances in the treatment of primary hyperlipidaemias. It has thus been recommended that clofibrate be given only when other dietary means are ineffective and only to patients with significant hyperlipidaemia and high risk of arterial disease.

2.2 Occurrence

Clofibrate is not known to occur in nature. Clofibric acid, the active form is a hydrolysis product of clofibrate and has been detected in effluents from sewage treatment plants as a result of human consumption. The average level detected was 7.09 μg/l (Hignite & Azarnoff, 1977).

2.3 Analysis

Typical methods of analysis for clofibrate in various matrices are summarized in Table 1. Abbreviations used are: GC/ECD, gas chromatography with electron capture detection; NMR, nuclear magnetic resonance spectrometry; UV, ultra-violet spectrometry.

Table 1. Analytical methods for clofibrate

Sample matrix	Sample preparation	Assay procedure	Limit of detection	Reference
Capsules and pure compound	Add internal standard and acetone-D_6	NMR	not given	Hassan & Loutfy, 1979
	Add methanol; pass through basic polystyrene anion-exchange resin; dilute with methanol	UV	not given	US Pharmacopeial Convention, Inc., 1975
Blood plasma	Acidify with hydrochloric acid; extract with benzene; evaporate; add acetonitrile, diisopropylethylamine and pentafluorobenzyl bromide; evaporate; add sodium bicarbonate; extract with hexane	GC/ECD	10 pg	Pellizzari & Seltzman, 1978

3. Biological Data Relevant to the Evaluation of Carcinogenic Risk to Humans

3.1 Carcinogenicity studies in animals

(a) Oral administration

Rat: A group of 15 male Fischer 344 rats, weighing 84-100 g, were fed clofibrate (purity not specified) at a dietary concentration of 0.5% (v/w) [about 250 mg/kg bw per day] in ground rat chow for up to 28 months. A group of 15 untreated controls was available. Of treated animals, 1 rat was killed at 13 months and 3 more between 17 and 21 months. The remaining 11 rats were killed between 24 and 28 months. One or more hepatocellular carcinomas developed in 10/11 rats, compared with 0/14 controls ($P < 0.001$); 5 of the animals with hepatocellular carcinomas showed metastases. In addition, pancreatic exocrine acinar carcinomas were found in 2/11 rats, a dermatofibrosarcoma in 1 rat and a leiomyoma of the intestine in 1 rat in the clofibrate-fed group. No such tumours were seen in controls (Reddy & Qureshi, 1979).

Clofibrate (purity not specified) was fed at a dietary concentration of 0.5% to 25 male Fischer 344 rats, weighing approximately 100 g, for 72-97 weeks, to give a total intake of 25-33 g clofibrate per rat. A group of 25 male rats were used as controls. The study was terminated at 129 weeks when all survivors were killed. Among the treated rats, 10 developed malignant tumours at various sites; the first tumour, a hepatocellular carcinoma, appeared at 72 weeks. Hepatocellular carcinomas were found in 4/25 rats; all 4 tumours were successfully transplanted. Among the other tumours observed were a pancreatic exocrine acinar carcinoma in 1 rat and pancreatic exocrine acinar adenomas in 3 rats; an adenocarcinoma of the stomach in 1 rat; a renal-cell carcinoma in 1 rat; a papillary carcinoma of the urinary bladder in 1 rat; a sarcoma of the urinary bladder in 1 rat; a sarcoma of the parotid in 1 rat; sarcomas of the lung in 2 rats; and a lymphosarcoma involving the pancreas in 1 rat. None of these tumours were encountered in the 25 control rats. Interstitial-cell tumours of the testes were seen in 5/25 treated and 5/25 control animals (Svoboda & Azarnoff, 1979).

(b) Other experimental systems

Administration in conjunction with a known carcinogen: Thirty male Fischer 344 rats that were pretreated with *N*-nitrosodiethylamine (NDEA) (100 mg/l in the drinking-water) for 2 weeks and given a control diet and water for 1 week were subsequently given clofibrate (purity not specified) at a dietary concentration of 0.5% [v/w] for 48 weeks, at which time the experiment was terminated. Clofibrate significantly ($P < 0.001$) enhanced the development of liver tumours in rats previously exposed to NDEA: 25/28 rats given NDEA plus clofibrate had liver-cell tumours (type not specified) *versus* 5/18 (3 hepatocellular carcinomas) in the group given NDEA alone (Reddy & Rao, 1978).

3.2 Other relevant biological data

(a) Experimental systems

Toxic effects

The oral LD_{50} of clofibrate in mice is 1280 mg/kg bw and that in rats 1650 mg/kg bw (Metz *et al.*, 1977).

Prenatal toxicity

Clofibrate has been tested in pregnant animals in several studies, and, although no fetal defects have been reported, relative enlargement of the liver in proportion to the body of newborn rats has been found (Chhabra & Kurup, 1978) as well as an abnormal postnatal fetal thrombosis syndrome. The postnatal thrombosis consisted of an extension of the normal thrombosis in the umbilical arteries, and this caused necrosis of the tail or parts of the hindlimbs (Dange *et al.*, 1975).

With doses of 200 mg/kg bw per day given to both male and female rats, both before and during gestation, a significant decrease in litter size was observed ($P < 0.05$). With doses of 500 mg/kg bw, the number of pregnancies was decreased from 7/8 to 0/8 ($P < 0.005$). No such effects were found when female rabbits were treated similarly (Pantaleoni & Valeri, 1974). In a preliminary report lacking details, no changes in litter size or fetal weight were reported in rats given 0.6-140 mg/kg bw/day clofibrate from day 6 to day 20 of gestation (Diener & Hsu, 1966).

Transfer across the placenta and into the milk and a postnatal increase in liver α-glycerophosphate dehydrogenase has been reported in newborn rats whose mothers were fed clofibrate (Chhabra & Kurup, 1978).

Clofibrate injected into pregnant mice induced a rise in catalase activity in the proximal portion of the embryonic intestine, but this rise was observed only after 17 days of gestation (Calvert *et al.*, 1979).

Absorption, distribution, excretion and metabolism

After oral administration, clofibrate is rapidly hydrolysed to clofibric acid, which is the pharmacologically active metabolite (Thorp, 1962; Thorp & Waring, 1962). The calculated half-life of clofibric acid in rats was 5.2 ± 0.16 hours. In rats, equimolar oral doses of ^{14}C-clofibrate and ^{14}C-clofibric acid produced essentially the same blood levels, tissue distribution and urinary excretion of radioactivity. The radioactivity found in the serum was mostly due to unconjugated clofibric acid; 5% of the radioactivity accumulated in the liver within 3 hours. In the urine, clofibric acid was present both free and conjugated with glucuronic acid (Cayen *et al.*, 1977).

When ^{14}C-clofibrate was perfused through rat liver *in vivo*, 42% of the radioactivity entered the bile during the 3-hour perfusion period, and only about 2% was retained in the liver. Subfractionation of the liver showed that most of the retained radioactivity was located in the cytosol (Laker & Mayes, 1978).

Effects on intermediary metabolism

Since the hypolipidaemic properties of aryloxyisobutyric acids and their esters were first reported (Thorp & Waring, 1962), several reviews have dealt with the hepatic and hypolipidaemic effects of clofibrate, the most effective compound of this series (Havel & Kane, 1973; Gear *et al.*, 1974; Svoboda & Reddy, 1974; Reddy & Krishnakantha, 1975; Yeshurun & Gotto, 1976).

Clofibrate-induced hepatomegaly and hepatic peroxisome proliferation in rodents have been extensively documented (Paget, 1963; Best & Duncan, 1964; Hess *et al.*, 1965; Platt & Thorp, 1966; Svoboda & Azarnoff, 1966; Svoboda *et al.*, 1967; Reddy *et al.*, 1969). In rats, dietary concentrations of 0.25-2% clofibrate caused a rapid and sustained increase in the number of peroxisomes in liver cells (Hess *et al.*, 1965; Svoboda *et al.*, 1967; Reddy & Kumar, 1979)

Clofibrate-induced hepatic peroxisome proliferation is associated with enhanced synthesis of the peroxisomal marker enzyme catalase in both male and female rats (Reddy *et al.*, 1971; Reddy & Kumar, 1979). Clofibrate also increases the activities of other hepatic peroxisome-associated enzymes, particularly carnitine acetyltransferase, in rats and mice (Solberg *et al.*, 1972; Kähönen & Ylikahri, 1974; Moody & Reddy, 1974, 1978; Markwell *et al.*, 1977; Reddy & Kumar, 1979). The enzymes involved in the β-oxidation of long-chain fatty acids are localized in the peroxisomes, and hypolipidaemic drugs which induce hepatic peroxisome proliferation stimulate the peroxisomal system of β-oxidation (Lazarow, 1978). Clofibrate-induced hepatic peroxisome proliferation in both male and female rats is associated with a marked increase in the liver content of an 80,000 mol. wt polypeptide (Reddy & Kumar, 1977, 1979).

In rats treated with clofibrate, there was a statistically significant increase ($P < 0.001$) in the capacity of their livers to oxidize palmitoyl-coenzyme A (CoA) (Lazarow & De Duve, 1976). Acute and chronic treatment with clofibrate increased the total CoA content of rat liver and altered the profile of the various CoA thioesters; there was a two- to three-fold elevation in the contents of long-chain acyl CoA, acetyl CoA and free CoA, whereas the contents of succinyl CoA, malonyl CoA and acetoacetyl CoA decreased significantly (Ball et al., 1979). Clofibrate caused a three-fold increase in hepatic carnitine levels as well as a 2 and 4.5-fold increase in the ketogenesis from octanoate and oleate in rats (Mannaerts et al., 1978).

Pretreatment of rats with clofibrate for 1 week increased hepatic uptake of lactate and of free fatty acids in the perfused liver. It induced a decrease in perfusate glucose and in the output of low-density lipoprotein triacylglycerol (Laker & Mayes, 1979).

The mitochondrial protein content in the liver increased by 50-100% in rats fed diets containing clofibrate (Kurup et al., 1970; Krishnakantha & Kurup, 1972; Gear et al., 1974). Clofibrate increased the activity of α-glycerol phosphate dehydrogenase in the liver mitochondria many-fold (Krishnakantha & Kurup, 1972). It decreased the hepatic microsomal β-hydroxy-β-methylglutaryl-CoA reductase (Cohen et al., 1974).

Administration of 0.4-0.8 mmol/kg bw clofibrate twice daily for 7 days to male rats induced hepatic Type-1 substrate drug-metabolizing enzymes and increased the P-450 cytochrome content of the liver (Lewis et al., 1974). Clofibrate significantly increased the rate of elimination of ethanol in female rats (Pösö & Hillbom, 1977).

Daily i.m. injections of doses ranging between 140-420 mg/kg bw clofibrate to rats suppressed the increase in certain plasma proteins that normally accompanies experimentally induced inflammation and produced decreases in plasma zinc, copper, transferin and seromucoid and an increase in hepatic amino acid uptake (Powanda et al., 1979).

Mutagenicity and other, related short-term tests

Clofibrate was not mutagenic to *Salmonella typhimurium* strains TA1535, TA1537, TA1538, TA98 or TA100, with or without metabolic activation by rat liver microsomes (Warren et al., 1980).

Although clofibrate suppressed the incorporation of ^{3}H-thymidine into replicating DNA in primary cultures of concanavalin-A-stimulated mouse splenic lymphocytes, both in the presence and absence of a rat liver microsomal preparation, the effect was reversible upon removal of the drug. This is in contrast to the action of several DNA-binding carcinogens. It was concluded that clofibrate did not cause DNA damage (Warren et al., 1980).

(b) Humans

The main effect of clofibrate is to decrease the serum concentrations of cholesterol and triglycerides (Oliver, 1962).

Toxic effects

A 69-year old woman, who was on clofibrate therapy for 3 months, developed painless jaundice and complained of fatigue, anorexia, nausea and vomiting; a liver biopsy revealed granulomatous hepatitis (Pierce & Chesler, 1978). In a study involving 17 haemodialysed patients treated with clofibrate, all complained of muscle pain, 12 (71%) complained of anorexia, 8 (47%) developed malaise, and 10 (59%) had gastrointestinal symptoms (Kijima et al., 1978).

A young male patient with nephrotic syndrome treated with clofibrate developed muscle pain, stiffness and very high serum levels of muscle enzymes, in particular creatine phosphokinase (Pokroy et al., 1977). Teräväinen & Mäkitie (1976) described the case of a patient given clofibrate for treatment of hyperlipidaemia who developed myokymia.

In a study on the hepatic effects of clofibrate in man, 40 patients with high plasma lipid levels had liver biopsies before and after 3 months of clofibrate treatment (1.5 g/day in 27 patients; 0.5 g/day in 13 patients). Under the light microscope, the liver tissue showed some tendency to decreased fatty infiltration; there was no evidence of liver damage (Schwandt et al., 1978).

The influence of clofibrate on fasting biliary lipids and on cholic acid kinetics was investigated in 10 recently cholecystectomized patients. Clofibrate increased the biliary cholesterol concentration and reduced bile acid levels (Pertsemlidis et al., 1974). Data from a coronary drug project (The Coronary Drug Project Research Group, 1975) and from a WHO cooperative study on clofibrate (Cooper et al., 1975; Committee of Principal Investigators, 1978) showed a significantly increased incidence ($P < 0.001$) of gall-stones in patients treated with clofibrate. A strong association between clofibrate therapy and gall-stones has also been documented by Bateson et al. (1978).

Absorption, distribution, excretion and metabolism

Clofibrate is rapidly and completely absorbed after oral administration (Thorp, 1962). In man, clofibric acid, a major metabolite of clofibrate, is excreted in the urine in the form of the glucuronide conjugate; the plasma elimination half-life of clofibric acid ranges between 12-25 hours (Chasseaud et al., 1974; Houin et al., 1975; Männistö et al., 1975; Harvengt & Desager, 1976; Gugler & Hartlapp, 1978).

Effects on intermediary metabolism

Clofibrate has substantial effects on hepatic intermediary metabolism, on excretion of cholesterol and bile acids and upon removal of triglycerides in extrahepatic tissues (Havel & Kane, 1973).

Oral administration of 1 g clofibrate daily for 13 days did not significantly alter the half-life of antipyrine and urinary glucaric acid excretion in 5 volunteers (Houin & Tillement, 1978).

No data were available on the mutagenic or prenatal toxic effects of clofibrate in humans.

3.3 Case reports and epidemiological studies of carcinogenicity in humans

One case report has been published (MacGregor, 1979) concerning a man who developed adenocarcinoma of the jejunum, which is rare, after having taken 1-1.5 g/day clofibrate for 15 years. He had also taken phenindione, propranolol and cholestyramine intermittently for 8 years.

Evidence also derives from a large, randomized clinical trial conducted in Budapest, Edinburgh and Prague under the auspices of the WHO to determine whether clofibrate treatment would lower the incidence of ischaemic heart disease in men (Committee of Principal Investigators, 1978). The subjects, 52, 519 men, aged 30-59 at entry to the study; were identified using lists of blood donors, tuberculosis screening registers, electoral rolls and community-wide advertisements; and their serum cholesterol levels were measured (Heady, 1973). Those who met specified screening and medical criteria and who agreed to participate (15, 745) were divided into three groups according to their cholesterol levels. Those in the upper third of the distribution were assigned at random to receive either 1.6 g clofibrate daily (5331 men) or an olive-oil placebo (5296 men). As an additional control group, half of the men in the lowest third of the distribution (5118) were assigned at random to receive the placebo. The average length of follow-up in the trial was 5.3 years, and ascertainment of deaths continued into the year following the trial. The numbers of men in the clofibrate and in the 2 control groups who completed the 5-year trial were 3586, 3608 and 3509, respectively. The incidence of nonfatal myocardial infarction was reduced in the clofibrate-treated group, but there were significantly more deaths from all causes in this group (162) than in the high-cholesterol control group (127; $P < 0.05$). Many of the excess deaths were due to malignant neoplasms [58 (40 during trial, 18 within 1 year after trial) compared with 42 (24 during trial, 18 within 1 year after trial); not statistically significant]. The numbers of deaths from cancer at various sites in the clofibrate-treated and high-cholesterol control groups were: oesophagus and stomach, 9 and 5, respectively; small intestine, colon and rectum, 11 and 6; liver, gall-bladder and pancreas, 7 and 5; larynx, bronchus and lung, 17 and 11; skin, 2 and 2; brain, 5 and 5; haematopoietic tissue, 2 and 3; other or not known, 5 and 5. [This presentation of the data in which certain sites were grouped rather than being given individually may have obscured increases in tumours at specific sites, such as the colon or stomach.] The two high-cholesterol groups were very similar in respect of certain known or suspected cancer risk factors, for example, smoking habits, age, height and weight, as well as several known or suspected cardiovascular risk factors. The average annual age-standardized (ages 40-59) cancer death rates per 1000 were 2.2 in the high-cholesterol-clofibrate group and 2.5 in the low-cholesterol-placebo group; these rates were similar to those of the male populations in the study areas, while the rate for the high-cholesterol-placebo group (1.7) was lower. [It has been suggested on the basis of this evidence that the cancer death rate in the high-cholesterol control group may have been abnormally low, thus influencing the comparison with the clofibrate-treated group. Comparisons with the general population rates, however, may be influenced by the selection factors for entry into the study; therefore, the comparison between the randomly assigned high-cholesterol groups is probably the most appropriate.]

Several other randomized controlled trials of clofibrate were undertaken previously. The Coronary Drug Project Research Group (1975) investigated the effects of lipid-lowering drugs on men aged 30-64 with a history of myocardial infarction. No increase in the cancer death rate was observed in the clofibrate-treated group (10 deaths in 1103 patients, 9/1000) as compared with a placebo-treated group (24 deaths in 2789 patients, 9/1000) during follow-up for 5-8.5 years.

Three other trials of clofibrate were carried out in men who had already developed ischaemic heart disease. In two of these (Group of Physicians of the Newcastle upon Tyne Region, 1971; Krasno & Kidera, 1972), there was no mention of cancer deaths. The third (Research Committee of the Scottish Society of Physicians, 1971) reported 8 cancer deaths, which were 'equally distributed' between the clofibrate and placebo groups.

4. Summary of Data Reported and Evaluation

4.1 Experimental data

Clofibrate has been tested in two studies by oral administration to male rats; it produced hepatocellular carcinomas. In addition, an increased incidence of tumours at sites other than the liver was observed in treated rats compared with controls.

Clofibrate is not mutagenic in *Salmonella typhimurium*. There is no evidence that it is teratogenic in rats and rabbits; however, some evidence of perinatal toxicity is provided by the finding of abnormal postnatal thrombosis in rats.

4.2 Human data

Clofibrate has been used for the long-term treatment of hyperlipidaemia.

Data relating to the carcinogenicity of clofibrate in humans are limited to a single case report and evidence of increased mortality from a variety of cancers, mainly gastrointestinal, in a randomized trial of clofibrate in men with elevated serum cholesterol levels.

4.3 Evaluation

There is *limited evidence*[1] for the carcinogenicity of clofibrate in experimental animals. The epidemiological data were insufficient. No evaluation of the carcinogenicity of clofibrate to humans could be made.

---

[1] See preamble, p. 18.

5. References

Ball, M.R., Gumaa, K.A. & McLean, P. (1979) Effect of clofibrate on the CoA thioester profile in rat liver. *Biochem. biophys. Res. Comm., 87,* 489-496

Bateson, M.C., Maclean, D., Ross, P.E. & Bouchier, I.A.D. (1978) Clofibrate therapy and gallstone induction. *Am. J. dig. Dis., 23,* 623-628

Best, M.M. & Duncan, C.H. (1964) Hypolipemia and hepatomegaly from ethyl chlorophenoxyisobutyrate (CPIB) in the rat. *J. Lab. clin. Med., 64,* 634-642

British Pharmacopoeia Commission (1973) *British Pharmacopoeia,* London, Her Majesty's Stationery Office, p. 115

Calvert, R., Malka, D. & Ménard, D. (1979) Effect of clofibrate on the small intestine of fetal mice. *Histochemistry, 63,* 7-14

Cayen, M.N., Ferdinandi, E.S., Greselin, E., Robinson, W.T. & Dvornik, D. (1977) Clofibrate and clofibric acid: comparison of the metabolic disposition in rats and dogs. *J. Pharmacol. exp. Ther., 200,* 33-43

Chasseaud, L.F., Cooper, A.J. & Saggers, V.H. (1974) Plasma concentrations and bioavailability of clofibrate after administration to human subjects. *J. clin. Pharmacol., 14,* 382-386

Chhabra, S. & Kurup, C.K.R. (1978) Maternal transport of chlorophenoxyisobutyrate at the foetal and neonatal stages of development. *Biochem. Pharmacol., 27,* 2063-2065

Cohen, B.I., Raicht, R.F., Shefer, S. & Mosbach, E.H. (1974) Effects of clofibrate on sterol metabolism in the rat. *Biochim. biophys. Acta, 369,* 79-85

Committee of Principal Investigators (1978) A cooperative trial in the primary prevention of ischaemic heart disease using clofibrate. *Br. Heart J., 40,* 1069-1118

Cooper, J., Geizerova, H. & Oliver, M.F. (1975) Clofibrate and gallstones. *Lancet, i,* 1083

The Coronary Drug Project Research Group (1975) Clofibrate and niacin in coronary heart disease. *J. Am. med. Assoc., 231,* 360-381

Dange, M., Junghani, J., Nachbaur, J., Perraud, J. & Reinert, H. (1975) Postnatal thrombosis (PNT) in newborn rats by hypolipemic agents. Preliminary results (Abstract). *Teratology, 12,* 328

Diener, R.M. & Hsu, B. (1966) Effects of certain aryloxisobutyrates on the rat fetus (Abstract no. 12). *Toxicol. appl. Pharmacol., 8,* 338

Gear, A.R.L., Albert, A.D. & Bednarek, J.M. (1974) The effect of the hypocholesterolemic drug clofibrate on liver mitochondrial biogenesis. A role for neutral mitochondrial proteases. *J. biol. Chem., 249,* 6495-6504

Goodman, L.S. & Gilman, A., eds (1975) *The Pharmacological Basis of Therapeutics,* 5th ed., New York, Macmillan, pp. 747-748, 857

Group of Physicians of the Newcastle upon Tyne Region (1971) Trial of clofibrate in the treatment of ischaemic heart disease. *Br. med. J., iv,* 767-775

Gugler, R. & Hartlapp, J. (1978) Clofibrate kinetics after single and multiple doses. *Clin. pharmacol. Ther., 24,* 432-438

Harvengt, C. & Desager, J.P. (1976) Pharmacokinetic study and bioavailability of three marketed compounds releasing *p*-chlorophenoxyisobutyric acid (CPIB) in volunteers. *Int. J. clin. Pharmacol., 14,* 113-118

Hassan, M.M.A. & Loutfy, M.A. (1979) PMR spectrometric analysis of clofibrate. *Spectros. Lett., 12,* 177-185

Havel, R.J. & Kane, J.P. (1973) Drugs and lipid metabolism. *Ann. Rev. Pharmacol., 13,* 287-308

Heady, J.A. (1973) A cooperative trial on the primary prevention of ischaemic heart disease using clofibrate: design, methods, and progress. *Bull. World Health Organ., 48,* 243-256

Hess, R., Stäubli, W. & Riess, W. (1965) Nature of the hepatomegalic effect produced by ethyl-chlorophenoxy-isobutyrate in the rat. *Nature, 208,* 856-858

Hignite, C. & Azarnoff, D.L. (1977) Drugs and drug metabolites as environmental contaminants: chlorophenoxyisobutyrate and salicylic acid in sewage water effluent. *Life Sci., 20,* 337-342

Houin, G. & Tillement, J.-P. (1978) Clofibrate and enzymatic induction in man. *Int. J. clin. Pharmacol., 16,* 15-154

Houin, G., Thébault, J.J., d'Athis, P., Tillement, J.-P. & Beaumont, J.-L. (1975) A GLC method for estimation of chlorophenoxyisobutyric acid in plasma. Pharmacokinetics of a single oral dose of clofibrate in man. *Eur. J. clin. Pharmacol., 8,* 433-437

Johansson, E. & Ryhage, R. (1976) Gas chromatographic-mass spectrometric identification and determination of residual by-products in clofibrate preparations. *J. Pharm. Pharmacol., 28,* 927-929

Kähönen, M.T. & Ylikahri, R.H. (1974) Effect of clofibrate treatment on the activity of carnitine acetyltransferase in rat tissues. *FEBS Lett., 43,* 297-299

Kijima, Y., Makise, J., Sasaoka, T., Kanayama, M. & Kubota, S. (1978) The adverse actions of clofibrate in chronic hemodialyzed patients. Acute muscular syndrome and others (Jpn.). *Jpn. J. Nephrol., 20,* 955-966

Krasno, L.R. & Kidera, G.J. (1972) Clofibrate in coronary heart disease. Effect on morbidity and mortality. *J. Am. med. Assoc., 219,* 845-851

Krishnakantha, T.P. & Kurup, C.K. R. (1972) Increase in hepatic catalase and glycerol phosphate dehydrogenase activities on administration of clofibrate and and clofenapate to the rat. *Biochem. J., 130,* 167-175

Kurup, C.K.R., Aithal, H.N. & Ramasarma, T. (1970) Increase in hepatic mitochondria on administration of ethyl α-p-chlorophenoxyisobutyrate to the rat. *Biochem. J., 116,* 773-779

Laker, M.E. & Mayes, P.A. (1978) The fate of clofibrate in the perfused rat liver. *Biomedicine, 29,* 88-90

Laker, M.E. & Mayes, P.A. (1979) The immediate and long term effects of clofibrate on the metabolism of the perfused rat liver. *Biochem. Pharmacol., 28,* 2813-2827

Lazarow, P.B. (1978) Rat liver peroxisomes catalyze the β oxidation of fatty acids. *J. biol. Chem., 253,* 1522-1528

Lazarow, P.B. & De Duve, C. (1976) A fatty acyl-CoA oxidizing system in rat liver peroxisomes; enhancement by clofibrate, a hypolidemic drug. *Proc. natl Acad. Sci. USA, 73,* 2043-2046

Lewis, N.J., Witiak, D.T. & Feller, D.R. (1974) Influence of clofibrate (ethyl-4-chlorophenoxyisobutyrate) on hepatic drug metabolism in male rats. *Proc. Soc. exp. Biol. Med., 145,* 281-285

MacGregor, G.A. (1979) Clofibrate and malignancy. *Lancet, i,* 445

Mannaerts, G.P., Thomas, J., Debeer, L.J., McGarry, J.D. & Foster, D.W. (1978) Hepatic fatty acid oxidation and ketogenesis after clofibrate treatment. *Biochim. biophys. Acta, 529,* 201-211

Männistö, P.T., Tuomisto, J., Jounela, A. & Penttilä, O. (1975) Pharmacokinetics of clofibrate and chlorophenoxy isobutyric acid. 1. Cross-over studies on human volunteers. *Acta pharmacol. toxicol., 36,* 353-365

Markwell, M.A.K., Bieber, L.L. & Tolbert, N.E. (1977) Differential increase of hepatic peroxisomal, mitochondrial and microsomal carnitine acyltransferases in clofibrate-fed rats. *Biochem. Pharmacol., 26,* 1697-1702

Metz, G., Specker, M., Sterher, W., Heisler, E. & Grahwit, G. (1977) 1-(Theophyllin-7-yl)-ethyl-2-[2-(*p*-chlorophenoxy)-2-methylpropionate] (ML 1024), a new hypolipemic agent. *Arzneimittelforsch., 27,* 1173-1177

Moody, D.E. & Reddy, J.K. (1974) Increase in hepatic carnitine acetyltransferase activity associated with peroxisomal (microbody) proliferation induced by the hypolipidemic drugs clofibrate, nafenopin, and methyl clofenapate. *Res. Commun. chem. Pathol. Pharmacol., 9,* 501-510

Moody, D.E. & Reddy, J.K. (1978) The hepatic effects of hypolipidemic drugs (clofibrate, nafenopin, fibric acid, and Wy-14, 643) on hepatic peroxisomes and peroxisome-associated enzymes. *Am. J. Pathol., 90,* 435-445

Oliver, M.F. (1962) Reduction of serum-lipid and uric-acid levels by an orally active androsterone. *Lancet, i,* 1321-1323

Paget, G.E. (1963) Experimental studies of the toxicity of atromid with particular reference to fine structural changes in the livers of rodents. *J. Atheroscler. Res., 3,* 729-736

Pantaleoni, G.C. & Valeri, P. (1974) Investigations on the interactions of clofibrate with reproductive function (Ital.). *Clin. Ter., 69,* 321-328

Pellizzari, E.D. & Seltzman, T.A. (1978) Two dimensional gas-liquid chromatography of clofibrate in plasma. *Analyt. Lett., B11,* 975-989

Pertsemlidis, D., Panveliwalla, D. & Ahrens, E.H., Jr (1974) Effects of clofibrate and of an estrogen-progestin combination on fasting biliary lipids and cholic acid kinetics in man. *Gastroenterology, 66,* 565-573

Pierce, E.H. & Chesler, D.L. (1978) Possible association of granulomatous hepatitis with clofibrate therapy. *New Engl. J. Med., 299,* 314

Platt, D.S. & Thorp, J.M. (1966) Changes in the weight and composition of the liver in the rat, dog and monkey treated with ethyl chlorophenoxyisobutyrate. *Biochem. Pharmacol., 15,* 915-925

Pokroy, N., Ress, S. & Gregory, M.C. (1977) Clofibrate-induced complications in renal disease. A case report. *S. Afr. med. J., 52,* 806-808

Pösö, A.R. & Hillbom, M.E. (1977) Metabolism of ethanol and sorbitol in clofibrate-treated rats. *Biochem. Pharmacol., 26,* 331-335

Powanda, M.C., Abeles, F.B., Bostian, K.A., Fowler, J.P. & Hauer, E.C. (1979) Differential effect of clofibrate on inflammation-induced alterations in plasma proteins in the rat. *Biochem. J., 178,* 633-641

Reddy, J.K. & Krishnakantha, T.P. (1975) Hepatic peroxisome proliferation: induction by two novel compounds structurally unrelated to clofibrate. *Science, 190,* 787-789

Reddy, J.K. & Kumar, N.S. (1977) The peroxisome proliferation-associated polypeptide in rat liver. *Biochem. biophys. Res. Commun., 77,* 824-829

Reddy, J.K. & Kumar, N.S. (1979) Stimulation of catalase synthesis and increase of carnitine acetyltransferase activity in the liver of intact female rats fed clofibrate. *J. Biochem., 85,* 847-856

Reddy, J.K. & Qureshi, S.A. (1979) Tumorigenicity of the hypolipidaemic peroxisome proliferator ethyl-α-p-chlorophenoxyisobutyrate (clofibrate) in rats. *Br. J. Cancer, 40,* 476-482

Reddy, J.K. & Rao, M.S. (1978) Enhancement by Wy-14,643, a hepatic peroxisome proliferator, of diethylnitrosamine-initiated hepatic tumorigenesis in the rat. *Br. J. Cancer, 38,* 537-543

Reddy, J., Bunyaratvej, S. & Svoboda, D. (1969) Microbodies in experimentally altered cells. IV. Acatalasemic (Cs^b) mice treated with CPIB. *J. Cell Biol., 42,* 587-596

Reddy, J., Chiga, M. & Svoboda, D. (1971) Stimulation of liver catalase synthesis in rats by ethyl-α-p-chlorophenoxyisobutyrate. *Biochem. biophys. Res. Commun., 43,* 318-324

Research Committee of the Scottish Society of Physicians (1971) Ischaemic heart disease: a secondary prevention trial using clofibrate. *Br. med. J., iv,* 775-784

Schwandt, P., Klinge, O. & Immich, H. (1978) Clofibrate and the liver. *Lancet, ii,* 325

Solberg, H.E., Aas, M. & Daae, L.N.W. (1972) The activity of the different carnitine acyltransferases in the liver of clofibrate-fed rats. *Biochem. biophys. Acta, 280,* 434-439

Svoboda, D.J. & Azarnoff, D.L. (1966) Response of hepatic microbodies to a hypolipidemic agent, ethyl chlorophenoxyisobutyrate (CPIB). *J. Cell Biol., 30,* 442-450

Svoboda, D.J. & Azarnoff, D.L. (1979) Tumors in male rats fed ethylchlorophenoxyisobutyrate, a hypolipidemic drug. *Cancer Res., 39,* 3419-3428

Svoboda, D.J. & Reddy, J.K. (1974) *Some biologic properties of microbodies (peroxisomes).* In: Ioachim, H.L., ed., *Pathobiology Annual,* Vol. 4, New York, Appleton-Century Crofts, pp. 1-32

Svoboda, D., Grady, H. & Azarnoff, D. (1967) Microbodies in experimentally altered cells. *J. Cell Biol., 35,* 127-152

Teräväinen, H. & Mäkitie, J. (1976) Myokymia, unusual side-effect of clofibrate. *Lancet, ii,* 1298

Thorp, J.M. (1962) Experimental evaluation of an orally active combination of androsterone with ethyl chlorophenoxyisobutyrate. *Lancet, i,* 1323-1326

Thorp, J.M. & Waring, W.S. (1962) Modification of metabolism and distribution of lipids by ethyl chlorophenoxyisobutyrate. *Nature, 194,* 948-949

US Food & Drug Administration (1979) *FDA Drug Bulletin,* Rockville, MD, August, p. 14

US International Trade Commission (1978) *Imports of Benzenoid Chemicals and Products, 1977,* USITC Publication 900, Washington DC, US Government Printing Office, p. 83

US International Trade Commission (1979) *Imports of Benzenoid Chemicals and Products, 1978,* USITC Publication 990, Washington DC, US Government Printing Office, p. 82

US Pharmacopeial Convention, Inc. (1975) *The US Pharmacopeia,* 19th rev., Rockville, MD, pp. 96-97

Wade, A., ed. (1977) *Martindale, The Extra Pharmacopoeia,* 27th ed., London, The Pharmaceutical Press, pp. 363-366

Warren, J.R., Simmon, V.F. & Reddy, J.K. (1980) Properties of hypolipidemic peroxisome proliferators in the lymphocyte [3H] thymidine and *Salmonella* mutagenesis assays. *Cancer Res., 40,* 36-41

WHO (1979) *Drug Information - July - September 1979,* PDT/DI/79.3, Geneva, p. 17

Windholz, M., ed. (1976) *The Merck Index,* 9th ed., Rahway, NJ, Merck & Co., Inc., p. 305

Yeshurun, D. & Gotto, A.M., Jr (1976) Drug treatment of hyperlipidemia. *Am. J. Med., 60,* 379-396

DAPSONE

1. Chemical and Physical Data

1.1 Synonyms and trade names

Chem. Abstr. Services Reg. No.: 80-08-0

Chem. Abstr. Name: Benzenamine, 4,4'-sulfonylbis-

IUPAC Systematic Name: Bis(4-aminophenyl)sulphone

Synonyms: Bis(4-aminophenyl)sulfone; bis(*para*-aminophenyl)sulfone; bis-(4-aminophenyl) sulphone; bis(*para*-aminophenyl)sulphone; DADPS; dapsonum; DDS; DDS [pharmaceutical]; diamino-4,4'-diphenyl sulfone; 4,4'-diaminodiphenyl sulfone; *para,para*-diaminodiphenyl sulfone; diamino-4,4'-diphenyl sulphone; 4,4'-diaminodiphenyl sulphone; *para,para*-diaminodiphenyl sulphone; di(4-aminophenyl) sulfone; di(*para*-aminophenyl)sulfone; di(4-aminophenyl)sulphone; di(*para*-aminophenyl)sulphone; diphenylsulfon; diphenylsulfone; diphenylsulphon; diphenylsulphone; 1,1'-sulfonylbis(4-aminobenzene); 4,4'sulfonylbisaniline; 4,4'-sulfonylbisbenzamine; *para,para*-sulfonylbisbenzamine; *para,para*-sulfonylbisbenzenamine; 4,4'sulfonyldianiline; *para,para*-sulfonyldianiline; 1,1'-sulphonylbis(4-aminobenzene); 4,4'-sulphonylbisbenzamine; *para,para*-sulphonylbisbenzamine; 4,4'-sulphonylbisbenzenamine; *para,para*-sulphonylbisbenzenamine; sulphonyldianiline; 4,4'-sulphonyldianiline; *para,para*-sulphonyldianiline

Trade names: Avlosulfon; Avlosulphone; Croysulfone; Croysulphone; Dapson; Diphenasone; Diphone; Disulone; DDS (VAN); Dubronax; Dumitone; Eporal; 1358F; F1358; Maloprim; Metabolite C; Novophone; Sulfona; Sulfona-Mae; Sulfone UCB; Sulphadione; Sulphon-mere; Tarimyl; Udolac

1.2 Structural and molecular formulae and molecular weight

$$H_2N-\underset{}{\underset{}{\bigcirc}}-\underset{O}{\overset{O}{\underset{\|}{S}}}-\underset{}{\underset{}{\bigcirc}}-NH_2$$

$C_{12}H_{12}N_2O_2S$ Mol. wt: 248.3

1.3 Chemical and physical properties of the pure substance

From Wade (1977) or Windholz (1976) unless otherwise specified

(a) *Description:* White or creamy-white crystalline powder with slightly bitter taste
(b) *Melting-point:* 175-176°C (also 180.5°C)
(c) *Spectroscopy data:* λ_{max} 260 nm, A(1%, 1 cm) = 73; and 295 nm, A(1%, 1cm) = 121 (in methanol). Infrared, nuclear magnetic resonance and mass spectral data have been tabulated (Orzech *et al.*, 1976).
(d) *Solubility:* Practically insoluble in water; soluble in ethanol (1 in 30 w/v), acetone, methanol and dilute mineral acids
(e) *Stability:* Sensitive to oxidation and light

1.4 Technical products and impurities

Various national and international pharmacopoeias give specifications for the purity of dapsone in pharmaceutical products. For example, dapsone is available in the US as a USP grade contining 99.0-101.0% active ingredient calculated on the dried basis. The weight loss on drying should not exceed 1.5%, residue on ignition should be less than 0.1%, and the amount of selenium should be less than 0.003%. It is available in 25 and 100 mg doses as tablets containing 92.5-107.5% of the stated amount of dapsone (US Pharmacopeial Convention Inc., 1975). In the British Pharmacopoeia, a test is available for impurities in dapsone, based on thin-layer chromatography (British Pharmacopoeia Commission, 1973).

In the UK, dapsone is available as injections containing 20% w/v or 5% w/v of dapsone. It is also available in 25 and 100 mg doses as tablets (Wade, 1977).

In Japan, dapsone is available in 25 mg doses as tablets.

A number of specifically identified related impurities [2,4'-sulphonylbis(benzenamine), 4-(phenylsulphonylbenzenamine) and 4-(4'-chlorophenylsulphonyl)benzenamine] have been reported in commercially available samples of dapsone (Cheung & Lim, 1977).

2. Production, Use, Occurrence and Analysis

2.1 Production and use

(a) Production

Dapsone was first synthesized from *para*-chloronitrobenzene by Weijlard and Messerly in 1945 (Windholz, 1976). A possible method for its manufacture is the condensation of benzene with sulphuric acid to yield diphenylsulphone, which can be nitrated to its 4,4'-dinitro derivative. Reduction of this compound (e.g., with tin and hydrochloric acid) yields dapsone (Harvey, 1975).

Dapsone was first marketed in the US in 1957, but it is apparently not presently manufactured in the US. US imports in 1978 amounted to 11,500 kg (US International Trade Commission, 1979). No data were available on US exports.

Dapsone is not produced commercially in Japan, but minor amounts (less than 1000 kg annually) are imported from France.

No data were available on its production in Europe or elsewhere in the world.

(b) Use

The antibacterial spectrum and mechanism of action of dapsone are similar to those of the sulphonamides.

In human medicine, it is used primarily in the long-term, chronic treatment of all forms of leprosy. The recommended dosage is 100 mg daily in adults for lepromatous forms and 50 mg daily for nonlepromatous forms (WHO, 1977).

Dapsone has also been used in the treatment of tuberculosis (Harvey, 1975) and is used as an antimalarial at a dose of 100 mg/week in conjunction with pyrimethamine when resistance to pyrimethamine, other antifolate preparations or chloroquine is known or suspected (Association of British Pharmaceutical Industry, 1979).

Dapsone has also been used in the treatment of dermatitis herpetiformis (Harvey, 1975).

Dapsone is also used in veterinary practice against coccidiosis in cattle. The usual dose is 100 mg/kg bw followed by one-half that amount daily for 4 to 5 days. As an intramammary infusion for bovine streptococcal mastitis, dapsone may be used alone or in combination with benzylpenicillin (Harvey, 1975).

A derivative of dapsone, 4,4'-diacetyldiaminodiphenyl sulphone, has been used in clinical trials as a long-acting repository sulphone: the slow release of dapsone is mediated through deacetylation of the drug. A single intramuscular dose of 225 mg given every 11 weeks produces the same response as a 50 mg dose of dapsone given daily. The disodium formaldehyde sulphoxylate substitution product of dapsone (sulphoxone sodium) is another derivative of dapsone used in the therapy of leprosy, especially in patients who suffer from gastric distress when treated with dapsone (Goodman & Gilman, 1975).

Dapsone has found some use as a hardening agent in the curing of epoxy resins (Windholz, 1976), but it is apparently not being used for this purpose now.

2.2 Occurrence

Dapsone is not known to occur in nature.

2.3 Analysis

Analytical methods for the determination of dapsone based on colorimetry, titration, fluorimetry, paper chromatography, high-pressure liquid chromatography, gas chromatography and thin-layer chromatography have been reviewed by Orzech *et al.* (1976).

Typical methods of analysis for dapsone in various matrices are summarized in Table 1. Abbreviations used are: EC-CG, electron capture-gas chromatography; HPLC, high-performance liquid chromatography; I, immunoassay; UV, ultra-violet spectrometry; and T, titration.

Table 1. Analytical methods for dapsone

Sample matrix	Sample preparation	Assay procedure	Sensitivity or limit of detection	Reference
Formulation	Powder sample; add hydrochloric acid and water	T (sodium nitrite)	not given	US Pharmacopeial Convention, Inc., 1975
Biological samples				
Plasma	Prepared for diazotization by several extractions; the diazotized product is processed through several additional steps prior to chromatography	EC-GC	1-10 µg/l	Burchfield et al., 1970
	Mix with water; add sodium hydroxide and diethyl ether; shake and centrifuge; evaporate organic phase; add water, acetonitrile and acetic acid	HPLC-UV	20 µg/l	Carr et al., 1978
Serum and urine	Adjust sample to pH 7.2	I	0.3 mg/l	Huikeshoven et al., 1978

3. Biological Data Relevant to the Evaluation of Carcinogenic Risk to Humans

3.1 Carcinogenicity studies in animals

(a) Oral administration

Mouse: Two groups of 35 male and 35 female B6C3F1 mice, 5 weeks of age, were fed a diet containing 500 or 1000 mg/kg diet dapsone (USP grade) on 5 days/week for 78 weeks and observed up to 106-108 weeks. A group of 14 male and 14 female matched controls were untreated. Seventy-three percent of the high-dose males and 67% of the low-dose males survived to the end of the study. Median survival rates were 92 weeks in treated females and 69 and 102 weeks in untreated male and female controls. There was no difference in the incidence or types of tumours between treated and control animals (National Cancer Institute, 1977).

Forty pregnant C57Bl/6 mice were given 100 mg/kg bw dapsone (purity not specified) by intragastric intubation on days 17 and 18 of gestation and when lactating, 5 times weekly from the 3rd day after the birth of their offspring. Of their offspring, 50 males and 37 females were subsequently given the same dose of dapsone 5 times weekly over 104 weeks starting 2 weeks after separation from their mothers; the total dose received after weaning was 52 g/kg bw (1.2-1.4 g/mouse). The animals were observed for lifetime; no difference in survival was observed between treated and control mice. No significant difference in the incidence or site of tumours was seen between the 50 males and 37 females of the experimental group that survived over 24 weeks and the 47 male and 47 female untreated controls that survived for similar times (28/50 *versus* 20/47 in males, and 23/37 *versus* 24/47 in females) (Griciute & Tomatis, 1980).

Rat: Twenty 50-55-day-old Sprague-Dawley female rats were given single doses of 100 mg of dapsone (purity not specified) in sesame oil by gastric intubation. At the end of the 6-month observation period, no tumours were reported in the 19 surviving rats. Another group of 20 Sprague-Dawley females, 40-days old at the beginning of the experiment, were given 30 mg/rat of dapsone in sesame oil by gastric intubation 10 times in a one-month period and then observed up to 9 months. No tumours were reported in the 19 surviving rats (Griswold *et al.*, 1966, 1968). [Attention is drawn to the short observation period due to the special design of the experiment.]

A group of 25 male Wistar rats were fed a diet containing increasing concentrations of dapsone (purity not stated). The experiment was started on 25-day-old rats with a concentration of 0.025%; the dose increased every 10th or 20th day, and from the 90th day after onset of the experiment until the 25th month the rats received 0.3% of dapsone in their food. During 17-25 months, 9 tumours were detected in 8/12 rats: 2 spleen tumours (fibrosarcoma and fibroangioma), 3 thyroid follicular adenocarcinomas, 1 fibrosarcoma of the retroperitoneum and 1 of the mesentery, 1 reticulosarcoma of the intestine and 1 liver cavernous angioma. One subcutaneous fibroma was observed in 13 control males observed up to 25 months (Bergel, 1973).

Two groups of 35 male and 35 female Fischer 344 rats (34 days of age) were fed a diet containing 600 or 1200 mg/kg diet dapsone (USP grade) on 5 days/week and control diets on 2 days/week for 78 weeks and observed for an additional 26-27 weeks. Mesenchymal tumours occurred in 13/35 males fed the lower concentration of dapsone, and in 22/33 males fed the higher concentration. In the low-dose group, the tumours were: 6 splenic fibromas, 4 sarcomas (not otherwise specified), 1 fibrosarcoma and 1 fibroma of the peritoneum, 1 fibroma of the pancreas and 1 of the abdominal cavity. In the high-dose group, there were 3 sarcomas (not otherwise specified), 3 fibrosarcomas and 10 fibromas of the spleen and 3 sarcomas (not otherwise specified) and 3 fibrosarcomas of the peritoneum. None of these types of tumours occurred in male controls. The incidence of spleen tumours in males was statistically significant in both experimental groups when compared with 43 pooled controls (low dose, $P = 0.006$; high dose, $P<0.001$) and in the high-dose group when compared with 14 matched controls ($P = 0.002$). The incidence of malignant mesenchymal tumours (sarcomas and fibrosarcomas) in the peritoneum was also significant in males of the 2 treated groups: $P = 0.014$ and $P = 0.005$, respectively, when compared with 44 pooled controls. The authors detected fibrosis and osseous metaplasia in the spleen and peritoneum of some tumour-free males. No tumours or fibrosis of the spleen or peritoneum were observed in females (National Cancer Institute, 1977).

Twenty pregnant BD IV rats were given 100 mg/kg bw dapsone (purity not specified) by intragastric intubation on days 18 and 19 of gestation and 5 times weekly when lactating from the third day after the birth of their offspring. Of their offspring, 76 males and 72 females were subsequently given dapsone 5 times weekly for 104 weeks, starting 2 weeks after separation from their mothers; the total dose received after weaning was 52 g/kg bw (10-16 g/rat). The animals were observed for lifetime. Malignant fibrosarcomas and angiosarcomas of the spleen occurred in 4/44 males ($P = 0.046$) and 1/63 females that survived over 34 weeks, compared with 0/49 male and 0/47 female control rats that received olive-oil by gastric intubation and which survived for similar times. Partial or complete fibrosation of the spleen, in some cases with calcification and bone formation, was observed in 47% of males and 1.2% of females. Spleen sarcomas were topographically related to the lesions. Malignant C (parafollicular)-cell tumours of the thyroid were observed in 8/44 males and 13/63 females of the treated group compared with 2/49 males and 3/47 females of the control group ($P = 0.014$). Areas of C-cell proliferation in the thyroid were observed equally in all groups of rats, including controls (Griciute & Tomatis, 1980).

(b) Intraperitoneal administration

Mouse: Three groups of 10 male and 10 female A/He mice, 6-8 weeks old, were given 12 i.p. injections (3 times weekly during 4 weeks) of dapsone (purity not specified) in steroid-suspending vehicle. Total doses were 0.525, 1.312 or 2.625 g/kg bw. All survivors (17, 15 and 13 mice of both sexes) were killed 24 weeks after the 1st injection. The numbers of mice with lung tumours (males and females combined) were 6, 7 and 4, and average numbers of tumours per mouse were 0.35 ± 0.09, 0.87 ± 0.2 and 0.38 ± 0.11. Of 30 male and 30 female control mice injected with steroid-suspending vehicle alone, 6/28 and 6/30 developed lung tumours; the average numbers of lung tumours per mouse were 0.22 ± 0.04 and 0.19 ± 0.04 (Stoner *et al.*, 1973). [Attention is drawn to the limitation of a negative result obtained in this test system.]

(c) Other experimental systems

Administration in conjunction with known carcinogens: Forty pregnant C57Bl/6 *mice* received 100 mg/kg bw dapsone by intragastric intubation on days 17 and 18 of gestation and 5 times weekly when lactating. Of their offspring, 35 males and 35 females were subsequently given i.p. injections of urethane (dose and duration unspecified). A control group of 30 male and 30 female young adult C57Bl mice received urethane only. Multiple pulmonary adenomas, lachrymal gland adenomas and liver-cell tumours occurred with the same frequency in the dapsone-plus-urethane-treated group and in the urethane-control group (Griciute & Tomatis, 1980).

A group of 15 male and 26 female BD IV *rats* were administered dapsone by gastric intubation 5 times a week during 104 weeks and benzo[a]pyrene by intratracheal instillations. The total dose of dapsone was 10-16 g/rat. A control group of 16 male and 29 female rats received only benzo[a]pyrene. Malignant tumours of the respiratory tract were observed in 8/14 male and 6/24 female rats in the group that received the combined treatment, and in 3/16 male and 12/29 female rats in the group that received benzo[a]pyrene only (Griciute & Tomatis, 1980).

3.2 Other relevant biological data

(a) Experimental systems

Toxic effects

In male rats, the i.p. LD_{50} is about 200 mg/kg bw and the oral LD_{50} about 630 mg/kg bw; in female rats, the oral LD_{50} is about 650 mg/kg bw; the i.p. LD_{50} in male mice is about 230 mg/kg bw (Wu & DuBois, 1970).

Daily i.p. doses to male rats of 50 mg/kg bw for 3 days resulted in lowered red blood cells counts and haemoglobin (Dhar & Mukherji, 1969). Daily doses of 30, 60 and 120 mg/kg bw over a period of 30 days decrease the red blood cell count by 8, 10 and 14% and haemoglobin by 8, 12 and 17%. It was therefore concluded that 20 mg/kg bw daily over a long period is the maximum tolerated i.p. dose in rats (Dhar & Mukherji, 1971). Studies of subacute toxicity indicated that rats can tolerate repeated daily oral doses of 150 mg/kg bw for 60 days (Wu & DuBois, 1970).

The toxic effects of dapsone in mice and rats were found by *in vitro* and *in vivo* experiments to be mediated by an inhibitory effect of the drug on the oxidation of pyruvate (Wu & DuBois, 1970).

No data on prenatal toxicity were available to the Working Group.

Absorption, distribution, excretion and metabolism

Much variation between species has been reported with regard to the kinetics of dapsone (Francis, 1953; Chang *et al.*, 1969; Biggs *et al.*, 1975). The half-life of dapsone in mice ranged between 2 and 4 hrs (Levy *et al.*, 1972) - very short in comparison with the 14-53 hrs in humans (Peters *et al.*, 1972). The shortest half-life for dapsone has been reported in rabbits (0.8 hrs), and in rats the half-life is about 6 hrs (Murray *et al.*, 1972); that in dogs is 11.7 hrs (Peters *et al.*, 1975a).

Rats fed a diet containing 50 mg/kg diet dapsone had similar plasma levels at 7 days and at 21 days. Similar results were found in mice fed a diet containing 25 mg/kg diet dapsone. In rats the tissue:plasma ratios ranged from 0.7 to 1.8, with a maximal ratio of 2.2 in foot pads and tail skin; in mice they ranged from 0.6 to 1.6, with a maximal ratio of 3.5 for liver (Gordon *et al.*, 1974). Dapsone has also been detected in nerves of mice fed a diet containing 0.01%, at the same concentration as in blood (Balakrishnan & Desikan, 1977).

In rats, after oral or i.p. administration, dapsone is excreted in the urine and faeces. Excretion in the bile was demonstrated directly in bile-duct-cannulated rats. The main metabolite in the urine was dapsone-*N*-sulphamate, with small amounts of acetyldapsone, *N*-acetyl dapsone *N'*-sulphamate and dapsone *N*-glucuronide. The latter was also found in the bile (Andoh *et al.*, 1974). There was no evidence of acetylation to monoacetyl dapsone in dogs (Peters *et al.*, 1975a).

Evidence of *N*-hydroxylation of dapsone and the possible formation of nitroso- and azoxy- analogues of dapsone was found *in vitro* with rat microsomes (Cucinell *et al.*, 1972). *N*-Hydroxylation of dapsone was also observed with rabbit liver microsomes (Tabarelli &

Uehleke, 1971). After oral doses of 50 mg/kg bw female dogs excreted 3-4% of the dose as 4-N-hydroxy-4'-aminodiphenylsulphone (Tabarelli & Uehleke, 1971). Comparative observations in humans, rats and guinea-pigs confirmed the formation of N-hydroxy metabolites (Israili et al., 1973).

Mutagenicity and other, related short-term tests

Neither dapsone nor its N-acetyl and N,N'-diacetyl metabolites were mutagenic in *Salmonella typhimurium* strains TA1535, TA1537, TA1538, TA98 or TA100 with or without liver microsomal fractions from Aroclor 1254-pretreated rats, mice or hamsters (Peters et al., 1978).

In an *in vitro* chromosome aberration study using human lymphocytes, Beiguelman et al. (1975) observed no differences in the proportion of metaphases between control and treated cultures (0.4 and 4 µg dapsone/ml). No effect on chromosomes was seen with the lower concentration, whereas with the higher concentration a significant increase in aneuploid metaphases and in achromatic gaps was observed.

(b) Humans

Toxic effects

The adverse effects and toxic reactions following chronic treatment with dapsone are well documented and have been reviewed by Graham (1975). A mild degree of haemolytic anaemia, together with methaemoglobin formation occurs commonly (Shelley & Goldwein, 1976; Wilson & Harris, 1977; Halmekoski et al., 1978; Elonen et al., 1979). Other reported, but much less common adverse reactions include the following: leucopenia, agranulocytosis, infectious mononucleosis syndrome, pseudo-leukaemia (Leiker, 1955; Levine & Weintraub, 1968; Wilson & Harris, 1977); dermatitis, phototoxicity, lupus erythematosus (Vandersteen & Jordon, 1974); urticaria (Verma et al., 1973); cholestatic hepatitis (Stone & Goodwin, 1978); abnormalities in liver function tests (Goette, 1977); psychosis (Verma et al., 1973); peripheral neuropathy (Hubler & Solomon, 1972; Epstein & Bohm, 1976; Koller et al., 1977); renal papillary necrosis (Hoffbrand, 1978); and hypoalbuminaemia (Kingham et al., 1979; Young & Marks, 1979). Excerbation of lepromatous leprosy may occur in malnourished persons 5-6 weeks after initiation of therapy (DeGowin, 1967).

Absorption, distribution, excretion and metabolism

Dapsone is mainly converted to monoacetyl and diacetyl derivatives under polymorphic genetic control (Gelber et al., 1971; Peters & Levy, 1971; Peters et al., 1972, 1975b).

Both dapsone and monoacetyldapsone are largely bound to serum protein; this could account for the long half-life of the drug in man (Biggs & Levy, 1971).

Dapsone is also metabolized by N-hydroxylation to form monohydroxydapsone; and a new metabolite, the monohydroxylamine of 4-acetylamino-4'-aminodiphenylsulphone,has also been identified in urine (Israili et al., 1973). After oral treatment (200 mg), N-hydroxy metabolites can comprise 50% of the dose in the urine (Uehleke & Tabarelli, 1973).

In a suicidal patient who ingested a large dose of dapsone, high levels of dapsone and monoacetyldapsone were found in the urine; trace amounts of azoxydapsone were found in urine but not in serum (Elonen et al., 1979).

The suggestion that generation of reactive N-hydroxy metabolites in the cells of various organs might explain the toxic symptoms due to dapsone (Uehleke, 1971) was confirmed in in vitro experiments in which human red cells were incubated with dapsone in the presence of rat liver microsomes; these showed that N-hydroxydapsone (and/or N-oxydapsone) was the cause of the methaemoglobinaemia observed in dapsone therapy (Cucinell et al., 1972).

No data on the prenatal toxicity or mutagenicity of this compound in humans were available.

3.3 Case reports and epidemiological studies of carcinogenicity in humans

Seven cases of cancer have been reported in patients treated with dapsone for dermatitis herpetiformis: one adenocarcinoma of the caecum, two lung carcinomas, one renal carcinoma, one prostatic cancer, one anaplastic tumour of uncertain histology and one Hodgkin's disease (Gjone & Nordöy, 1970; Mänsson, 1971). Five of these cancers were found in 9 patients during the three years following gastrointestinal investigations which were carried out either because of anaemia [in some cases possibly indicating pre-existing cancer] or because of their need for high doses of dapsone (Mänsson, 1971).

Two studies of the relative frequency of cancer at autopsy in patients with leprosy, some of whom would have been treated with dapsone (Furuta et al., 1972; Purtilo & Pangi, 1975), and a cohort study of 848 leprosy patients yielding 21 cancer deaths (19.7 expected) (Oleinick, 1969) have not suggested an increased mortality from cancer in these patients. [These studies were not designed to study the carcinogenicity of dapsone, and no data on dapsone use were provided.]

4. Summary of Data Reported and Evaluation

4.1 Experimental data

Dapsone has been tested by oral administration in mice and rats, by intraperitoneal administration in mice and by prenatal and lifetime oral exposure in mice and rats. In three different studies in rats, high doses of dapsone induced mesenchymal tumours of the spleen in males (and of the peritoneum in two studies). An increased incidence of tumours of the thyroid was found in rats of both sexes in one study and in males in another study.

In mice, the experiment involving intraperitoneal administration of dapsone could not be evaluated. The other two experiments did not provide evidence of carcinogenicity.

Dapsone and its acetylated metabolites were not mutagenic to *Salmonella typhimurium*. Attention is drawn to the absence of studies on the teratogenicity of this compound.

4.2 Human data

Dapsone is used mainly in the treatment of leprosy.

Several cases of cancer have been reported in patients with dermatitis herpetiformis treated with dapsone. There was no evidence of an increased rate of cancer in patients with leprosy, many of whom would also have been treated with the drug.

4.3 Evaluation

There is *limited evidence*[1] for the carcinogenicity of dapsone in experimental animals. The epidemiological data were insufficient. No evaluation of the carcinogenicity of dapsone to humans can be made.

---

[1] See preamble, p. 18.

5. References

Andoh, B.Y.A., Renwick, A.G. & Williams, R.T. (1974) The excretion of [^{35}S] dapsone and its metabolites in the urine, faeces and bile of the rat. *Xenobiotica, 4,* 571-583

Association of the British Pharmaceutical Industry (1979) *Data Sheet Compendium, 1979-80,* London, Pharmind Publications Ltd, p. 1104

Balakrishnan, S. & Desikan, K.V. (1977) Blood and tissue levels of diamino diphenyl sulphone (DDS) in experimental mice. *Indian J. med. Res., 65,* 201-205

Beiguelman, B., Pisani, R.C.B. & El Guindy, M.M. (1975) *In vitro* effect of dapsone on human chromosomes. *Int. J. Lepr., 43,* 41-44

Bergel, M. (1973) Carcinogenic activity of diaminodiphenylsulphone (DDS) (Span.). *Publ. Cent. Est. Leprol., 13,* 30-41

Biggs, J.T. & Levy, L. (1971) Binding of dapsone and monoacetyldapsone by human plasma proteins. *Proc. Soc. exp. Biol. Med., 137,* 692-695

Biggs, J.T., Jr, Uher, A.K., Levy, L., Gordon, G.R. & Peters, J.H. (1975) Renal and biliary disposition of dapsone in the dog. *Antimicrob. Agents Chemother., 7,* 816-824

British Pharmacopoeia Commission (1973) *British Pharmacopoeia,* London, Her Majesty's Stationery Office, p. 140

Burchfield, H.P., Storrs, E.E. & Bhat, V.K. (1970) *Annual Contract Progress Report to the National Institute of Allergy and Infectious Diseases. Analytical Methods for Analysis of DDS, MADDS, DADDS and B663,* PB196817, Gulf South Research Institute for National Institutes of Health, Springfield, VA, National Technical Information Service

Carr, K., Oates, J.A., Nies, A.S. & Woosley, R.L. (1978) Simultaneous analysis of dapsone and monoacetyldapsone employing high performance liquid chromatography: a rapid method for determination of acetylator phenotype. *Br. J. clin. Pharmacol., 6,* 421-427

Chang, T., Chang, S.F., Baukema, J., Savory, A., Dill, W.A. & Glazko, A.J. (1969) Metabolic disposition of dapsone (4,4'-diamino-diphenyl sulfone; DDS) (Abstract no. 168). *Fed. Proc., 28,* 289

Cheung, A.P. & Lim, P. (1977) Contaminants in commercial dapsone. *J. pharm. Sci., 66,* 1723-1726

Cucinell, S.A., Israili, Z.H. & Dayton, P.G. (1972) Microsomal N-oxidation of dapsone as a cause of methemoglobin formation in human red cells. *Am. J. trop. Med. Hyg., 21*, 322-331

DeGowin, R.L. (1967) A review of the therapeutic and hemolytic effects of dapsone. *Arch. intern. Med., 120*, 242-248

Dhar, D.C. & Mukherji, A. (1969) Anaemia in subacute toxicity with DDS in white rats. *Indian J. med. Res., 57*, 1028-1031

Dhar, D.C. & Mukherji, A. (1971) Effect of long-term administration of 4,4'-diamino diphenyl sulphone (DDS) in white rats. *Indian J. exp. Biol., 9*, 388-390

Elonen, E., Neuvonen, P.J., Halmekoski, J. & Mattila, M.J. (1979) Acute dapsone intoxication : a case with prolonged symptoms. *Clin. Toxicol., 14*, 79-85

Epstein, F.W. & Bohm, M. (1976) Dapsone-induced peripheral neuropathy. *Arch. Dermatol., 112*, 1761-1762

Francis, J. (1953) The distribution of sulphone in the tissues of various animals. *J. comp. Pathol., 63*, 1-6

Furuta, M., Ozaki, M., Hakada, M., Takahashi, S., Matsumoto, S. & Murakami, M. (1972) Malignant tumours in leprosy patients. Autopsy reports from Oku-Komyo-En (Jpn.). *Repura. La Lepr. (Tokyo), 41*, 76-77

Gelber, R., Peters, J.H., Gordon, G.R., Glazko, A.J. & Levy, L. (1971) The polymorphic acetylation of dapsone in man. *Clin. Pharmacol. Ther., 12*, 225-238

Gjone, E. & Nordöy, A. (1970) Dermatitis herpetiformis, steatorrhoea, and malignancy. *Br. med. J., i*, 610

Goette, D.K. (1977) Dapsone-induced hepatic changes. *Arch. Dermatol., 113*, 1616-1617

Goodman, L.S. & Gilman, A., eds (1975) *The Pharmacological Basis of Therapeutics*, 5th ed., New York, Macmillan, pp. 1216-1218

Gordon, G.R., Ghoul, D.C., Murray, J.F., Jr, Peters, J.H. & Levy, L. (1974) Tissue levels of dapsone and monoacetyldapsone in rats and mice receiving dietary dapsone. *Int. J. Lepr., 42*, 373-374

Graham, W.R., Jr (1975) Adverse effects of dapsone. *Int. J. Dermatol., 14*, 494-500

Griciute, L. & Tomatis, L. (1980) Carcinogenicity of dapsone in mice and rats. *Int. J. Cancer, 25,* 123-129

Griswold, D.P., Jr, Casey, A.E., Weisburger, E.K., Weisburger, J.H. & Schabel, F.M., Jr (1966) On the carcinogenicity of a single intragastric dose of hydrocarbons, nitrosamines, aromatic amines, dyes, coumarins, and miscellaneous chemicals in female Sprague-Dawley rats. *Cancer Res., 26,* 619-625

Griswold, D.P., Jr, Casey, A.E., Weisburger, E.K. & Weisburger, J.H. (1968) The carcinogenicity of multiple intragastric doses of aromatic and heterocyclic nitro or amino derivatives in young female Sprague-Dawley rats. *Cancer Res., 28,* 924-933

Halmekoski, J., Mattila, M.J. & Mustakallio, K.K. (1978) Metabolism and haemolytic effect of dapsone and its metabolites in man. *Med. Biol., 56,* 216-221

Harvey, S.C. (1975) *Antimicrobial drugs.* In: Osol, A., ed., *Remington's Pharmaceutical Sciences,* 15th ed., Easton, PA, Mack Publishing Co., pp. 1150-1151

Hoffbrand, B.I. (1978) Dapsone and renal papillary necrosis. *Br. med. J., i,* 78

Hubler, W.R., Jr & Solomon, H. (1972) Neurotoxicity of sulfones. *Arch. Dermatol., 106,* 598

Huikeshoven, H., Landheer, J.E., van Denderen, A.C., Vlasman, M., Leiker, D.L., Das, P.K., Goldring, O.L. & Pondman, K.W. (1978) Demonstration of dapsone in urine and serum by ELISA inhibition. *Lancet, i,* 280-281

Israili, Z.H., Cucinell, S.A., Vaught, J., Davis, E., Lesser, J.M. & Dayton, P.G. (1973) Studies of the metabolism of dapsone in man and experimental animals : formation of *N*-hydroxy metabolites. *J. Pharmacol. exp. Ther., 187,* 138-151

Kingham, J.G.C., Swain, P., Swarbrick, E.T., Walker, J.G. & Dawson, A.M. (1979) Dapsone and severe hypoalbuminaemia. A report of two cases. *Lancet, ii,* 662-664

Koller, W.C., Gehlmann, L.K., Malkinson, F.D. & Davis, F.A. (1977) Dapsone-induced peripheral neuropathy. *Arch. Neurol., 34,* 644-646

Leiker, D.L. (1955) The mononucleosis syndrome in leprosy patients treated with sulfones. *Int. J. Lepr., 24,* 402-405

Levine, P.H. & Weintraub, L.R. (1968) Pseudoleukemia during recovery from dapsone-induced agranulocytosis. *Ann. intern. Med., 68*, 1060-1065

Levy, L., Biggs, J.T., Jr, Gordon, G.R. & Peters, J.H. (1972) Disposition of the antileprosy drug, dapsone, in the mouse. *Proc. Soc. exp. Biol. Med., 140*, 937-943

Mänsson, T. (1971) Malignant disease in dermatitis herpetiformis. *Acta dermatovenerol. (Stockholm), 51*, 379-382

Murray, J.F., Jr, Gordon, G.R., Ghoul, D.C. & Peters, J.H. (1972) Metabolic disposition of the antileprotic sulfone, dapsone, in Buffalo and Lewis rats. *Proc. west. pharmacol. Soc., 15*, 100-103

National Cancer Institute (1977) *Bioassay of Dapsone for Possible Carcinogenicity (Technical Report Series No. 20)*, DHEW Publication No. (NIH) 77-820, Washington DC, US Department of Health, Education, & Welfare

Oleinick, A. (1969) Altered immunity and cancer risk: a review of the problem and analysis of the cancer mortality experience of leprosy patients. *J. natl Cancer Inst., 43*, 775-771

Orzech, C.E., Nash, N.G. & Daley, R.D. (1976) Dapsone. In: Florey, K., ed., *Analytical Profiles of Drug Substances*, Vol. 5, New York, Academic Press, pp. 87-114

Peters, J.H. & Levy, L. (1971) Dapsone acetylation in man: another example of polymorphic acetylation. *Ann. N.Y. Acad. Sci., 179*, 660-666

Peters, J.H., Gordon, G.R., Ghoul, D.C., Tolentino, J.G., Walsh, G.P. & Levy, L. (1972) The disposition of the antileprotic drug dapsone (DDS) in Philippine subjects. *Am. J. trop. Med. Hyg., 21*, 450-457

Peters, J.H., Gordon, G.R., Biggs, J.T., Jr & Levy, L. (1975a) The disposition of dapsone and monoacetyldapsone in the dog. *Proc. Soc. exp. Biol. Med., 148*, 251-255

Peters, J.H., Gordon, G.R. & Karat, A.B.A. (1975b) Polymorphic acetylation of the antibacterials, sulfamethazine and dapsone, in South Indian subjects. *Am. J. trop. Med. Hyg., 24*, 641-648

Peters, J.H., Gordon, G.R., Simmon, V.F. & Tanaka, W. (1978) Mutagenesis of dapsone and its derivatives in *Salmonella typhimurium* (Abstract no. 1266). *Fed. Proc., 37*, 450

Purtilo, D.T. & Pangi, C. (1975) Incidence of cancer in patients with leprosy. *Cancer, 35*, 1259-1261

Shelley, W.B. & Goldwein, M.I. (1976) High dose dapsone toxicity. *Br. J. Dermatol., 95*, 79-82

Stone, S.P. & Goodwin, R.M. (1979) Dapsone-induced jaundice. *Arch. Dermatol., 114*, 947

Stoner, G.D., Shimkin, M.B., Kniazeff, A.J., Weisburger, J.H., Weisburger, E.K. & Gori, G.B. (1973) Test for carcinogenicity of food additives and chemotherapeutic agents by the pulmonary tumor response in strain A mice. *Cancer Res., 33*, 3069-3085

Tabarelli, S. & Uehleke, H. (1971) N-Hydroxylation of 4,4'-diaminodiphenylsulphone in liver microsomes and *in vivo*. *Xenobiotica, 1*, 501-502

Uehleke, H. (1971) Mode of action, secondary effects and toxicity of drugs due to their metabolism (Ger.). *Progr. Drug Res., 15*, 147-203

Uehleke, H. & Tabarelli, S. (1973) N-Hydroxylation of 4,4'-diaminodiphenylsulphone (dapsone) by liver microsomes, and in dogs and humans. *Naunyn-Schmiedeberg's Arch. Pharmacol., 278*, 55-68

US International Trade Commission (1979) *Imports of Benzenoid Chemicals and Products, 1978*, USITC Publication 990, Washington DC, US Government Printing Office, p. 82

US Pharmacopeial Convention, Inc. (1975) *The US Pharmacopeia*, 19th rev., Rockville, MD, pp. 118-119, 626

Vandersteen, P.R. & Jordon, R.E. (1974) Dermatitis herpetiformis with discoid lupus erythematosus. Occurrence of sulfone-induced discoid lupus erythematosus. *Arch. Dermatol., 110*, 95-98

Verma, K.C., Singh, K. & Chowdhary, S.D. (1973) Dapsone toxicity. *J. Indian med. Assoc., 60*, 255

Wade, A., ed. (1977) *Martindale, The Extra Pharmacopoeia*, 27th ed., London, The Pharmaceutical Press, pp. 1499-1503

WHO (1977) WHO Expert Committee on Leprosy. Fifth Report. *Tech. Rep. Ser., No. 607*, pp. 20-22

Wilson, J.R. & Harris, J.W. (1977) Hematologic side-effects of dapsone. *Ohio State med. J., 73*, 557-560

Windholz, M., ed. (1976) *The Merck Index*, 9th ed., Rahway, NJ, Merck & Co., Inc., p. 370

Wu, D.L. & DuBois, K.P. (1970) Studies on the mechanism of the toxic action of di-aminodiphenylsulfone (DDS) to mammals. *Arch. int. Pharmacodyn., 183*, 36-45

Young, S. & Marks, J.M. (1979) Dapsone and severe hypoalbuminaemia. *Lancet, ii*, 908-909

DIHYDROXYMETHYLFURATRIZINE

1. Chemical and Physical Data

1.1 Synonyms and trade names

Chem. Abstr. Services Reg. No.: 794-93-4

Chem. Abstr. Name: Methanol,{ [6- [2-(5-nitro-2-furanyl)ethenyl] -1,2,4-triazin-3-yl] imino} bis-

IUPAC Systematic Name: N-{6-[2-(5-nitro-2-furyl)vinyl]-1,2,4-triazin-3-yl} imino-dimethanol

Synonyms: 3-Bis(hydroxymethyl)amino-6-(5-nitro-2-furylethenyl)-1,2,4-triazine; bis(hydroxymethyl)furatrizine; {[6- 2-(5-nitro-2-furyl)vinyl] as-triazin-3-yl] -imino}dimethanol; N-[6-(5-nitrofurfurylidenemethyl)-1,2,4-triazin-3-yl] imino-dimethanol

Trade names: Furatone; Furatone-S; Panfuran-S

1.2 Structural and molecular formulae and molecular weight

$C_{11}H_{11}N_5O_5$ Mol. wt: 293.2

1.3 Chemical and physical properties of the pure substance

From Wade (1977)

(a) *Description:* Yellow crystalline powder
(b) *Melting-point:* ~ 157°C (dec.)
(c) *Solubility:* Practically insoluble in water and most organic solvents; soluble in dimethylformamide

1.4 Technical products and impurities

No specifications for this material have been published. Panfuran-S, a commercial formulation, contains 200 g/kg dihydroxymethylfuratrizine, sucrose, sodium saccharin, methylcellulose and spices (Konishi et al., 1978).

2. Production, Use, Occurrence and Analysis

2.1 Production and use

(a) Production

Dihydroxymethylfuratrizine can be prepared from 3-amino-6-(5-nitro-2-furylethenyl)-1,2,4-triazine by treatment with formaldehyde in dimethylformamide at 80-90°C (Takai et al., 1965).

No evidence was found that dihydroxymethylfuratrizine has ever been produced in the US or Europe. It was produced by two companies in Japan, but the last one ceased production and sales in 1977.

(b) Use

Dihydroxymethylfuratrizine is an antibacterial agent which was claimed to be effective against a wide range of gram-negative and gram-positive organisms. It was used in bacillary dysentery and acute colitis when resistance to antibiotics was a problem (Iyakuhin Yoran, 1979). The usual recommended dose was 20 mg/kg bw every 4-6 hours (Wade, 1977). It was withdrawn from use in Japan in July 1977, following an evaluation of its comparative efficacy and safety in relation to alternative drugs.

2.2 Occurrence

Dihydroxymethylfuratrizine is not known to occur in nature.

2.3 Analysis

The content of dihydroxymethylfuratrizine in a sample can be determined by ultraviolet and visible spectrometry after heating a solution in aqueous sodium hydroxide (Kanno et al., 1966). Gas chromatography can also be used (Nakamura et al., 1966).

3. Biological Data Relevant to the Evaluation of Carcinogenic Risk to Humans

3.1 Carcinogenicity studies in animals

(a) Oral administration

Rat: Two groups of 55 female Wistar rats were fed a diet containing 0 or 1000 mg/kg diet dihydroxymethylfuratrizine for 80 weeks, at which time the study was terminated: 41 controls and 48 treated rats survived at least for 29 weeks. No difference in overall tumour incidence was found; however, 2 sarcomas and 1 adenocarcinoma of the small intestine were observed in the treated group, while no intestinal tumour occurred in controls (Takai et al., 1974a).

(b) Oral administration in a mixture[1]

Mouse: Groups of 17 to 29 male dd mice were fed Panfuran-S in the diet, corresponding to doses of 0 (control), 175, 350, 700, 1750 or 3500 mg/kg diet dihydroxymethylfuratrizine for 35 weeks, at which time they were killed. No tumours were observed in the 28 controls that survived up to 35 weeks. The tumour incidences in animals in the 5 treated groups that survived up to that time (in order of increasing dietary concentration) were as follows: oesophageal papillomas: 0/20, 0/29, 0/26, 2/28, 4/17; oesophageal squamous-cell carcinomas: 0/20, 0/29, 0/26, 3/28, 0/17; forestomach papillomas: 5/20, 15/29, 13/26, 4/28, 0/17; forestomach squamous-cell carcinomas: 0/20, 3/29, 9/26, 20/28, 17/17; duodenal/jejunal adenocarcinomas: 0/20, 0/29, 0/26, 8/28, 10/17; and urinary bladder transitional-cell carcinomas: 0/20, 0/29, 0/26, 2/28, 1/17 (Konishi et al., 1979).

Rat: Groups of 15-20 male Wistar rats, 7 weeks-old, were fed Panfuran-S in the diet, corresponding to doses of 0 (control), 350, 1750 or 3500 mg/kg diet dihydroxymethylfuratrizine, for 35-37 weeks, at which time they were killed, with the exception of 7 animals given the lowest dose that were killed at 52 weeks. No tumours were observed in the controls or in the lowest-dose group. The tumour incidences in the medium- and high-dose groups were as follows: forestomach papillomas: 8/18, 11/19; duodenal adenocarcinomas: 2/18, 11/19; and jejunal adenocarcinomas: 10/18, 16/19 (Konishi et al., 1978).

---

[1] In these experiments, animals were treated with commercial Panfuran-S, which contains 200 g/kg dihydroxymethylfuratrizine, sucrose, sodium saccharin, methylcellulose and spices.

3.2 Other relevant biological data

(a) Experimental systems

Toxic effects

The subcutaneous LD_{50} of Panfuran-S in male Swiss ICR/Ha mice is 2.8 g/kg bw. After daily injections of 7 mg/mouse for 7 days, the animals developed diarrhoea and lost weight (Ichihashi et al., 1969).

No data on the prenatal toxicity of this compound were available.

Absorption, distribution, excretion and metabolism

Following an oral dose of 10 mg/kg bw ^{14}C-labelled dihydroxymethylfuratrizine to rats, absorption was estimated to be 40-50%, and a maximum plasma level of about 1.3 µg/ml was reached after 2 hours. ^{14}C-Label was higher in kidney, liver, bladder, stomach and intestine. All radioactivity was cleared from the body within 120 hours (Takai et al., 1974b).

Mutagenicity and other, related short-term tests

Dihydroxymethylfuratrizine inhibited the growth of *Staphylococcus aureus* and of *Escherichia coli*. The much higher sensitivity of different repair-deficient mutants of *E. coli* as compared with repair-proficient ones indicates that this compound induces DNA damage (Yamagishi et al., 1974; Iida & Koike, 1977).

(b) Humans

No data were available to the Working Group.

3.3 Case reports and epidemiological studies of carcinogenicity in humans

No data were available to the Working Group.

DIHYDROXYMETHYLFURATRIZINE

4. Summary of Data Reported and Evaluation

4.1 Experimental data

Dihydroxymethylfuratrizine was tested alone in female rats by oral administration. Although a few tumours of the small intestine were observed in treated animals, there was no difference in overall tumour incidence as compared with controls. Panfuran-S, a commercial formulation which contains dihydroxymethylfuratrizine, was also tested in male mice and male rats by oral administration; it induced benign and malignant tumours of the forestomach and small intestine in animals of both species and of the oesophagus in mice.

Attention is drawn to the absence of studies on the teratogenicity of this compound.

4.2 Human data

Dihydroxymethylfuratrizine in the form of Panfuran-S has been used in the past for treatment of acute gastrointestinal infections.

No case reports or epidemiological studies were available to the Working Group.

4.3 Evaluation

There are insufficient data to evaluate the carcinogenicity of dihydroxymethylfuratrizine alone in experimental animals. There is *sufficient evidence*[1] that Panfuran-S, a commercial formulation which contains dihydroxymethylfuratrizine and several other compounds, is carcinogenic in experimental animals.

---

[1] See preamble, p. 18.

5. References

Ichihashi, H., Muragishi, H., Kanemitsu, T. & Kondo, T. (1969) Cytotoxic effects of a nitrofuran derivative on ascites carcinoma cells. *Nagoya J. Med., 32*, 103-112

Iida, K. & Koike, M. (1977) Effect of dihydroxymethyl furatrizine on cell division of *Escherichia coli*. *Microbiol. Immunol., 21*, 481-494

Iyakuhin Yoran (1979) *Drug Index,* Osaka Prefecture, Association of Pharmacists, pp. 1128-1129

Kanno, S., Watanabe, S. & Murai, A. (1966) Analysis of pharmaceutical drugs. VI. Assay and identification of dihydroxymethylfuratrizine (Jpn.). *Yakuzaigaku, 26*, 275-279 [*Chem. Abstr., 70*, 31717p]

Konishi, Y., Denda, A., Takahashi, S., Inui, S., & Aoki, Y. (1978) Production of adenocarcinomas of the small intestines of Wistar rats fed Panfuran-S containing 3-di-(hydroxymethyl)amino-6-(5-nitro-2-furylethenyl)-1,2,4-triazine. *J. natl Cancer Inst., 60*, 1339-1343

Konishi, Y., Aoki, Y., Takahashi, S., Inui, S., Denda, A. & Takita, M. (1979) Carcinogenic activity of Panfuran-S containing 3-di-(hydroxymethyl)-amino-6-(5-nitro-2-furylethenyl)-1,2,4-triazine in mice (Ger.). *Onkologie, 2*, 41-42

Nakamura, K., Utsui, Y. & Ninomiya, Y. (1966) Gas chromatography of some nitrofuran derivatives (Jpn.). *Yakagaku Zasshi, 86*, 404-409 [*Chem. Abstr., 65*, 18429h]

Takai, A., Kodama, Y., Saikawa, I. & Tamatsukuri, H. (1965) 1,2,4-Triazine derivative. *Japan Patent 20,393,* 10 September to Toyama Chemical Industry Co. [*Chem. Abstr., 63*, 16370c]

Takai, A., Yoneda, T., Nakada, H. & Ohta, G. (1974a) Evaluation of the carcinogenic activity of 3-di(hydroxymethyl)amino-6-(5-nitro-2-furylethenyl)-1,2,4-triazine (dihydroxymethyl-furatrizine, Panfuran-S) in female rats (Jpn.). *Chemotherapy (Tokyo), 22*, 1171-1179

Takai, A., Nakashima, Y., Simizu, E. & Terashima, N. (1974b) Absorption, distribution and excretion of nitrofuran compounds (Jpn.). *Chemotherapy (Tokyo), 22*, 1165-1170

Wade, A., ed. (1977) *Martindale, The Extra Pharmacopoeia,* 27th ed., London, The Pharmaceutical Press, p. 1750

Yamagishi, S., Nakajima, Y., Ishikawa, Y. & Fujii, K. (1974) The mode of antibacterial action of nitrofuran compounds (Jpn). *Chemotherapy (Tokyo), 22,* 1159-1164

HYDRALAZINE and HYDRALAZINE HYDROCHLORIDE

1. Chemical and Physical Data

HYDRALAZINE

1.1 Synonyms and trade names

Chem. Abstr. Services Reg. No.: 86-54-4

Chem. Abstr. Name: 1(2H)-Phthalazinone hydrazone

IUPAC Systematic Name: 1-Hydrazinophthalazine

Synonyms: 1-Hydrazinophthalazine; hydralazin; hydrallazine

1.2 Structural and molecular formulae and molecular weight

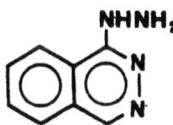

$C_8H_8N_4$ Mol. wt: 160.2

1.3 Chemical and physical properties of the pure substance

From Windholz (1976)

(a) *Description:* Yellow needles from methanol
(b) *Melting-point:* 172-173°C (rapid heating)
(c) *Solubility:* Soluble in 2N acetic acid (1 in 3) and warm methanol (1 in 12)

1.4 Technical products and impurities

There are no technical products or pharmaceutical preparations containing the free base. It is used in the preparation of the hydrochloride salt.

HYDRALAZINE HYDROCHLORIDE

1.1 Synonyms and trade names

Chem. Abstr. Services Reg. No.: 304-20-1

Chem. Abstr. Name: 1(2H)-Phthalazinone hydrazone, monohydrochloride

IUPAC Systematic Name: 1-Hydrazinophthalazine hydrochloride

Synonyms: Hydralazine chloride; hydralazine HCl; hydrallazine hydrochloride; 1-hydrazinophthalazine monohydrochloride; 1(2H)-phthalazinone hydrazone hydrochloride

Trade names: Aiselazine; Appresinum; Aprelazine; Apresazide; Apresine; Apresolin; Apresoline; Apresoline-Esidrix; Apresoline HCl; Apresoline hydrochloride; Apressin; Apressoline; Aprezolin; Ba 5968; C-5968; Ciba 5968; Dralzine; Hidralazin; Hipoftalin; Hydrapress; Hyperazin; Hyperazine; Hypophthalin; Hypos; Ipolina; Lopres; Lopress; Nor-Press 25; Präparat 5968; Rolazine; Serpasil Apresoline No. 2

1.2 Structural and molecular formulae and molecular weight

$C_8H_8N_4$, HCl   Mol. wt: 196.6

1.3 Chemical and physical properties of the pure substance

From Wade (1977) or Windholz (1976) unless otherwise specified

(a) *Description:* White to off-white odourless crystalline powder with a bitter saline taste

(b) *Melting-point:* 273°C (dec.)

(c) *Spectroscopy data*: λ_{max} (in water): 211 nm, A(1%, 1 cm) = 172; 239 nm, A(1%, 1cm) = 56; 260 nm, A(1%, 1 cm) = 54; 303 nm, A(1%, 1 cm) = 26; 315 nm, A(1%, 1 cm) = 21. Infrared, nuclear magnetic resonance and mass spectral data have been tabulated (Orzech *et al.*, 1979)

(d) *Solubility*: Soluble in water (1 in 25), ethanol (1 in 500) and methanol (1 in 150); practically insoluble in chloroform, diethyl ether, ethyl acetate, and acetonitrile (Orzech *et al.*, 1979)

(e) *Stability*: Sensitive to oxidation and light

1.4 Technical products and impurities

Various national and international pharmacopoeias give specifications for the purity of hydralazine hydrochloride in pharmaceutical products. For example, it is available in the US as a USP grade containing 98.0-100.5% active ingredient calculated on the dried basis. The loss on drying should be less than 0.5%, the residue on ignition less than 0.1% and water-insoluble substances no more than 0.5%. It is also available in doses of 20 mg/ml as injections and in 10, 25, 50 and 100 mg doses as tablets containing 95.0-105.0% of the stated amount of hydralazine hydrochloride (US Pharmacopeial Convention, Inc., 1975).

Pharmaceutical preparations in the UK are the same as in the US (Wade, 1977).

Hydralazine hydrochloride is available in Japan as powders, granules and tablets in 30-200 mg doses. It is also available as injections.

Hydrazine (see IARC, 1974) is regarded as a potentially toxic, possible impurity in hydralazine, and sensitive tests have been developed to detect it at low levels; none of the current compendial specifications include such a test but it may be expected to be added in future revisions.

2. Production, Use, Occurrence and Analysis

2.1 Production and use

(a) *Production*

In the first synthesis, reported in 1949, phthalazone was converted to 1-chlorophthalazine, and this compound was treated first with ethanol and hydrazine hydrate and then with hydrochloric acid to give hydralazine hydrochloride (Harvey, 1975; Windholz, 1976; Orzech *et al.*, 1979). This is the process used for commercial production.

Hydralazine (free base) is produced by one company in the US in an undisclosed amount (see preamble, p. 21). In 1978, US imports of hydralazine hydrochloride amounted to 8000 kg (US International Trade Commission, 1979); separate data on US exports are not available.

Hydralazine hydrochloride was first marketed in Japan in 1967. It is presently produced by at least three companies there, and imports amounted to 700 kg in 1976, 1900 kg in 1977 and 1400 kg in 1978.

No data were available on whether it is produced elsewhere.

(b) Use

Hydralazine hydrochloride is an antihypertensive agent used in the treatment of essential hypertension and in the treatment of hypertension of toxaemia during pregnancy (Harvey, 1975).

The oral dose is 10 mg taken 4 times per day for 2 - 4 days, then 25 mg 4 times per day for the rest of the first week; the total dose can then be increased to 200 mg per day. The daily dose should not exceed 200 mg, except in preeclampsia, where the daily dose may be as high as 400 mg. When fast response is needed, hydralazine hydrochloride is given parenterally (i.m. or i.v.) in 20 - 40 mg doses repeated as necessary (Harvey, 1975; Nickerson & Ruedy, 1975; Wade, 1977).

2.2 Occurrence

Hydralazine and its hydrochloride are not known to occur in nature.

2.3 Analysis

Analytical methods for the determination of hydralazine hydrochloride based on spectrometry, fluorescence, titration, gasometry, polarography and chromatography have been reviewed (Orzech *et al.*, 1979).

Typical methods for the analysis of hydralazine and hydralazine hydrochloride are summarized in Table 1. Abbreviations used are: GC/ECD, gas chromatography with electron capture detection; GC/FID, gas chromatography with flame-ionization detection; GC/MS, gas chromatography with mass spectrometry; and T, titration.

Table 1. Analytical methods for hydralazine and hydralazine hydrochloride

Sample matrix	Sample preparation	Assay	Limit of detection	Reference
Formulations				
Hydralazine hydrochloride	Dissolve in water; add hydrochloric acid and chloroform; titrate with potassium iodide	T	not given	US Pharmacopeial Convention, Inc., 1975
Hydralazine[1] tablets	Powder; dissolve in water; add to 2,4-pentanedione; shake; add internal standard solution of phenanthrene and ethyl acetate; separate ethyl acetate layer	GC/FID	not given	Smith et al., 1977
Plasma				
Hydralazine	Oxidize in dilute hydrochloric acid with manganese oxide; centrifuge; add sodium nitrite; adjust pH with sodium hydroxide and borax buffer; extract into benzene; centrifuge; evaporate; dissolve in ethyl acetate	GC/ECD	10 ng/ml	Zak et al., 1977
Urine				
Rat (hydralazine)	Add EDTA, hydrochloric acid and sodium nitrite; extract with chloroform and isopropanol; dry over anhydrous sodium sulphate; redissolve in acetonitrile	GC/MS	not given	Haegele et al., 1976
Human (hydralazine)	Extract with chloroform; evaporate; dissolve in ethyl acetate; apply to silica gel plate; develop with n-propanol-ammonium hydroxide; extract with chloroform and water; evaporate; dissolve in n-hexane and ethyl acetate	GC/FID	not given	Talseth, 1976
Liver				
Rat (hydralazine)	Place immediately in potassium phosphate buffer; homogenize; react with sodium nitrite; extract with chloroform and isopropanol; evaporate	GC/MS	not given	Haegele et al., 1976

[1] Probably the hydrochloride

3. Biological Data Relevant to the Evaluation of Carcinogenic Risk to Humans

3.1 Carcinogenicity studies in animals

Oral administration

Mouse: An aqueous solution of 0.125% hydralazine hydrochloride (93% pure) was given continuously as drinking-water for life to 50 male and 50 female random-bred Swiss mice, from 6 weeks of age. The average daily intake of hydralazine hydrochloride was 7.4 mg for males and 5.4 mg for females. A control group consisted of 50 females and 50 males. Whenever a treated mouse died, a corresponding untreated control mouse was killed on the same day. Of the treated females, 30 (60%) developed 81 lung tumours; 19 mice had 40 adenomas, 2 had 2 adenocarcinomas, and 9 had 28 adenomas plus 11 adenocarcinomas. Their average age at death was 78 weeks; the first tumour was found at the 49th week and the last at the 98th week. In untreated females, 18 (36%) developed 20 lung tumours; 15 mice had 17 adenomas, and 3 mice had 3 adenocarcinomas. Their average age at death was 78 weeks; the first tumour was found at the 55th week and the last at the 92nd week. The increased incidence of lung tumours in females was statistically significant ($P<0.014$). In treated males, 23 (46%) developed 58 lung neoplasms; 14 mice had 21 adenomas; 1 mouse had an adenocarcinoma; and 8 had 24 adenomas plus 12 adenocarcinomas. Their average age at death was 79 weeks; the first tumour was found at the 60th week and the last at the 96th week of age. In untreated males, 13 (26%) developed 16 lung tumours; 9 mice had 9 adenomas; 4 had 4 adenocarcinomas; and 1 had 1 adenoma plus 2 adenocarcinomas. Their average age at death was 75 weeks; the first tumour was found at the 54th week and the last at the 95th week of age ($P<0.032$) (Toth, 1978). [Attention is drawn to the fact that the unusual design of the experiment, whereby a control mouse was killed each time a treated mouse died, was not followed by an appropriate analysis of the results. The fact that the purity of the compound (93%) was lower than USP standards (98%) was also noted.]

3.2 Other relevant biological data

(a) Experimental systems

Toxic effects

The i.p. LD_{50} of hydralazine hydrochloride in rats is 35 mg/kg bw (McIsaac & Kanda, 1964). The oral LD_{50} is, respectively, 260 and 210 mg/kg bw in male and female mice and 320 and 280 mg/kg bw in male and female rats. Chronic treatment with 60 and 120 mg/kg bw per day for 1-6 months induced anaemia. Autopsy revealed slight renal tubular degeneration in male rats and haemosiderosis of the spleen (Onodera *et al.*, 1978).

Lupus erythematosus cells were found in the blood of 7 out of 8 dogs administered hydralazine hydrochloride at daily doses of 200 mg/dog for 2-8 months. The kidneys showed changes consistent with those found in disseminated lupus erythematosus (Comens, 1956). In other studies in dogs, daily doses of 20 mg/kg bw hydralazine (unspecified) daily for 2-12.5 months produced anaemia, which the authors said was 'probably haemolytic'; no lupus erythematosus cells were found (Dubois et al., 1957). Daily doses of 50-200 mg/dog for 29 weeks caused multifocal hepatic necrosis but no symptoms that showed a clear relationship with disseminated lupus erythematosus (Gardner, 1957). The presence of antinuclear antibodies, an indicator of disseminated lupus erythematosus, was not detected in rats given 60 mg/kg bw hydralazine hydrochloride daily for 6 months (Onodera et al., 1978). Antinuclear antibodies were detected in 30% of guinea-pigs after daily administration of 100 mg/animal of dihydralazine sulphate, a hydralazine derivative, for 7 months (Monier et al., 1968).

Hydralazine (not otherwise specified) inhibited hydroxylation steps in collagen synthesis in *in vitro* studies on chick tibia (Rapaka et al., 1977).

No published data on the prenatal toxicity of this compound were available, but it has been reported that oral doses ranging from 20-120 mg/kg hydralazine hydrochloride produce a low incidence of cleft palate and minor bone malformations (Association of the British Pharmaceutical Industry, 1979).

Absorption, distribution, excretion and metabolism

In rats given an oral dose of 12 mg/kg bw hydralazine hydrochloride, maximum levels of about 100 ng/ml unchanged hydralazine were observed in plasma 30 minutes after ingestion; the levels of unchanged hydralazine declined to zero within 24 hours (Degen, 1979).

Acetyl hydralazine 1-(2-acetylhydrazino)phthalazine was reported to be a major metabolic product in rats, guinea-pigs and pigeons (Douglass & Hogan, 1959). In rats and rabbits, excretion of hydralazine and its metabolites is rapid (75% of the administered dose in the urine in 24 hrs); 40-50% was 1-hydralazine-*O*-glucuronide, 15% unchanged hydralazine and 25-30% *N*-acetyl-1-hydralazine (McIsaac & Kanda, 1964). It was later demonstrated that the actual acetylation metabolite was 3-methyl-*s*-triazolo(3,4-*a*)phthalazine (Edwards & Marquardt, 1969; Haegele et al., 1976).

Mutagenicity and other, related short-term tests

Hydralazine (form and purity unspecified) is mutagenic in *Salmonella typhimurium* TA1530 and TA1537 (Tosk *et al.*, 1979; Williams *et al.*, 1980) and TA100 with or without rat liver S-9 activation (Shaw *et al.*, 1979; Williams *et al.*, 1980). The compound was also active in the *Escherichia coli pol* A^+/A^- test, indicating an interaction with DNA (Shaw *et al.*, 1979).

3-Methyl-*s*-triazolo(3,4-*a*)phthalazine and 3-hydroxymethyl-*s*-triazolo(3,4-*a*)phthalazine, metabolites in humas and animals were not mutagenic to *S. typhimurium* TA1535, TA1537, TA1538, TA98 or TA100 in the presence or absence of a metabolic activation system (Shaw *et al.*, 1979).

Hydralazine, at a dose of 1 mg/ml, elicited DNA repair in rat hepatocytes in primary culture (Williams *et al.*, 1980).

(b) Humans[1]

Hydralazine hydrochloride is an antihypertensive agent, which acts by depressing the vasomotor centre and by peripheral actions (Harvey, 1975).

Toxic effects

The onset of a syndrome resembling disseminated lupus erythematosus related to the long-term use of hydralazine is well documented (Bendersky & Ramirez, 1960). This has also been termed 'rheumatic syndrome' or the 'rheumatogenic action' of hydralazine. Lupus erythematosus cells have been found repeatedly in hydralazine-treated patients (Dustan *et al.*, 1954). This abnormality is said to occur very rarely with doses under 200 mg/day; however, in a 39-year-old woman who had taken 150 mg/day for 3 years, lupus erythematosus cells were present, antinuclear factor was weakly positive and antideoxyribonucleic acid antibodies were found in significant amounts. The syndrome regressed completely when the drug was withdrawn (Berkowitz, 1976).

---

[1] In most of these studies, the authors did not specify whether hydralazine was used as the free base or as the hydrochloride, although since there are no technical products or pharmaceutical preparations that contain the free base, it was probably given as the hydrochloride.

A case was described of a 72-year-old woman treated with 100 mg hydralazine daily for 2 years who died in shock with gastrointestinal bleeding. Autopsy revealed proliferative and fibronoid necroses of the arterioles and arteries of many organs and the appearance of wire-looping in the renal glomeruli (Bendersky & Ramirez, 1960).

Previous industrial exposure to hydrazine compounds which gives rise to contact dermatitis may produce hypersensitivity to hydralazine (Malten, 1962).

Prenatal toxicity

In reports in which patients with toxaemia or chronic hypertension during pregnancy were treated with hydralazine hydrochloride (Curet & Olson, 1979) or with hydralazine in combination with other antihypertensive agents (Arias & Zamora, 1979), no malformations were observed in the offspring. The intrauterine growth retardation often seen could have been associated with the maternal disease.

Heinonen *et al.* (1977) reported 8 cases of malformation in the children of 136 women who took hydralazine during pregnancy; this incidence was not statistically significantly different from the expected rate of 3.8.

Absorption, distribution, excretion and metabolism

Orally administered hydralazine hydrochloride is eliminated rapidly; the main route of excretion is the urine (more than 70% of the absorbed dose); the faeces represent a minor route of elimination (less than 10%) (Lesser *et al.*, 1974). In man, hydralazine undergoes extensive metabolism; acetylation was proposed as the major pathway for hydralazine clearance (Zimmer *et al.*, 1970; Zacest & Koch-Weser, 1972; Reidenberg *et al.*, 1973). Aceylation *via* hepatic *N*-acetyl transferase of hydralazine, as of sulphamethazine or isoniazid, is subject to genetic polymorphism (Evans, 1968). The plasma half-life of hydralazine ranges from 2.0 to 7.8 hrs in both rapid and slow acetylators; and plasma concentrations following i.v. administration were similar in the two groups (Reidenberg *et al.*, 1973), while they were lower in rapid than in slow acetylators following oral administration (Zacest & Koch-Weser, 1972; Reidenberg *et al.*, 1973). Therefore, slow acetylators can be identified by their higher plasma levels and rapid acetylators by their lower hydralazine plasma concentrations after an oral intake (Zacest & Koch-Weser, 1972; Reidenberg *et al.*, 1973). Most or nearly all cases of the so-called 'hydralazine syndrome' have been observed among slow acetylators (Tester-Dalderup, 1978, 1979).

Another major plasma metabolite in humans is the hydralazine pyruvic acid hydrazone (Reece et al., 1978). The mean plasma half-life of this metabolite is 156 min (Shepherd et al., 1979). Urine of patients treated with hydralazine contains 3-methyl-s-triazolo (3,4-a)phthalazine (Zimmer et al., 1973) and 3-hydroxymethyl-s-triazolo(3,4-a)phthalazine (Zimmer et al., 1975).

3.3 Case reports and epidemiological studies of carcinogenicity in humans[1]

Two studies relevant to the carcinogenicity of hydralazine in humans were available to the Working Group. In the first (Perry, 1963), patients with malignant hypertension who developed hydralazine toxicity were compared with other hydralazine recipients who did not; 4 of 24 (17%) with toxicity but only 1 of 92 (1%) without toxicity developed cancer: 2 of the recipients with toxicity had breast carcinomas and 2 had lung carcinomas; the recipient without toxicity had a rectal carcinoma. [Apart from the small numbers, only some of the potentially important confounding variables were taken into account. For example, there were more females among the patients with hydralazine toxicity and hence a greater likelihood of observing breast cancer among them. Smoking status, of relevance to lung cancer, was not mentioned.]

Williams et al. (1978), on the basis of a large study in which cases and controls were identified in the course of the National Breast-Cancer Screening Project, reported elevated relative risk estimates for breast cancer in relation to hydralazine use. These estimates varied but were as high as 2.0, depending upon the specific comparison. The highest relative risk was found for use which had lasted at least 5 years. The estimates were adjusted for confounding by age, ethnic group and geographical location, but only to a limited extent for the concomitant use of other drugs. The results were not statistically significant. [In addition, in the monograph dealing with reserpine (p. 211), which was the main focus of the study by Williams et al. (1978), reasons are given to suggest that there may have been a general bias arising from the nature of the population selected for study. If this bias were present, it could apply to all drugs, including hydralazine, found to be associated with breast cancer.]

[Various workers (e.g., Henderson, 1977; Labarthe, 1979) have suggested that the associations reported for drugs, such as hydralazine, with breast cancer, may be explained if hypertension increases the risk. There is good evidence, however (e.g., Labarthe & O'Fallon, 1980), that hypertension *per se* is not related to the risk for breast cancer.]

---

[1] See footnote on p. 92.

HYDRALAZINE and HYDRALAZINE HYDROCHLORIDE

4. Summary of Data Reported and Evaluation

4.1 Experimental data

Hydralazine hydrochloride was tested in one experiment in mice by oral administration. A significant increase in the incidence of lung tumours was reported.

Hydralazine is mutagenic for *Salmonella typhimurium*. Attention is drawn to the absence of published studies on the teratogenicity of this compound.

4.2 Human data

Hydralazine is used in the long-term treatment of essential and early malignant hypertension.

Two studies have suggested an association between hydralazine and human cancer. One was confined to patients with and without hydralazine toxicity, and potential confounding factors were not controlled for. The other involved a small number of subjects exposed to hydralazine, and the possibility of selection bias could not be excluded.

4.3 Evaluation

The experimental data, while providing *limited evidence*[1] for the carcinogenicity of hydralazine hydrochloride, were difficult to interpret due to certain aspects of experimental design and analysis. The epidemiological data were insufficient. In view of the extensive use of this drug, further studies should be undertaken.

---

[1] See preamble, p. 18.

5. References

Arias, F. & Zamora, J. (1979) Antihypertensive treatment and pregnancy outcome in patients with mild chronic hypertension. *Obstet. Gynecol., 53,* 489-494

Association of the British Pharmaceutical Industry (1979) *Data Sheet Compendium, 1979-80, Apresoline,* London, Pharmind Publications Ltd

Bendersky, G. & Ramirez, C. (1960) Hydralazine poisoning. Review of the literature and autopsy study of person with massive intestinal bleeding. *J. Am. med. Assoc., 173,* 1789-1794

Berkowitz, H.S. (1976) Disseminated lupus erythematosus syndrome associated with hydralazine. *S. Afr. med. J., 50,* 797

Comens, P. (1956) Experimental hydralazine disease and its similarity to disseminated lupus erythematosus. *J. Lab. clin. Med., 47,* 444-454

Curet, L.B. & Olson, R.W. (1979) Evaluation of a program of bed rest in the treatment of chronic hypertension in pregnancy. *Obstet. Gynecol., 53,* 336-340

Degen, P.H. (1979) Determination of unchanged hydralazine in plasma by gas-liquid chromatography using nitrogen-specific detection. *J. Chromatogr., 176,* 375-380

Douglass, C.D. & Hogan, R. (1959) A metabolite of 1-hydrazino-phthalazine (hydralazine). *Proc. Soc. exp. Biol. Med., 100,* 446-448

Dubois, E.L., Katz, Y.J., Freeman, V. & Garbak, F. (1957) Chronic toxicity studies of hydralazine (Apresoline) in dogs with particular reference to the production of the 'hydralazine syndrome'. *J. lab. clin. Med., 50,* 119-126

Dustan, H.P., Taylor, R.D., Corcoran, A.C. & Page, I.H. (1954) Rheumatic and febrile syndrome during prolonged hydralazine treatment. *J. Am. med. Assoc., 154,* 23-29

Edwards, S. & Marquardt, F.H. (1969) The metabolism of 1-hydrazinophthalazine: the correct structure of the pseudo- 'N-acetyl-1-hydrazinophthalazine'. *Hoppe-Seyler's Z. Physiol. Chem., 350,* 85-86

Evans, D.A.P. (1968) Genetic variations in the acetylation of isoniazid and other drugs. *Ann. N.Y. Acad. Sci., 151,* 723-733

Gardner, D.L. (1957) The response of the dog to oral 1-hydrazinophthalazine (hydralazine). *Br. J. exp. Pathol., 38,* 227-235

Haegele, K.D., Skrdlant, H.B., Robie, N.W., Lalka, D. & McNay, J.L., Jr (1976) Determination of hydralazine and its metabolites by gas chromatography-mass spectrometry. *J. Chromatogr., 126,* 517-534

Harvey, S.C. (1975) *Cardiovascular drugs.* In: Osol, A., ed., *Remington's Pharmaceutical Sciences,* 15th ed., Easton, PA, Mack Publishing Co., p. 784

Heinonen, O.P., Slone, D. & Shapiro, S. (1977) *Birth Defects and Drugs in Pregnancy,* Littleton, MA, Publishing Sciences Group, Inc., p. 441

Henderson, M. (1977) *Reserpine and breast cancer. A review.* In: Colombo, F., Shapiro, S., Slone, D. & Tognoni, G., eds, *Epidemiological Evaluation of Drugs, Proceedings of the International Symposium on Epidemiological Evaluation of Drugs, Milano, Italy,* Amsterdam, Elsevier, pp. 211-227

IARC (1974) *IARC Monographs on the Evaluation of the Carcinogenic Risk of Chemicals to Man,* Vol. 4, *Some aromatic amines, hydrazine and related substances,* N-*nitroso compounds and miscellaneous alkylating agents,* Lyon, pp. 127-136

Labarthe, D.R. (1979) Methodologic variation in case-control studies of reserpine and breast cancer. *J. chronic Dis., 32,* 95-104

Labarthe, D.R. & O'Fallon, W.M. (1980) Reserpine and breast cancer: a community-based longitudinal study of 2000 hypertensive women. *J. Am. med. Assoc.* (in press)

Lesser, J.M., Israili, Z.H., Davis, D.C. & Dayton, P.G. (1974) Metabolism and disposition of hydralazine-^{14}C in man and dog. *Drug Metab. Disposition, 2,* 351-360

Malten, K.E. (1962) Industrial contact dermatitis caused by hydrazine derivatives, with group hypersensitivity to hydralazine and isoniazid (Neth). *Ned. T. Geneesk., 106,* 2219-2222

McIsaac, W.M. & Kanda, M. (1964) The metabolism of 1-hydrazinophthalazine. *J. Pharmacol. exp. Ther., 143,* 7-13

Monier, J.C., Richard, M.H. & Thivolet, J. (1968) Long-term administration of hydralazine to guinea-pigs. Serological and clinicopathological evaluation (Fr.). *Rev. franc. Etud. clin. biol., 13,* 67-71

Nickerson, M. & Ruedy, J. (1975) *Antihypertensive agents and the drug therapy of hypertension.* In: Goodman, L.S. & Gilman, A., eds, *The Pharmacological Basis of Therapeutics,* 5th ed., New York, Macmillan, pp. 705-707

Onodera, T., Takayama, S., Yamada, A., Ono, Y. & Akimoto, T. (1978) Toxicological studies of 1-[2-(1,3-dimethyl-2-butenylidene)hydrazino]-phthalazine, a new antihypertensive drug, in mice and rats. *Toxicol. appl. Pharmacol., 44,* 431-439

Orzech, C.E., Nash, N.G. & Daley, R.D. (1979) *Hydralazine hydrochloride.* In: Florey, K., ed., *Analytical Profiles of Drug Substances.* Vol. 8, New York, Academic Press, pp. 283-314

Perry, H.M., Jr (1963) Carcinoma and hydralazine toxicity in patients with malignant hypertension. *J. Am. med. Assoc., 186,* 1020-1022

Rapaka, R.S., Parr, R.W., Liu, T.-Z. & Bhatnagar, R.S. (1977) Biochemical basis of skeletal defects induced by hydralazine: inhibition of collagen synthesis and secretion in embryonic chicken cartilage *in vitro. Teratology, 15,* 185-193

Reece, P.A., Stanley, P.E. & Zacest, R. (1978) Interference in assays for hydralazine in humans by a major plasma metabolite, hydralazine pyruvic acid hydrazone. *J. pharm. Sci., 67,* 1150-1153

Reidenberg, M.M., Drayer, D., DeMarco, A.L. & Bello, C.T. (1973) Hydralazine elimination in man. *Clin. pharmacol. Ther., 14,* 970-977

Shaw, C.R., Butler, M.A., Thenot, J.-P., Haegle, K.D. & Matney, T.S. (1979) Genetic effects of hydralazine. *Mutat. Res., 68,* 79-84

Shepherd, A.M.M., Ludden, T.M., Haegele, K.D., Talseth, T. & McNay, J.L. (1979) Pharmacokinetics of hydralazine, apparent hydralazine and hydralazine pyruvic acid hydrazone in humans. *Res. Commun. chem. Pathol. Pharmacol., 26,* 129-144

Smith, K.M., Johnson, R.N. & Kho, B.T. (1977) Determination of hydralazine in tablets by gas chromatography. *J. Chromatogr., 137,* 431-437

Talseth, T. (1976) Studies on hydralazine. III. Bioavailability of hydralazine in man. *Eur. J. clin. Pharmacol., 10,* 395-401

Tester-Dalderup, C.B.M. (1978) *Hypotensive drugs.* In: Dukes, M.N.G., ed., *Side Effects of Drugs Annual 2. A Worldwide Yearly Survey of New Data and Trends,* Amsterdam, Excerpta Medica, p. 193

Tester-Dalderup, C.B.M. (1979) *Hypotensive drugs.* In: Dukes, M.N.G., ed., *Side Effects of Drugs Annual 3. A Worldwide Yearly Survey of New Data and Trends,* Amsterdam, Excerpta Medica, p. 192

Tosk, J., Schmeltz, I. & Hoffmann, D. (1979) Hydrazines as mutagens in a histidine-requiring auxotroph of *Salmonella typhimurium. Mutat. Res., 66,* 247-252

Toth, B. (1978) Tumorigenic effect of 1-hydrazinophthalazine hydrochloride in mice. *J. natl Cancer Inst., 61,* 1363-1365

US International Trade Commission (1979) *Imports of Benzenoid Chemicals and Products, 1978,* USITC Publication 990, Washington DC, US Government Printing Office, p. 85

US Pharmacopeial Convention, Inc. (1975) *The US Pharmacopoeia,* 19th rev., Rockville, MD, pp. 234-235

Wade, A., ed. (1977) *Martindale, The Extra Pharmacopoeia,* 27th ed., London, The Pharmaceutical Press, pp. 664-665

Williams, G.M., Masué, G., McQueen, C. & Shimada, T. (1980) Genotoxicity of the antihypertensive drug hydralazine. *Science* (in press)

Williams, R.R., Feinleib, M., Connor, R.J. & Stegens, N.L. (1978) Case-control study of antihypertensive and diuretic use by women with malignant and benign breast lesions detected in a mammography screening program. *J. natl Cancer Inst., 61,* 327-335

Windholz, M., ed. (1976) *The Merck Index,* 9th ed., Rahway, NJ, Merck & Co., p. 625

Zacest, R. & Koch-Weser, J. (1972) Relation of hydralazine plasma concentration to dosage and hypotensive action. *Clin. Pharmacol. Ther., 13,* 420-425

Zak, S.B., Lukas, G. & Gilleran, T.G. (1977) Plasma levels of real and 'apparent' hydralazine in man and rat. *Drug Metab. Disposition, 5,* 116-121

Zimmer, H., McManus, J., Novinson, T., Hess, E.V. & Litwin, A.H. (1970) A major metabolite of 1-hydrazinophthalazine. *Arzneimittel. forsch., 20,* 1586-1587

Zimmer, H., Kokosa, J. & Garteiz, D.A. (1973) Identification of 3-methyl-s-triazolo[3,4-a]phthalazine, a human hydralazine metabolite, by gas chromatography-mass spectrometry. *Arzneimittel. forsch., 23,* 1028-1029

Zimmer, H., Glaser, R., Kokosa, J., Garteiz, D.A., Hess, E.V. & Litwin, A. (1975) 3-Hydroxymethyl-s-triazolo[3,4-a]phthalazine, a novel urinary hydralazine metabolite in man. *J. med. Chem., 18,* 1031-1033

METHOXSALEN

1. Chemical and Physical Data

1.1 Synonyms and trade names

Chem. Abstr. Services Reg. No.: 298-81-7

Chem. Abstr. Name: 7H-Furo[3,2-g] [1] benzopyran-7-one, 9-methoxy-

IUPAC Systematic Name: 9-Methoxy-7H-furo[3,2-g]benzopyran-7-one

Synonyms: 6-Hydroxy-7-methoxy-5-benzofuranacrylic acid δ-lactone; 8-MP; 8-MOP; 8-methoxy-(furano-3',2':6,7-coumarin); 8-methoxy-4'-5':6,7-furocoumarin; 8-methoxypsoralen; 9-methoxypsoralen; 8-methoxypsoralene; oxypsoralen

Trade names: Ammoidin; Meladinin (VAN); Meladinine; Meladoxen; Meloxine; Methoxa-Dome; Mopsoralen; Oxsoralen; Soloxsalen; Trioxun; Xanthotoxin; Xanthotoxine

1.2 Structural and molecular formulae and molecular weight

$C_{12}H_8O_4$ Mol. wt: 216.2

1.3 Chemical and physical properties of the pure substance

From Wade (1977) or Windholz (1976)

(a) *Description:* White to cream-coloured, odourless, fluffy, needle-like crystals
(b) *Melting-point:* 143-148°C
(c) *Spectroscopy data:* λ_{max} 219 nm, A(1%, 1cm) = 97; 249 nm, A(1%, 1cm) = 104; 300 nm, A(1%, 1cm) = 53

(d) Solubility: Practically insoluble in cold water; sparingly soluble in boiling-water and diethyl ether; soluble in boiling ethanol, acetone, acetic acid, vegetable oils, propylene glycol, benzene and chloroform

(e) Stability: Easily hydrolysed, whereby the lactone ring is opened; however, this is closed with acid. Unstable to air and light

1.4 Technical products and impurities

Various national and international pharmacopoeias give specifications for the purity of methoxsalen in pharmaceutical products. For example, it is available in the US as a USP grade containing 98.0-102.0% active ingredient calculated on the dried basis; the melting-range is 143° to 148°, the loss on drying should not exceed 0.5%, the residue on ignition should be less than 0.1%, and the content of heavy metals should not exceed 0.002%. The pharmacopoeia also includes a paper chromatographic test to limit the presence of the possible impurities ammidin and bergapten. It is available in a topical solution containing 9.2-10.8 mg/ml methoxsalen (US Pharmacopeial Convention, Inc., 1975).

In the UK, it is available in a 1% topical solution and in a skin paint containing 0.75% methoxsalen in combination with 0.25% pentosalen. It is also available as tablets containing 10 mg methoxsalen in combination with 5 mg pentosalen (Wade, 1977).

It is available in Japan in 10 mg doses as tablets.

2. Production, Use, Occurrence and Analysis

2.1 Production and use

(a) Production

Methoxsalen is a naturally occurring compound that can be isolated from a variety of plants (see section 2.2). It was first synthesized by Späth and Pailer in 1936 (Windholz, 1976). In one procedure (Stanley & Vannier, 1957), geranoxypsoralen, obtained from fractionation of lemon oil, was treated with sulphuric acid to give 8-hydroxypsoralen, which, on treatment with diazomethane in methanol, gave methoxsalen. It is not known whether this is the process used for its commercial production.

Methoxsalen was first marketed in the US in 1955. There is believed to be only one producer in the US at present, and no data are available on the amount produced (see preamble, p. 21).

The compound was introduced in Japan in 1967. One company is believed to manufacture it currently but no data are available on the amount produced.

(b) Use

Methoxsalen is used to increase skin tolerance to sunlight and to facilitate repigmentation in the treatment of the skin disease, vitiligo. For treatment of vitiligo, the daily oral dose is 20 mg followed within 2-4 hours by a 5-minute exposure to sunlight or long-wave ultra-violet light (exposure to light may be gradually increased to 30 minutes). When the 1% topical solution is used, it is applied weekly to well-defined affected areas, followed by a 1-minute exposure to long-wave ultra-violet light (Goodman & Gilman, 1975).

Methoxsalen is also used with long-wave ultra-violet light to produce a phototoxic reaction in the treatment of psoriasis. It is applied as a 0.1-0.15% topical solution or in 20-50 mg doses by mouth, followed by irradiation (Wade, 1977).

2.2 Occurrence

Methoxsalen is a naturally occurring substance, produced by several plants, e.g., *Psoralea corylifolia* L., *Ammi majus* L., *Ruta chalepensis* L., *Ruta graveolens* L., and others (Windholz, 1976; Shawl & Vishwapaul, 1977), which are found in both temperate and tropical regions. *Ammi majus* is a white umbellifer related to the wild carrot (*Daucus carota*); plants of the genus *Ruta* include rue, a perennial evergreen shrub with bitter, strong-scented leaves, once widely used as a medicine. It is also produced by the fungus *Sclerotinia sclerotiorum*, which causes 'pink rot' disease in celery (Scheel *et al.*, 1963).

2.3 Analysis

Typical methods for the analysis of methoxsalen in various matrices are summarized in Table 1. Abbreviations used are: UV, ultra-violet spectrometry, HPLC/UV, high-performance liquid chromatography with ultra-violet spectrometry; TLC/FL, thin-layer chromatography with fluorimetry; GC/FID, gas chromatography with flame-ionization detection; TLC/FD, thin-layer chromatography with fluorescence densitometry; and GC/MS, gas chromatography with mass spectrometry.

Table 1. Analytical methods for methoxsalen

Sample matrix	Sample preparation	Assay procedure	Limit of detection	Reference
Formulation	Dissolve in ethanol	UV	not given	US Pharmacopeial Convention, Inc., 1975
Biological samples				
Ammi majus seeds	Extract with ethanol; add hydrochloric acid; reflux; dilute with ethanol	TLC/UV	not given	Shawl & Vishwapaul, 1977
Plasma	Add water, potassium hydroxide and methanolic trimethylpsoralen solution (internal standard); extract with ethyl acetate; evaporate; redissolve in methanol	HPLC/UV	10 µg/l	Fincham et al., 1978
	Add water and hydrochloric acid; heat; extract with benzene-ethyl acetate mixture; evaporate; redissolve in dichloromethane	TLC/FL	20 ng	Chakrabarti et al., 1978
	Equilibrate with trimethylpsoralen in potassium hydroxide; extract with ethyl acetate; evaporate; redissolve in methanol	HPLC/UV GC/MS	10 µg/l	Hensby, 1978
Serum	Add hydrochloric acid, acetone and chloroform; evaporate; redissolve in toluene	TLC/FD	not given	Herfst et al., 1978
	Add benzene; centrifuge; evaporate; redissolve in benzene	GC/FID	10 µg/l	Gazith & Schaefer, 1977

3. Biological Data Relevant to the Evaluation of Carcinogenic Risk to Humans

3.1 Carcinogenicity studies in animals[1]

(a) Oral administration

Mouse: No statistically significant increase in the incidence of skin tumours or tumours of internal organs was observed in either sex of mice of various strains given methoxsalen orally (0.6-40 mg/kg bw or 200-1000 mg/kg diet daily) for 4-12 months alone or in combination with ultra-violet irradiation (250-400 nm) (O'Neal & Griffin, 1957; Griffin et al., 1958; Pathak et al., 1959; Langner et al., 1977; Pathak & Molica, 1978). [Attention is drawn to the short duration of these experiments.]

Groups of 40 female Swiss mice were given oral doses of 500 mg/kg of diet methoxsalen for 100 days in combination with various exposures to ultra-violet light. When the ultra-violet light was given for 2 hours daily for 3 months, 35% of the mice had skin tumours; when given for 30 minutes daily for 3 months, 25% of the mice had skin tumours; and when given for 10 minutes daily for 6 weeks, 20% of the mice had skin tumours. No skin tumours were seen in 3 groups of 40 control mice that received ultra-violet light only (Griffin, 1959).

(b) Skin application

Mouse: A group of 24 female ICR Swiss mice were given applications of a 0.1% solution of methoxsalen in ethanol on the ears and exposed to whole-body ultra-violet irradiation (280-360 nm) on 5 days a week for 25 weeks, at which time the incidence of ear tumours (epidermal papillomas and carcinomas) was 52% *versus* 20% in a control group exposed to ultra-violet light only (Urbach, 1959).

Two groups of 20 SKH:hairless mice were given daily skin applications of 40 μg of a 0.01% solution of methoxsalen in methanol, or of 40 μg of methanol only, 30-60 minutes before a whole-body 10-minute exposure to ultra-violet light (300-400 nm) on 5 days a week. Skin tumours, most of which developed at the site of application near the midline of the back, were seen in 15/30 and 12/24 animals (i.e., 50%) in the two groups at 14 and 30 weeks, respectively. The number of tumours per mouse was significantly higher in animals given methoxsalen plus ultra-violet light. Most of the tumours were squamous-cell carcinomas; others were fibrosarcomas, lymphosarcomas, sebaceous adenomas and haemangiomas (Forbes & Urbach, 1975).

---

[1] The Working Group was aware of a bioassay in progress in which methoxsalen was administered without ultra-violet light to mice and rats (Anon., 1980).

Two groups of 24 SKH:hairless-1 outbred stock mice were given applications of 40 µg of a 0.1 g/l solution of methoxsalen in methanol, or of methanol alone, prior to a 2-hour local exposure to ultra-violet light (300-400 nm) on 5 days a week for 38 weeks. Fifty percent of animals developed skin tumours at the site of application near the midline of the back, at 20 weeks in the treated group and at 27 weeks in the vehicle-control group ($P<0.01$). From 18 to 28 weeks, the numbers of tumour-bearing animals and of tumours per animal were significantly higher in treated animals than in controls ($P<0.05$ and $P<0.01$); 45/50 histologically analysed tumours were squamous-cell carcinomas; other tumours were sarcomas, haemangiomas and spindle-cell tumours of the skin (Forbes et al., 1976).

Groups of 20-25 female SKH:hairless-1 and HRS/J/An1 mice were given applications of 250 µg methoxsalen in ethanol 60 minutes prior to a whole-body exposure to 3 different wavelengths of ultra-violet light (300-400 nm, 320-400 nm or 365 nm) 5 times weekly for 24 weeks. Of the SKH:hairless-1 mice exposed to either 300-400 nm or 320-400 nm plus methoxsalen, 17/20 and 15/19 developed squamous-cell or basal-cell carcinomas within 90 weeks, some of which metastasized, compared with 8/19 in the group exposed to 365 nm. Of HRS/J/An1 mice exposed to the 3 wavelengths, 0/25, 4/23 and 9/23 animals developed squamous-cell and basal-cell carcinomas of the skin, one of which metastasized. Treated mice also developed fibrosarcomas: in SKH:hairless-1 mice, the respective incidences were 6/20, 5/19 and 2/19; in HRS/J/An1 mice, the incidences were 5/25, 1/23 and 4/23. In a second experiment in which groups of 30 mice of each strain were exposed to ultra-violet light from a fluorescent sun lamp prior to skin application of methoxsalen and subsequently exposed to 365 nm ultra-violet light, a high (almost 100%) incidence of skin carcinomas was observed in SKH:hairless-1 mice and a 30% incidence in HRS/J/An1 mice, compared with a 0 incidence in mice exposed only to 365 nm ultra-violet light (Grube et al., 1977).

Of 40 XVIInc/Z mice given 115 topical applications of 15 µg/cm^2 methoxsalen in acetone on each ear and irradiated with 1.68×10^4 J/m^2 of 365 nm ultra-violet light, 92% developed skin tumours, compared with none in 20 irradiated controls (Dubertret et al., 1979).

Four groups of 25 female Swiss albino mice received twice-weekly skin paintings of 5 µg methoxsalen in 0.05 ml ethanol together with subsequent exposures to ultra-violet light (300-400 nm) for 15, 30, 45 or 60 minutes, respectively. Subcutaneous malignant tumours (mammary adenocarcinomas, skin carcinomas and carcino-mixo-sarcomas) and lymphomas were seen in 43% of the treated animals from all groups combined at the 60th week after initial exposure, compared with 15% of control mice exposed to ultra-violet light alone (Santamaria et al., 1979).

(c) Intraperitoneal administration

Mouse: Two groups of twenty 8-10-week-old female Swiss mice were given i.p. injections of 0.4 mg methoxsalen on 6 days a week for 10 months and were observed for an additional month. In one group, each injection was followed 1 hour later by a 20-60-minute ultra-violet irradiation (250 nm). A third group of 20 mice was exposed to ultra-violet irradiation (250 nm) alone. No epidermal tumours were observed in the group that received methoxsalen alone; the epidermal tumour incidences in the two groups exposed to ultra-violet light, with and without methoxsalen, were 10-20% and 20%, respectively. In a concomitant experiment, 20 female Swiss mice were injected intraperitoneally with methoxsalen (0.4 mg/day, 6 days a week for 6 weeks) 1 hour before a 10-minute exposure to long-wave ultra-violet light (>320 nm). All animals developed epidermal tumours, whereas none were observed in 20 control mice exposed only to the ultra-violet light. The tumours were fibrosarcomas and squamous carcinomas of the ears and the eye region (Griffin *et al.*, 1958).

A group of 40 female Swiss albino mice were exposed to ultra-violet light (<320 nm) for 15 minutes per day for 90 days and received daily i.p. injections of 0.4 mg/mouse methoxsalen in gum arabic. A control group of 40 mice were exposed only to the ultra-violet light for 100 days. Ear tumours were observed in 60% of treated and 12% of control mice at 100 days, and in 97% and 68%, respectively, at 210 days. In a concomitant experiment, 2 groups of 40 Swiss albino mice received daily i.p injections of 0.1 mg/mouse methoxsalen 1 hour before a 15-minute ultra-violet irradiation, or 0.4 mg/mouse methoxsalen 20-22 hours before the ultra-violet irradiation, for 110 days. A control group of 40 mice were exposed only to ultra-violet irradiation. At 180 days, ear tumours were observed in 89% and 66% of the treated mice and in 62% of the control mice. The tumours were fibrosarcomas and squamous-cell carcinomas (O'Neal & Griffin, 1957).

Daily i.p. injections of 0.4 mg methoxsalen to 24 female ICR Swiss mice 1 hour before exposure to ultra-violet light (280-360 nm) on 5 days a week for 25 weeks resulted in an increased incidence of ear tumours (epidermal papillomas and carcinomas): 68% of mice developed tumours *versus* 20% of controls exposed only to ultra-violet light (Urbach, 1959).

Of 40 Swiss mice given 36 i.p. injections of 0.4 mg methoxsalen per animal and irradiated with 1.68×10^4 J/m^2 of 365 nm ultra-violet light, 90% developed skin tumours. No controls were available for this strain of mice (Dubertret *et al.*, 1979).

3.2 Other relevant biological data

(a) Experimental systems

Toxic effects

The oral LD_{50} of micronized methoxsalen was 791 mg/kg bw in male Sprague-Dawley rats, 699 mg/kg bw and 556 mg/kg bw in male and female CD-1 mice and 449 and 423 mg/kg bw in male and female Swiss-Webster mice. The i.p. LD_{50} of micronized methoxsalen was 189 and 158 mg/kg bw in male and female Sprague-Dawley rats and about 250 mg/kg bw in male and female CD-1 mice (Apostolou et al., 1979). [In the suspensions used in these studies, 90% of the particles were <50 μm in diameter and 80% were <20 μm.]

Chronic toxicity studies in mice revealed that small i.p. doses (12 mg/kg bw daily for 1 year) of a suspension (of unspecified particle size) of methoxsalen in saline induced no detectable changes; however, i.p. injection of 4 mg/kg bw methoxsalen in saline followed by exposure to long-wave ultra-violet irradiation (320-400 nm) resulted in severe toxic effects including erythema, burns and liver damage (Hakim et al., 1961).

In guinea-pigs, skin treatment with methoxsalen and ultraviolet irradiation blocked delayed hypersensitivity responses in exposed areas and, to a lesser but quite significant extent, at unexposed sites (Morison et al., 1979). Mice given topical applications of methoxsalen and ultra-violet light (320-400 nm) supported the growth of transplanted tumours irradiated with ultra-violet light (Spellman, 1979). These two studies suggest that methoxsalen and ultra-violet light suppress immunological surveillance of the skin.

No data on the prenatal toxicity of this compound were available.

Absorption, distribution, excretion and metabolism

After oral administration to dogs (0.5 mg/kg bw) and rats (40 mg/kg bw), absorption was rapid. After administration of ^{14}C-methoxsalen, maximum levels of radioactivity in the plasma occurred within 2 hrs after dosing in rats and within 30 minutes in dogs (Busch et al., 1978).

The distribution of ^{3}H-methoxsalen was studied by whole-body radiography in albino and pigmented rats after oral and i.v. treatment. The total radioactivity present in the various organs was estimated semiquantitatively: the higher accumulation of radioactivity (approximately 6 times higher than blood) occurred in the liver, kidneys and adrenal cortices. Skin concentrations of radioactivity were comparable with blood levels and were similar in albino and pigmented rats; ultra-violet light (10^5 J/m^2) increased the s.c. concentrations of radioactivity (Wulf & Hart, 1979). After oral administration (3 mg/kg bw), pigmented rats had a very high concentration of ^{3}H-methoxsalen (or its metabolites) in the pigmentary layer of the retina, ciliary body and iris, which were not comparable with those in albino rats (Wulf & Hart, 1978).

Single i.v. doses of 5 mg/kg bw ^{14}C-methoxsalen to dogs disappeared rapidly from plasma, although small levels of radioactivity persisted for 5 weeks after administration. Evidence suggested that the persistent plasma radioactivity was due to a metabolite bound to plasma protein. Elimination occurred in both urine and bile; 45% of the dose appeared in the urine and 40% in the faeces within 72 hrs of administration. Methoxsalen is extensively metabolized, and less than 2% of the drug is excreted unchanged in the urine. Four urinary metabolites were isolated; 3 of them resulted from opening of the furan ring: these are 7-hydroxy-8-methoxy-2-oxo-2*H*-1-benzopyran-6-acetic acid, α,7-dihydroxy-8-methoxy-2-oxo-2*H*-1-benzopyran-6-acetic acid, and an unknown conjugate of the former at the 7-hydroxy position. The fourth metabolite, formed by opening of the pyrone ring, is an unknown conjugate of (Z)-3-(6-hydroxy-7-methoxybenzofuran-5-yl)-2-propenoic acid (Kolis *et al.*, 1979).

Methoxsalen administered orally to mice at high dosages (80 mg/kg bw daily for 6 days) increased microsomal enzyme activity and cytochrome P450 content in the liver (Bickers *et al.*, 1977). Prolonged treatment (1,2 and 4 weeks) with 0.6 mg/kg bw per day did not modify this activity in rats although administration of 6 and 12 mg/kg bw per day did so to a statistically significant degree (Tsambaos *et al.*, 1978).

Mutagenicity and other, related short-term tests

Methoxsalen forms cyclobutane mono- and di-adducts with pyrimidine bases of DNA, by photoaddition under ultra-violet radiation, crosslinking 2 pyrimidine bases in the latter case (Parrish *et al.*, 1974; Dubertret *et al.*, 1979; Dall'Acqua *et al.*, 1979). The monoadducts produced by treatment with methoxsalen plus near ultra-violet light are converted to crosslinks by further irradiation (Seki *et al.*, 1978). This binding has been measured and found to increase in a dose-dependent manner (Bredberg *et al.*, 1977). A review on the photobiology of psoralens is available (Song & Tappley, 1979).

The covalent photobinding to DNA does not occur at random along the macromolecule: the regions with alternate sequence of A-T appear to be the best receptor sites for the formation of monoadducts, while the regions containing an alternate sequence of A-T and C-G appear to be the preferential sites for the crosslinkage formation (Dall'Acqua *et al.*, 1979).

Methoxsalen in combination with long-wave ultra-violet irradiation (320-400 nm, maximum at 340-360 nm) has been found to induce mutagenic effects in a variety of test systems. In most of the studies, methoxsalen alone, without ultra-violet light, had no detectable mutagenic effect on the frequencies of the mutagenic events (reviewed by Scott et al., 1976). Mutations were observed with methoxsalen plus ultra-violet light in some strains of *Escherichia coli* (Igali et al., 1970; Fujita et al., 1978; Bridges & Mottershead, 1979), *Serratia marcescens* (Joseph et al., 1974), *Aspergillus nidulans* (Alderson & Scott, 1970), *Streptomyces* species (Townsend et al., 1971) and *Saccharomyces cerevisiae* (Swanbeck & Thyresson, 1974; Henriques et al., 1977; Averbeck & Moustacchi, 1979). In *E. coli*, the induced mutation frequency per lethal hit was highest with 298 nm, decreased to a minimum with 345 nm and increased again with higher wavelengths (Fujita & Suzuki, 1978). In studies with different strains of *E. coli*, it was suggested that crosslinks are more mutagenic than monoadducts in wild-type bacteria and that mutations may arise as rare events during excision repair (Seki et al., 1978; Bridges et al., 1979). Methoxsalen has furthermore been shown to act as a weak frameshift mutagen in the absence of ultra-violet light in *E. coli* K-12 and in *Salmonella typhimurium* TA1538 and TA98 (Clarke & Wade, 1975; Ashwood-Smith, 1978; Bridges & Mottershead, 1977).

In *Saccharomyces cerevisiae*, at least two pathways are involved in the repair of damage induced by methoxsalen plus 365 nm ultra-violet light (Averbeck & Moustacchi, 1975). The DNA interstrand crosslinks induced in *S. cerevisiae* by such damage may be repaired by an error-prone process which may be the chief step in the mutagenic effect (Averbeck & Moustacchi, 1980).

Mouse, rat and hamster embryo cultures, as well as several established cell lines (BHK_{21}/Cl_{13}, NIH/3T3, Balb/c 3T3), were transformed by treatment with methoxsalen-ultra-violet light, as judged by morphological and growth criteria. When hamster embryo fibroblasts transformed by methoxsalen-ultra-violet light were injected into hamsters, spindle-cell sarcomas were produced in the cheek pouches of adult animals, and palpable tumours in 2-day animals, 3 days after s.c. injection (Evans & Morrow, 1979).

A significant increase in sister chromatid exchanges has been described in Chinese hamster ovary cells under the influence of 6-50 μM methoxsalen plus 560 J/m^2 ultra-violet light (Latt & Loveday, 1978).

In the dark, methoxsalen induced mutations in V-79 Chinese hamster cells (Bridges et al., 1978) and sperm morphology abnormalities in mice (Bridges, 1979).

The interaction of methoxsalen plus ultra-violet light with DNA leads to an inhibition of semiconservative DNA synthesis in mouse, hamster and human cells (Epstein & Fukuyama, 1970,1975; Baden et al., 1972; Pohl & Christophers, 1978) and evokes unscheduled DNA synthesis in cultured normal human fibroblasts (Baden et al., 1972).

Treatment with methoxsalen plus ultra-violet light was first shown to induce mutations in V-79 Chinese hamster cells by Arlett (1973). The induction of point mutations has also been studied on a quantitative basis with V-79 Chinese hamster cells: after treatment with 10 μg/ml methoxsalen plus 0-800 J/m^2 ultra-violet light, an increased number of hypoxanthineguanine phosphoribosyl transferase (HGPRT) mutants was found. This would result in an expected maximum number of 12.4×10^{-5} mutations in human skin during a photochemotherapy session (Burger & Simons, 1979a); however, a similar study in cultured human skin fibroblasts showed a 10-fold lower number of mutations in human cells as compared with rodent cells (Burger & Simons, 1979b).

Human cells have been used extensively for assessing possible genetic damage produced by photochemotherapy. Sister chromatid exchanges increased in frequency when human lymphocytes were irradiated with 365-400 nm in the presence of 0.06-0.5 μM methoxsalen (Carter et al., 1976; Gaynor & Carter, 1978; Wulf, 1978; Waksvik et al., 1977). Fibroblast cells also exhibited chromosome damage concomitant with an inhibition of cell proliferation; the proliferation rate gradually normalized during subsequent passages, whereas chromosome aberrations increased (Omar et al., 1977). Shuler & Latt (1979) observed an increase in sister chromatid exchanges after methoxsalen-ultra-violet light treatment of Chinese hamster pouch cells *in vivo*.

(b) Humans

Methoxsalen increases skin tolerance to sunlight (Goodman & Gilman, 1975).

Toxic effects

Nater (1979) has summarized the side effects from 41,000 courses of treatment with methoxsalen plus ultra-violet light; erythema or burns occurred in about 10%, pruritis in 14% and nausea in 3%; headache and dizziness were also recorded. In a similar study (Mackey, 1979), reactivation of peptic ulcer symptoms was reported in 3 patients who had a history of previous ulceration.

A significant decrease in the number and function of T-cells has been reported in patients undergoing therapy with a combination of psoralen drugs and ultra-violet irradiation (Cormane et al., 1977).

Damage to the nail-beds was induced by methoxsalen and sunlight in 2 patients. Histological examination of the nail-beds showed that the photosensitizing effect of the drug induced the generation of many multinucleated epithelial cells and fibroblasts in the dermis (Zala et al., 1977).

Three of 20 healthy volunteers given increasing doses of topically applied 1% methoxsalen in hydrophilic ointment 3 times a week plus ultra-violet light developed photoallergy (Fulton & Willis, 1968).

No data on prenatal toxicity of methoxsalen were available.

Absorption, distribution, excretion and metabolism

Methoxsalen is rapidly absorbed after an oral dose of 40-50 mg (Schalla et al., 1976; Gazith & Schaefer, 1977). Following an oral dose of 50 mg, maximum serum concentrations ranged between 1-1.5 µg/ml (Gazith & Schaefer, 1977).

After an oral dose of 40 mg ^{14}C-methoxsalen, the peak concentration of radio-activity in the plasma occurred at 2 hours; 50% could be accounted for by unchanged drug (Busch et al., 1978). Among 9 psoriasis patients given oral doses of 0.57-0.70 mg/kg bw methoxsalen, peak serum concentrations occurred 2-6 hours later, although individual variations were observed (Steiner et al., 1977).

Following topical application, methoxsalen penetrates rapidly into the epidermis and dermis. Penetration was dependent on the polarity of the vehicle. The drug transport rate from the skin is a function of the flow rate from the horny reservoir (Kammerau et al., 1976).

Methoxsalen is extensively metabolized, and no unchanged drug is excreted in the urine (Schalla et al., 1976; Busch et al., 1978); 80% of a dose of 40 mg was excreted in the urine within 8 hours as hydroxylated and glucuronide derivatives (Pathak et al., 1974).

Mutagenicity and other, related short-term tests

Treatment with methoxsalen plus ultra-violet irradiation resulted in a significant increase of aberrations in lymphocyte chromosomes of 1/8 patients, slight but nonsignificant increases in 6 and no increase in 1 patient (Swanbeck et al., 1975); sister chromatid exchanges were also observed (Mourelatos et al., 1977a). No chromosome aberrations or sister chromatid exchanges were observed in psoriasis patients treated with the combination (Wolff-Schreiner et al., 1977; Brøgger & Waksvik, 1978; Lambert et al., 1978);

but when white blood cells removed from patients after treatment were reirradiated with ultra-violet light *in vitro*, there was a significant increase in sister chromatid exchanges (Mourelatos *et al.*, 1977b; Wolff-Schreiner *et al.*, 1977; Lambert *et al.*, 1978).

The methoxsalen concentrations and ultra-violet irradiation conditions to which human lymphocytes are exposed therapeutically *in vivo* have been shown to be too low to induce observable numbers of sister chromatid exchanges (Burger & Simons, 1979b). However, more point mutations, as indicated by the increased incidence of 6-thioguanine-resistant lymphocytes, were observed in patients treated with psoralen drugs and ultra-violet irradiation than in healthy controls (Strauss *et al.*, 1979).

3.3 Case reports and epidemiological studies of carcinogenicity in humans

Møller & Howitz (1976) reported on a 41-year-old woman with vitiligo treated with sunlight and 20-30 mg/day (0.5 mg/kg bw) methoxsalen orally for 91 days. She developed multiple basal-cell carcinomas on the trunk about 2 months after treatment. She had received 1g arsenic trioxide (a known carcinogen, see IARC, 1980) for one year 8 years previously, had had therapy with sunlight for several years, and had received a placebo and sunlight in a clinical trial 1 year before receiving methoxsalen therapy.

Two further case reports described patients who developed haematological malignancies after receiving methoxsalen and long-wave ultra-violet irradiation for psoriasis. In one (Wagner *et al.*, 1978), a 73-year-old man who received two series of such treatment (30 mg methoxsalen/day plus ultra-violet light) 4 times a week for a total of 30 weeks developed haematological abnormalities described as 'preleukemia or hematopoietic dysplasia' with 'excess myeloblasts' in the marrow. Previous treatment had included topical steroids, Bucky rays [grenz rays (~200 nm)], tar paste and petroleum jelly with salicylic acid. He had also received hydroflumethiazide, potassium chloride, theophyllamine, phenylbutazone (see IARC, 1977), indomethacin and allopurinol, some of which have been associated with blood dyscrasias. In the other report, Hansen (1979) described a 70-year-old woman with psoriasis who received 20 mg methoxsalen/day plus ultra-violet irradiation for 109 days. Therapy was stopped when she developed spinocellular carcinomas on both elbows. Two years later she developed acute myeloid leukaemia. Previous treatment had included alpha rays, Bucky rays and local ointments, including steroids.

Two randomized clinical trials were carried out to determine whether methoxsalen would protect against sunlight-induced skin cancer by increasing pigmentation and cornification of the skin (Hopkins *et al.*, 1963; MacDonald *et al.*, 1963). Patients with a history of skin cancer (173 in El Paso, USA and 92 in Sydney, Australia) were entered into the trials and randomly assigned to receive either 20 mg/day methoxsalen or placebo.

The dose used was sufficient to produce a statistically significant increase in skin tanning in the methoxsalen-treated group. There was no significant difference in the incidence of new skin cancer over 2 years in either study, but the numbers of patients and skin cancers were small.

In a cohort study of 1373 patients treated with methoxsalen plus ultra-violet light for psoriasis (Stern et al., 1979), 30 patients developed 19 basal-cell carcinomas and 29 squamous-cell carcinomas of the skin over a 2.1-year follow-up period. On the basis of age, sex and geographic location-specific incidence rates, 11.4 patients would have been expected to develop skin tumours (relative risk, 2.6; 95% confidence interval, 1.9-3.9). In support of a causal interpretation of the data, the authors noted that: (1) The proportion of squamous-cell cancers occurring more than 1 year after the treatment was much higher (24 of 30 cancers, 80%) than either before the treatments began (5 of 30, 17%) or within the first year of treatment (5 of 18, 28%). (2) The squamous-cell cancers occurred more often (86%) on areas of the body not normally exposed to sunlight than did the basal-cell carcinomas (32%). (3) In the 2 years prior to treatment with methoxsalen plus ultra-violet light, the patients in the study showed no excess of new skin cancers: 12 patients reported new skin cancers, while the expected number was 11.3 (relative risk, 1.05; 95% confidence interval, 0.6-2.5). [The study subjects were examined annually by a dermatologist and were thus more likely to have skin cancers noted than would the general population, from which the expected number of cases was derived. This ascertainment bias would artefactually increase the relative risk. Additionally, even if the observed excess of cancers were due to the treatment, all patients received both methoxsalen and ultra-violet light; thus, the effect cannot be attributed to either agent alone.]

4. Summary of Data Reported and Evaluation

4.1 Experimental data

Methoxsalen alone has not been tested by skin application and was inadequately tested in mice by oral and by intraperitoneal administration.

It was tested in combination with long-wave ultra-violet light in mice by oral and intraperitoneal administration and by skin application: it increased the incidence of epidermal and dermal tumours.

Methoxsalen, mainly in combination with long-wave ultra-violet light, but also in the dark, was mutagenic in a variety of prokaryotic and eukaryotic cells.

Attention is drawn to the absence of studies on the teratogenicity of this compound.

4.2 Human data

Methoxsalen is mainly used in combination with long-wave ultra-violet light in the treatment of vitiligo and severe psoriasis.

Methoxsalen and long-wave ultra-violet light together have been associated with haematopoietic neoplasms in two patients, with basal-cell skin cancer in another, and with squamous-cell skin cancer in a cohort study of patients with psoriasis. In the cohort study, increased surveillance of study subjects may have biased comparisons with the general population. However, a change in the ratio of squamous- to basal-cell tumours, the appearance of tumours in body areas not normally exposed to sunlight, and a change in tumour incidence within the cohort would support a causal interpretation. In none of these reports could the possible effects of methoxsalen alone be distinguished from those of long-wave ultra-violet light or of the combination of the two. Methoxsalen alone did not alter the incidence of skin cancer over two years in two small controlled trials of its use as a putative prophylactic for this disease.

These data are insufficient to allow a conclusion as to the carcinogenicity of methoxsalen in humans.

4.3 Evaluation

The available experimental and epidemiological data on methoxsalen alone were inadequate to make an evaluation of its carcinogenicity.

There is *sufficient evidence*[1] that methoxsalen increases the carcinogenic effects of long-wave ultra-violet light in mouse skin. In view of the combined use of these agents in the treatment of skin disorders in humans, further studies should be undertaken of humans who have been exposed to them.

---

[1] See preamble, p. 18.

5. References

Alderson, T. & Scott, B.R. (1970) The photosensitising effect of 8-methoxypsoralen on the inactivation and mutation of *Aspergillus conidia* by near ultraviolet light. *Mutat. Res., 9*, 569-578

Anon. (1980) Prechronic studies for the bioassay of 8-methoxypsoralen and related psoralen derivatives. *Cancer Lett., 6*, 7

Apostolou, A., Williams, R.E. & Comereski, C.R. (1979) Acute toxicity of micronized 8-methoxypsoralen in rodents. *Drug Chem. Toxicol., 2*, 309-313

Arlett, C.F. (1973) Mutagenesis in cultured mammalian cells. *Studia biophys. (Berlin), 36/37*, 139-147

Ashwood-Smith, M.J. (1978) Frameshift mutations in bacteria produced in the dark by several furocoumarins; absence of activity of 4,5',8-trimethylpsoralen. *Mutat. Res., 58*, 23-27

Averbeck, D. & Moustacchi, E. (1975) 8-Methoxypsoralen plus 365 nm light effects and repair in yeast. *Biochim. biophys. Acta, 395*, 393-404

Averbeck, D. & Moustacchi, E. (1979) Genetic effect of 3-carbethoxypsoralen, angelicin, psoralen and 8-methoxypsoralen plus 365 nm irradiation in *Saccharomyces cerevisiae*. Induction of reversions, mitotic crossing-over, gene conversion and cytoplasmic 'petite' mutations. *Mutat. Res., 68*, 133-148

Averbeck, D. & Moustacchi, E. (1980) Decreased photo-induced mutagenicity of monofunctional as opposed to bi-functional furocoumarins in yeast. *Photochem. Photobiol., 31*, 475-478

Baden, H.P., Parrington, J.M., Delhanty, J.D.A. & Pathak, M.A. (1972) DNA synthesis in normal and xeroderma pigmentosum fibroblasts following treatment with 8-methoxypsoralen and long wave ultraviolet light. *Biochim. biophys. Acta, 262*, 247-255

Bickers, D.R., Pathak, M.A. & Molica, S.J., Jr (1977) Induction of hepatic drug-metabolising enzymes and cytochrome P-450 by 8-methoxypsoralen (Abstract). *Clin. Res., 25*, 279A

Bredberg, A., Lambert, B., Swanbeck, G. & Thyresson-Hök, M. (1977) The binding of 8-methoxypsoralen to nuclear DNA of UVA irradiated human fibroblasts *in vitro*. *Acta dermatovener. (Stockholm), 57,* 389-391

Bridges, B.A. (1979) An estimate of genetic risk from 8-methoxypsoralen photochemotherapy. *Human Genet., 49,* 91-96

Bridges, B.A. & Mottershead, R.P. (1977) Frameshift mutagenesis in bacteria by 8-methoxypsoralen (methoxalen) in the dark. *Mutat. Res., 44,* 305-312

Bridges, B.A. & Mottershead, R.P. (1979) Inactivation of *Escherichia coli* by near-ultraviolet light and 8-methoxypsoralen: different responses of strains B/r and K-12. *J. Bacteriol., 139,* 454-459

Bridges, B.A., Mottershead, R.P. & Arlett, C.F. (1978) 8-Methoxypsoralen as a frameshift mutagen in bacteria and Chinese hamster cells in the dark - implications for genetic risk in man (Abstract no. 25). *Mutat. Res., 53,* 156

Bridges, B.A., Mottershead, R.P. & Knowles, A. (1979) Mutation induction and killing of *Escherichia coli* by DNA adducts and crosslinks: a photobiological study with 8-methoxypsoralen. *Chem.-biol. Interactions, 27,* 221-233

Brøgger, A. & Waksvik, H. (1978) Chromosomes after psoralen/UVA treatment *in vitro* and *in vivo* (psoriasis patients) (Abstract no. 27). *Mutat. Res., 53,* 157-158

Burger, P.M. & Simons, J.W.I.M. (1979a) Mutagenicity of 8-methoxypsoralen and long-wave ultraviolet irradiation in V-79 Chinese hamster cells. A first approach to a risk estimate in photochemotherapy. *Mutat. Res., 60,* 381-389

Burger, P.M. & Simons, J.W.I.M. (1979b) Mutagenicity of 8-methoxypsoralen and long-wave ultraviolet irradiation in diploid human skin fibroblasts. An improved risk estimate in photochemotherapy. *Mutat. Res., 63,* 371-380

Busch, U., Schmid, J., Koss, F.W., Zipp, H. & Zimmer, A. (1978) Pharmacokinetics and metabolite-pattern of 8-methoxypsoralen in man following oral administration as compared to the pharmacokinetics in rat and dog. *Arch. dermatol. Res., 262,* 255-265

Carter, D.M., Wolff, K. & Schnedl, W. (1976) 8-Methoxypsoralen and UVA promote sister-chromatid exchanges. *J. invest. Dermatol., 67,* 548-551

Chakrabarti, S.G., Gooray, D.A. & Kenney, J.A., Jr (1978) Determination of 8-methoxypsoralen in plasma by scanning fluorometry after thin-layer chromatography. *Clin. Chem., 24*, 1155-1157

Clarke, C.H. & Wade, M.J. (1975) Evidence that caffeine, 8-methoxypsoralen and steroidal diamines are frameshift mutagens for *E. coli* K-12. *Mutat. Res., 28*, 123-125

Cormane, R.H., Hamerlinck, F., Simon, M. & Siddiqui, A.H. (1977) Photoimmunology in psoriasis (Abstract). *J. invest. Dermatol., 68*, 253

Dall'Acqua, F., Vedaldi, D., Bordin, F. & Rodighiero, G. (1979) New studies on the interaction between 8-methoxypsoralen and DNA *in vitro*. *J. invest. Dermatol., 73*, 191-197

Dubertret, L., Averbeck, D., Zajdela, F., Bisagni, E., Moustacchi, E., Touraine, R. & Latarjet, R. (1979) Photochemotherapy (PUVA) of psoriasis using 3-carbethoxypsoralen, a non-carcinogenic compound in mice. *Br. J. Dermatol., 101*, 379-389

Epstein, J.H. & Fukuyama, K. (1970) A study of 8-methoxypsoralen (8-MOP)-induced phototoxic effects on mammalian epidermal macromolecule synthesis *in vivo* (Abstract no. 3). *J. invest. Dermatol., 54*, 350-351

Epstein, J.H. & Fukuyama, K. (1975) Effects of 8-methoxypsoralen-induced phototoxic effects on mammalian epidermal macromolecule synthesis *in vivo*. *Photochem. Photobiol., 21*, 325-330

Evans, D.L. & Morrow, K.J. (1979) 8-Methoxypsoralen induced alterations of mammalian cells. *J. invest. Dermatol., 72*, 35-41

Fincham, N., Greaves, M.W., Hensby, C.N. & Briffa, D.V. (1978) The quantitative analysis of 8-MOP in human plasma by HPLC-UV. *Br. J. Pharmacol., 63*, 373P

Forbes, P.D. & Urbach, F. (1975) Experimental modification of photocarcinogenesis. II. Fluorescent whitening agents and simulated solar UVR. *Food Cosmet. Toxicol., 13*, 339-342

Forbes, P.D., Davies, R.E. & Urbach, F. (1976) Phototoxicity and photocarcinogenesis: comparative effects of anthracene and 8-methoxypsoralen in the skin of mice. *Food Cosmet. Toxicol., 14*, 303-306

Fujita, H. & Suzuki, K. (1978) Effect of near-UV light on *Escherichia coli* in the presence of 8-methoxypsoralen: wavelength dependency of killing, induction of prophage, and mutation. *J. Bacteriol., 135*, 345-362

Fujita, H., Sano, M. & Suzuki, K. (1978) Effect of near ultraviolet light on *Escherichia coli* sensitized with 8-methoxypsoralen: mutagenic effect and induction of lambda prophage. *Tokai J. exp. clin. Med., 3*, 35-42

Fulton, J.E., Jr & Willis, I. (1968) Photoallergy to methoxsalen. *Arch. Dermatol., 98*, 445-450

Gaynor, A.L. & Carter, D.M. (1978) Greater promotion in sister chromatid exchanges by trimethylpsoralen than by 8-methoxypsoralen in the presence of UV-light. *J. invest. Dermatol., 71*, 257-259

Gazith, J. & Schaefer, H. (1977) 8-Methoxypsoralen: its isolation and gas chromatographic determination for aqueous solutions and serum. *Biochem. Med., 18*, 102-109

Goodman, L.S. & Gilman, A., eds (1975) *The Pharmacological Basis of Therapeutics*, 5th ed., New York, Macmillan, p. 954

Griffin, A.C. (1959) Methoxsalen in ultraviolet carcingenesis in the mouse. *J. invest. Dermatol., 32*, 367-372

Griffin, A.C., Hakim, R.E. & Knox, J. (1958) The wave length effect upon erythemal and carcinogenic response in psoralen treated mice. *J. invest. Dermatol., 31*, 289-295

Grube, D.D., Ley, R.D. & Fry, R.J.M. (1977) Photosensitizing effects of 8-methoxypsoralen on the skin of hairless mice. II. Strain and spectral differences for tumorigenesis. *Photochem. Photobiol., 25*, 269-276

Hakim, R.E., Freeman, R.G., Griffin, A.C. & Knox, J.M. (1961) Experimental toxicologic studies on 8-methoxypsoralen in animals exposed to the long ultraviolet. *J. Pharmacol. exp. Ther., 131*, 394-399

Hansen, N.E. (1979) Development of acute myeloid leukaemia in a patient with psoriasis treated with oral 8-methoxypsoralen and longwave ultraviolet light. *Scand. J. Haematol., 22*, 57-60

Henriques, J.A.P., Chanet, R., Averbeck, D. & Moustacchi, E. (1977) Lethality and 'petite' mutation induced by the photoaddition of 8-methoxypsoralen in yeast. Influence of ploidy, growth phases and stages in the cell cycle. *Molec. gen. Genet., 158,* 63-72

Hensby, C.N. (1978) The qualitative and quantitative analysis of 8-methoxypsoralen by HPLC-UV and GLC-MS. *Clin. exp. Dermatol., 3,* 355-366

Herfst, M.J., Koot-Gronsveld, E.A.M. & de Wolff, F.A. (1978) Serum levels of 8-methoxypsoralen in psoriasis patients using a new fluorodensitometric method. *Arch. dermatol. Res., 262,* 1-6

Hopkins, C.E., Belisario, J.C., MacDonald, E.J. & Davis, C.T. (1963) Psoralen prophylaxis against skin cancer: report of clinical trial. II. *J. invest. Dermatol., 41,* 219-223

IARC (1977) *IARC Monographs on the Evaluation of Carcinogenic Risk of Chemicals to Man*, Vol. 13, *Some miscellaneous pharmaceutical substances*, Lyon, pp. 183-199

IARC (1980) *IARC Monographs on the Evaluation of the Carcinogenic Risk of Chemicals to Humans*, Vol. 23, *Some metals and metallic compounds*, Lyon, pp. 39-141

Igali, S., Bridges, B.A., Ashwood-Smith, M.J. & Scott, B.R. (1970) Mutagenesis in *Escherichia coli*. IV. Photosensitization to near ultraviolet light by 8-methoxypsoralen. *Mutat. Res., 9,* 21-30

Joseph, R., Shanthamma, M.S., Rehana, F. & Nand, K. (1974) Induced mutations in *Serratia marcescens* by near UV-light in presence of psoralen. *Experientia, 30,* 360-361

Kammerau, B., Klebe, U., Zesch, A. & Schaefer, H. (1976) Penetration, permeation, and resorption of 8-methoxypsoralen. Comparative *in vitro* and *in vivo* studies after topical application of four standard preparations. *Arch. dermatol. Res., 255,* 31-42

Kolis, S.J., Williams, T.H., Postma, E.J., Sasso, G.J., Confalone, P.N. & Schwartz, M.A. (1979) The metabolism of ^{14}C-methoxsalen by the dog. *Drug Metab. Disposition, 7,* 220-225

Lambert, B., Morad, M., Bredberg, A., Swanbeck, G. & Thyresson-Hök, M. (1978) Sister chromatid exchanges in lymphocytes from psoriasis patients treated with 8-methoxypsoralen and longwave ultraviolet light. *Acta dermatovener. (Stockholm), 58,* 13-16

Langner, A., Wolska, H., Marzulli, F.N., Jablonska, S., Jarzabek-Chorzelska, M., Glinski, W. & Pawinska, M. (1977) Dermal toxicity of 8-methoxypsoralen administered (by gavage) to hairless mice irradiated with long-wave ultraviolet light. *J. invest Dermatol., 69*, 451-457

Latt, S.A. & Loveday, K.S. (1978) Characterization of sister chromatid exchange induction by 8-methoxypsoralen plus near UV light. *Cytogenet. Cell Genet., 21*, 184-200

MacDonald, E.J., Griffin, A.C., Hopkins, C.E., Smith, L., Garrett, H. & Black, G.L. (1963) Psoralen prophylaxis against skin cancer: report of clinical trial. I. *J. invest Dermatol., 41*, 213-217

Mackey, J.P. (1979) Clinical side-effects of long-wave ultraviolet light and oral 8-methoxypsoralen in patients treated for psoriasis. *Ir. J. med. Sci., 148*, 36-38

Møller, R. & Howitz, J. (1976) Methoxsalen and multiple basal cell carcinomas. *Arch. Dermatol., 112*, 1613-1614

Morison, W.L., Woehler, M.E. & Parrish, J.A. (1979) PUVA and systemic immunosuppression in guinea pigs (Abstract). *J. invest Dermatol., 72*, 273

Mourelatos, D., Faed, M.J.W. & Johnson, B.E. (1977a) Sister chromatid exchanges in human lymphocytes exposed to 8-methoxypsoralen and long wave UV radiation prior to incorporation of bromodeoxyuridine. *Experientia, 33*, 1091-1093

Mourelatos, D., Faed, M.J.W., Gould, P.W., Johnson, B.E. & Frain-Bell, W. (1977b) Sister chromatid exchanges in lymphocytes of psoriatics after treatment with 8-methoxypsoralen and long wave ultraviolet radiation. *Br. J. Dermatol., 97*, 649-654

Nater, J.P. (1979) *Drugs used on the skin.* In: Dukes, M.N.G., ed., *Side Effects of Drugs Annual 3*, Amsterdam, Excerpta Medica, pp. 132-133

Omar, A., Wiesmann, U.N. & Krebs, A. (1977) Induction of multinucleate cells by 8-MOP and UV treatment *in vitro* and *in vivo*. *Dermatologica, 155*, 65-79

O'Neal, M.A. & Griffin, A.C. (1957) The effect of oxypsoralen upon ultraviolet carcinogenesis in albino mice. *Cancer Res., 17*, 911-916

Parrish, J.A., Fitzpatrick, T.B., Tanenbaum, L. & Pathak, M.A. (1974) Photochemotherapy of psoriasis with oral methoxsalen and longwave ultraviolet light. *New Engl. J. Med., 291*, 1207-1211

Pathak, M.A. & Molica, S.J. (1978) Ultraviolet carcinogenesis in mice and the effect of oral 8-methoxypsoralen (8-MOP) (Abstract). *Clin. Res., 26*, 300A

Pathak, M.A., Daniels, F., Hopkins, C.E. & Fitzpatrick, T.B. (1959) Ultra-violet carcinogenesis in albino and pigmented mice receiving furocoumarins: psoralen and 8-methoxypsoralen. *Nature, 183*, 728-730

Pathak, M.A., Dall'Acqua, F., Rodighiero, G. & Parrish, J.A. (1974) Metabolism of psoralens. *J. invest. Dermatol., 62*, 347

Pohl, J. & Christophers, E. (1978) Photoinactivation of cultured skin fibroblasts by sublethal doses of 8-methoxypsoralen and long wave ultraviolet light. *J. invest. Dermatol., 71*, 316-319

Santamaria, L., Arnaboldi, A., Daffara, P. & Bianchi, A. (1979) Photocarcinogenesis by methoxypsoralen, neutral red and proflavine. *Boll. Chim. Farm., 118*, 356-362

Schalla, W., Schaefer, H., Kammerau, B. & Zesch, A. (1976) Pharmacokinetics of 8-methoxypsoralen (8-MOP) after oral and local application (Abstract). *J. invest. Dermatol., 66*, 258

Scheel, L.D., Perone, V.B., Larkin, R.L. & Kupel, R.E. (1963) The isolation and characterization of two phototoxic furanocoumarins (psoralens) from diseased celery. *Biochemistry, 2*, 1127-1131

Scott, B.R., Pathak, M.A. & Mohn, G.R. (1976) Molecular and genetic basis of furocoumarin reactions. *Mutat. Res., 39*, 29-74

Seki, T., Nozu, K. & Kondo, S. (1978) Differential causes of mutation and killing in *Escherichia coli* after psoralen plus light treatment: monoadducts and cross-links. *Photochem. Photobiol., 27*, 19-24

Shawl, A.S. & Vishwapaul, A. (1977) Thin-layer chromatographic-spectrophotometric determination of methoxsalen (xanthotoxin) in *Ammi majus* seed. *Analyst, 102*, 779-782

Shuler, C.F. & Latt, S.A. (1979) *In vivo* mutagenic effect of 8-methoxypsoralen and ultraviolet light (Abstract no. 885). *J. Dent. Res., 58* (special), 313

Song, P.S. & Tappley, K.J. (1979) The photochemistry and photobiology of psoralens. *Photochem. Photobiol., 29*, 1177-1197

Spellman, C.W. (1979) Skin cancer after PUVA treatment for psoriasis. *New Engl. J. Med., 301*, 554-555

Stanley, W.L. & Vannier, S.H. (1957) Chemical composition of lemon oil. I. Isolation of a series of substituted coumarins. *J. Am. chem. Soc., 79*, 3488-3491

Steiner, I., Prey, T., Schnait, F., Washüttl, J. & Greiter, F. (1977) Serum level profiles of 8-methoxypsoralen after oral administration. *Arch. dermatol Res., 259*, 299-301

Stern, R.S., Thibodeau, L.A., Kleinerman, R.A., Parrish, J.A., Fitzpatrick, T.B. & 22 participating investigators (1979) Risk of cutaneous carcinoma in patients treated with oral methoxsalen photochemotherapy for psoriasis. *New Engl. J. Med., 300*, 809-813

Strauss, G.H., Albertini, R.J., Krusinski, P.A. & Baughman, R.D. (1979) 6-Thioguanine resistant peripheral blood lymphocytes in humans following psoralen, long-wave ultraviolet light (PUVA) therapy. *J. invest. Dermatol., 73*, 211-216

Swanbeck, G. & Thyresson, M. (1974) Induction of respiration-deficient mutants in yeast by psoralen and light. *J. invest. Dermatol., 63*, 242-244

Swanbeck, G., Thyresson-Hök, M., Bredberg, A. & Lambert, B. (1975) Treatment of psoriasis with oral psoralens and longwave ultraviolet light. Therapeutic results and cytogenetic hazards. *Acta dermatovener. (Stockholm), 55*, 367-376

Townsend, M.E., Wright, H.M. & Hopwood, D.A. (1971) Efficient mutagenesis by near ultraviolet light in the presence of 8-methoxypsoralen in *Streptomyces*. *J. appl. Bacteriol., 34*, 799-801

Tsambaos, D., Vizethum, W. & Goerz, G. (1978) Effect of oral 8-methoxypsoralen on rat liver microsomal cytochrome P-450. *Arch. dermatol. Res., 263*, 339-342

Urbach, F. (1959) Modification of ultraviolet carcinogenesis by photoactive agents. *J. invest. Dermatol., 32*, 373-378

US Pharmacopeial Convention, Inc. (1975) *The US Pharmacopeia*, 19th rev., Rockville, MD, pp. 317-318

Wade, A., ed. (1977) *Martindale, The Extra Pharmacopoeia*, 27th ed., London, The Pharmaceutical Press, pp. 446-447

Wagner, J., Manthorpe, R., Philip, P. & Frost, F. (1978) Preleukaemia (haemopoietic dysplasia) developing in a patient with psoriasis treated with 8-methoxypsoralen and ultraviolet light (PUVA treatment). *Scand. J. Haematol., 21*, 299-304

Waksvik, H., Brøgger, A. & Stene, J. (1977) Psoralen/UVA treatment and chromosomes. I. Aberrations and sister chromatid exchange in human lymphocytes *in vitro* and synergism with caffeine. *Human Genet., 38*, 195-207

Windholz, M., ed. (1976) *The Merck Index*, 9th ed., Rahway, NJ, Merck & Co., p. 783

Wolff-Schreiner, E.C., Carter, D.M., Schwarzacher, H.G. & Wolff, K. (1977) Sister chromatid exchanges in photochemotherapy. *J. invest. Dermatol., 69*, 387-391

Wulf, H.C. (1978) Acute effect of 8-methoxypsoralen and ultraviolet light on sister chromatid exchange. *Arch. dermatol. Res., 263*, 37-46

Wulf, H.C. & Hart, J. (1978) Accumulation of 8-methoxypsoralen in the rat retina. *Acta ophthalmol., 56*, 284-290

Wulf, H.C. & Hart, J. (1979) Distribution of tritium-labelled 8-methoxypsoralen in the rat, studied by whole body autoradiography. *Acta dermatovener. (Stockholm), 59*, 97-103

Zala, L., Omar, A. & Krebs, A. (1977) Photo-onycholysis induced by 8-methoxypsoralen. *Dermatologica, 154*, 203-215

NAFENOPIN

1. Chemical and Physical Data

1.1 Synonyms and trade names

Chem. Abstr. Services Reg. No.: 3771-19-5

Chem. Abstr. Name: Propanoic acid, 2-methyl-2-[4-(1,2,3,4-tetrahydro-1-naphthalenyl)phenoxy]-

IUPAC Systematic name: 2-Methyl-2-[4-(1,2,3,4-tetrahydro-1-naphthyl)phenoxy]-propanoic acid

Synonyms: 2-Methyl-2-[4-(1,2,3,4-tetrahydro-1-naphthalenyl)phenoxy] propanoic acid; 2-methyl-2-[*para*-(1,2,3,4-tetrahydro-1-naphthyl)phenoxy] propionic acid; α-methyl-α-(*para*-1,2,3,4-tetrahydronaphth-1-ylphenoxy)propionic acid; nafenoic acid

Trade names: CH 13-437; CH 13437; CIBA 13437 Su; CIBA 13,437 Su; C 13437 Su; Melipan; Su 13437; Su 13.437; TPIA

1.2 Structural and molecular formulae and molecular weight

$C_{20}H_{22}O_3$ Mol. wt: 310.4

1.3 Chemical and physical properties of the pure substance

Melting-point: 127-128°C (Hess & Bencze, 1968)

1.4 Technical products and impurities

No information was available to the Working Group.

2. Production, Use, Occurrence and Analysis

2.1 Production and use

(a) Production

Nafenopin was first prepared in 1963. Hess & Bencze (1968) described the following method of preparation: phenol was alkylated with 1,2,3,4-tetrahydro-1-naphthol by a Friedel-Crafts reaction, and the resulting *para*-substituted phenol was converted to its sodium salt and etherified with ethyl α-bromoisobutyrate. Hydrolysis of the resulting ethyl ester in methanolic potassium hydroxide solution furnished nafenopin. It is not known whether this is the process used in its manufacture.

It is believed that nafenopin is produced only as an investigative drug by one company in Switzerland. No data are available on the quantitites produced.

(b) Use

Nafenopin has been studied for use in the treatment of hypercholesterolaemia (Wade, 1977) or hypertriglyceridaemia at doses of 400-600 mg per day for 2-6 weeks.

2.2 Occurrence

Nafenopin is not known to occur in nature.

2.3 Analysis

No data were available to the Working Group.

3. Biological Data Relevant to the Evaluation of Carcinogenic Risk to Humans

3.1 Carcinogenicity studies in animals

Oral administration

Mouse: Nafenopin was administered in the diet of groups of 20 male and 20 female 5-8-week-old acatalasemic (Cs^b strain with unstable catalase gene) and wild-type (Cs^a strain) mice at a concentration of 0.1% (w/w) for one year, after which the surviving animals were fed this drug at a dietary concentration of 0.05% until termination of the experiment at 20 months. Exploratory laparotomies were performed at 6, 12, 18, 26, 35, 48, 60 and 70 weeks, and liver biopsies were obtained for light and electron microscopic examination. By 56 weeks, all male and female wild-type (Cs^a) mice had died, and no liver tumours were detected; the mortality rate in acatalasemic (Cs^b) mice at that time was about 50% (effective numbers: 9 males and 12 females). At between 18 and 20 months of the experiment, 9/9 male and 12/12 female acatalasemic mice developed multiple hepatocellular carcinomas; 5 of these metastasized to the lungs. None of the 15 male and 15 female acatalasemic mice that served as controls developed tumours of any type within 20 months (Reddy et al., 1976). [Attention is drawn to the unusual absence of tumours in the control mice.]

Rat: A group of male Fischer 344 rats, weighing 80-100 g, were administered nafenopin in the diet at a concentration of 0.1% (w/w) for up to 25 months. Of the treated rats, 12/15 developed tumours: 11 hepatocellular carcinomas, 1 pancreatic acinar-cell carcinoma and 2 pancreatic acinar-cell adenomas. None of the 10 control rats developed liver or pancreatic tumours; however, 6/10 controls and 10/15 nafenopin-treated rats developed Leydig-cell tumours of the testis. The hepatocellular carcinomas, as well as the acinar-cell carcinoma of the pancreas, that developed in nafenopin-treated rats were successfully transplanted (Reddy & Rao, 1977 a,b).

3.2 Other relevant biological data

(a) Experimental systems

No data on the toxicity, prenatal toxicity or absorption, distribution, excretion or metabolism of nafenopin were available.

Effects on intermediary metabolism

In rats and beagle dogs, oral administration of 1 or 2 mg/kg bw nafenopin daily for 7 days caused a significant reduction in serum cholesterol and triglyceride levels (Hess & Bencze, 1968). Reduction in serum triglycerides was also observed in mice fed diets containing 0.125% nafenopin for 8 weeks (Reddy et al., 1974).

Feeding of 0.01-0.25% (w/w) nafenopin produced a marked increase in liver weight in both male and female rats and mice (Best & Duncan, 1970; Beckett et al., 1972; Reddy et al., 1973, 1974; Leighton et al., 1975). In mice, after 1, 6 and 32 weeks of treatment with 0.125 or 0.1% nafenopin in the diet, the total hepatic DNA and mitotic and ^{3}H-thymidine-labelling indices in liver increased significantly compared with controls (Moody et al., 1977). After a single oral or i.p. dose to rats of 200 mg/kg bw nafenopin, a marked stimulation of hepatic ornithine decarboxylase activity occurred; peak activity was found 19-24 hours after the oral dose and 10 hours after i.p. administration (Levine et al., 1977).

Duration of zoxazolamine-induced paralysis after pretreatment with nafenopin was used as an index of drug-metabolizing enzyme induction in the rat liver. Three days' pretreatment with 250 mg/kg bw given orally twice daily significantly reduced ($P<0.005$) the duration of zoxazolamine paralysis in female rats but caused a significant increase ($P<0.005$) in males. Pretreatment for 14 days caused a similar, pronounced decrease in paralysis duration in animals of both sexes (Tuchweber et al., 1976).

Nafenopin, like other potent hypolipidaemic drugs (Reddy & Krishnakantha, 1975), induced proliferation of peroxisomes in liver parenchymal cells of rats and mice (Reddy et al., 1974; Leighton et al., 1975) and increased several peroxisome-associated enzymes, such as catalase, short- and medium-chain carnitine acyl-transferase and fatty acyl-coenzyme A oxidase in the livers (Reddy et al., 1973, 1974; Moody & Reddy, 1974, 1978; Inestrosa et al., 1979).

A marked increase in the content of an 80,000 mol. wt polypeptide that is associated with peroxisome proliferation occurred in the livers of rats fed nafenopin (see monograph on clofibrate, p. 39) (Reddy & Kumar, 1977).

Mutagenicity and other, related short-term tests

Nafenopin was not mutagenic to *Salmonella typhimurium* strains TA98, TA100, TA1535, TA1537 or TA1538, with or without metabolic activation by rat liver microsomes (Warren et al., 1980).

Although nafenopin suppressed the incorporation of ^{3}H-thymidine into replicating DNA in primary cultures of concanavalin A-stimulated mouse splenic lymphocytes, both in the presence and absence of a rat liver microsomal preparation, the effect was reversible upon removal of the drug. This is in contrast to the action of several DNA-binding carcinogens. It was concluded that nafenopin did not cause DNA damage (Warren et al., 1980).

(b) Humans

Nafenopin decreases serum triglycerides (Dujovne et al., 1971; Russo & Mendlowitz, 1971; Beaumont et al., 1974).

Toxic effects

In a clinical trial of 17 patients, nafenopin caused marked increases in both serum glutamic-oxaloacetic transaminase and glutamic-pyruvic transaminase (SGOT and SGPT) in two patients; the effect was reversible (Dujovne et al., 1971).

Absorption, distribution, excretion and metabolism

It was reported in an abstract that healthy, adult male subjects who ingested 200 mg nafenopin (^{14}C-labelled in the carboxyl position) excreted approximately 50% of the dose in the urine as polar metabolites, which were not characterized. No ^{14}C-activity was detected in expired air (Bianchine et al., 1969).

Effects on intermediary metabolism

Although serum lipid and vitamin E levels are reduced, nafenopin has no effect on serum carotene levels (Weiss & Bianchine, 1969).

No data were available on the prenatal toxicity or mutagenicity of nafenopin in humans.

3.3 Case reports and epidemiological studies of carcinogenicity in humans

No data were available to the Working Group.

4. Summary of Data Reported and Evaluation

4.1 Experimental data

Nafenopin was tested in acatalasemic mice (a strain with an unstable catalase gene) and in male rats by oral administration: it produced hepatocellular carcinomas in both species. A low incidence of pancreatic tumours was also observed in rats.

It was not mutagenic in *Salmonella typhimurium*.

Attention is drawn to the absence of studies on the teratogenicity of this compound.

4.2 Human data

Nafenopin has been suggested for use as a hypolipidaemic agent.

No case reports or epidemiological studies were available to the Working Group.

4.3 Evaluation

There is *sufficient evidence*[1] for the carcinogenicity of nafenopin in experimental animals. For practical purposes, nafenopin should be regarded as if it presented a carcinogenic risk to humans.

---

[1] See preamble, p. 18.

5. References

Beaumont, V., Buxtorf, J.C., Jacotot, B. & Beaumont, J.-L. (1974) Comparative study of several hypolipidemic agents related to clofibrate. *Atherosclerosis, 20*, 141-153

Beckett, R.B., Weiss, R., Stitzel, R.E. & Cenedella, R.J. (1972) Studies on the hepatomegaly caused by the hypolipidemic drugs nafenopin and clofibrate. *Toxicol. appl. Pharmacol., 23*, 42-53

Best, M.M. & Duncan, C.H. (1970) Lipid effects of a phenolic ether (Su-13437) in the rat: comparison with CPIB. *Atherosclerosis, 12*, 185-192

Bianchine, J.R., Weiss, O., Hersey, R.M. & Peaston, M.J.T. (1969) Metabolism of 2-methyl-2-[*p*-(1,2,3,4-tetrahydro-1-naphthyl)-phenoxy]-propionic acid (SU-13437) in man (Abstract). *Clin. Res., 17*, 378

Dujovne, C.A., Weiss, P. & Bianchine, J.R. (1971) Comparative clinical therapeutic trial with two hypolipidemic drugs: clofibrate and nafenopin. *Clin. Pharmacol. Ther., 12*, 117-125

Hess, R. & Bencze, W.L. (1968) Hypolipidaemic properties of a new tetralin derivative (CIBA 13,437-Su). *Experientia, 24*, 418-419

Inestrosa, N.C., Bronfman, M. & Leighton, F. (1979) Detection of peroxisomal fatty acyl-coenzyme A oxidase activity. *Biochem. J., 182*, 779-788

Leighton, F., Coloma, L. & Koenig, C. (1975) Structure, composition, physical properties, and turnover of proliferated peroxisomes. A study of the trophic effects of Su-13437 on rat liver. *J. Cell Biol., 67*, 281-309

Levine, W.G., Ord, M.G. & Stocken, L.A. (1977) Some biochemical changes associated with nafenopin-induced liver growth in the rat. *Biochem. Pharmacol., 26*, 939-942

Moody, D.E. & Reddy, J.K. (1974) Increase in hepatic carnitine acetyltransferase activity associated with peroxisomal (microbody) proliferation induced by the hypolipidemic drugs clofibrate, nafenopin, and methyl clofenapate. *Res. Commun. Chem. Pathol. Pharmacol., 9*, 501-510

Moody, D.E. & Reddy, J.K. (1978) The hepatic effects of hypolipidemic drugs (clofibrate, nafenopin, fibric acid, and Wy-14,643) on hepatic peroxisomes and peroxisome-associated enzymes. *Am. J. Pathol., 90*, 435-445

Moody, D.E., Rao, M.S. & Reddy, J.K. (1977) Mitogenic effect in mouse liver induced by a hypolipidemic drug, nafenopin. *Virchows Arch. B Cell Pathol., 23*, 291-296

Reddy, J.K. & Krishnakantha, T.P. (1975) Hepatic peroxisome proliferation: induction by two novel compounds structurally unrelated to clofibrate. *Science, 190*, 787-789

Reddy, J.K. & Kumar, N.S. (1977) The peroxisome proliferation-association polypeptide in rat liver. *Biochem. biophys. Res. Commun., 77*, 824-829

Reddy, J.K. & Rao, M.S. (1977a) Malignant tumors in rats fed nafenopin, a hepatic peroxisome proliferator. *J. natl Cancer Inst., 59*, 1645-1650

Reddy, J.K. & Rao, M.S. (1977b) Transplantable pancreatic carcinoma of the rat. *Science, 198*, 78-80

Reddy, J., Svoboda, D. & Azarnoff, D. (1973) Microbody proliferation in liver induced by nafenopin, a new hypolipidemic drug: comparison with CPIB. *Biochem. biophys. Res. Commun., 52*, 537-543

Reddy, J.K., Azarnoff, D.L., Svoboda, D.J. & Prasad, J.D. (1974) Nafenopin-induced hepatic microbody (peroxisome) proliferation and catalase synthesis in rats and mice. Absence of sex difference in response. *J. Cell Biol., 61*, 344-358

Reddy, J.K., Rao, M.S. & Moody, D.E. (1976) Hepatocellular carcinomas in acatalasemic mice treated with nafenopin, a hypolipidemic peroxisome proliferator. *Cancer Res., 36*, 1211-1217

Russo, C. & Mendlowitz, M. (1971) Antilipidemic effect of nafenoic acid. *Clin. Pharmacol. Ther., 12*, 676-677

Tuchweber, B., Kourounakis, P. & Latour, J.G. (1976) Drug metabolism and morphologic changes in the liver of nafenopin-treated rats. *Arch. intern. Pharmacodyn., 222*, 309-321

Wade, A., ed. (1977) *Martindale, The Extra Pharmacopoeia*, 27th ed., London, The Pharmaceutical Press, p. 368

Warren, J.R., Simmon, V.F. & Reddy, J.K. (1980) Properties of hypolipidemic peroxisome proliferators in the lymphocyte [^{3}H] thymidine and *Salmonella* mutagenesis assays. *Cancer Res., 40*, 36-41

Weiss, P. & Bianchine, J.R. (1969) Effect on serum tocopherol levels of drug-induced decrease in serum lipids. *Am. J. med. Sci., 258*, 275-281 [*Chem. Abstr., 71*, 100294h]

PHENACETIN

This substance was considered by a previous working group, in October 1976 (IARC, 1977). Since that time, new data have become available, and these have been incorporated into the monograph and taken into account in the present evaluation.

1. Chemical and Physical Data

1.1 Synonyms and trade names

Chem. Abstr. Services Reg. No.: 62-44-2

Chem. Abstr. Name: Acetamide, *N*-(4-ethoxyphenyl)-

IUPAC Systematic Name: Acetyl-phenetidine

Synonyms: 1-Acetamido-4-ethoxybenzene; *para*-acetophenetide; *para*-acetophenetidide; aceto-*para*-phenetidide; acetophenetidin; acetophenetidine; *para*-acetophenetidine; aceto-4-phenetidine; acetophenetin; aceto-*para*-phenalide; acetphenetidin; *para*-acetphenetidin; acet-*para*-phenetidin; acetylphenetidin; *N*-acetyl-*para*-phenetidine; *para*-ethoxy-acetanilid; 4-ethoxyacetanilide; 4'-ethoxyacetanilide; *para*-ethoxyacetanilide; *N-para*-ethoxyphenylacetamide; paracetophenetidin; *para*-phenacetin; phenacetine; phenacitin; phenazetin

Trade names: Achrocidin; Anapac; APC; ASA Compound; Bromo Seltzer; Buff-A-comp; Citra-Fort; Clistanol; Codempiral; Commotional; Contradol; Contradouleur; Coricidin; Coriforte; Coryban-D; Daprisal; Darvon Compound; Dasikon; Dasin; Dasin CH; Dolostop; Dolviran; Edrisal; Empiral; Empirin Compound; Emprazil; Emprazil-C; Epragen; Fenacetina; Fenedina; Fenidina; Fenina; Fiorinal; Fortacyl; Gelonida; Gewodin; Helvagit; Hjorton's powder; Hocophen; Kafa; Kalmin; Malex; Melabon; Melaforte; Norgesic; Pamprin; Paramette; Paratodol; Percobarb; Percodan; Pertonal; Phenacet; Phenacetinum; Phenacon; Phenalgin; Phenaphen; Phenaphen Plus; Phenazetina; Phenedina; Phenidin; Phenin; Phenodyne; Pyrroxate; Quadronal; Reformin; Robaxisal-PH; Salgydal; Sanalgine; Saridon; Seranex; Sinedal; Sinubid; Sinutab; Sinutab II; Soma; Stellacyl; Super Anahist; Supralgin; Synalogos; Synalgos-DC; Tacol; Terracydin; Tetracydin; Thephorin A-C; Treupel; Veganine; Viden; Wigraine; Xaril; Zactirin Compound -100

1.2 Structural and molecular formulae and molecular weight

$C_{10}H_{13}NO_2$ Mol. wt: 179.2

1.3 Chemical and physical properties of the pure substance

From Wade (1977) or Windholz (1976), unless otherwise specified

(a) *Description:* White, glistening, crystalline scales or fine, white, crystalline powder with a slightly bitter taste
(b) *Melting-point:* 134-137°C
(c) *Spectroscopy data:* λ_{max} 250 nm (in ethanol) (US Pharmacopeial Convention, Inc., 1970); 285 nm (in chloroform and isooctane) (National Formulary Board, 1970)
(d) *Solubility:* Slightly soluble in water (1 in 1,300); soluble in boiling-water (1 in 82), ethanol (1 in 15), chloroform (1 in 14) and diethyl ether (1 in 90); slightly soluble in glycerol
(e) *Stability:* Unstable to oxidizing agents, iodine and nitrating agents

1.4 Technical products and impurities

Various national and international pharmacopoeias give specifications for the purity of phenacetin in pharmaceutical products. For example, phenacetin is available in the US as a USP grade containing 98-101% active ingredient on a dried basis and a maximum of 0.03% *para*-chloroacetanilide (US Pharmacopeial Convention, Inc., 1970). In the *European Pharmacopoeia* (Council of Europe, 1969) specifications, sulphated ash is limited to 0.1%.

It is available in 300 mg doses as tablets containing 94-106% of the stated amount of phenacetin (US Pharmacopeial Convention Inc., 1970) and is also available in the US as tablets containing 150 mg phenacetin in combination with 230 mg aspirin and 15 or 30 mg caffeine, or with 230 mg aspirin, 30 mg caffeine, and 8, 15, 30 or 60 mg codeine phosphate and containing 90-110% of the stated amount of phenacetin (National Formulary Board, 1970). Phenacetin was omitted from the 19th edition of the *US Pharmacopeia* but was reinstated in the 20th edition.

In the UK, phenacetin was available as such in 250 and 300 mg doses as tablets or in combination with caffeine and also in a mixture containing 300 mg phenacetin and 50 mg caffeine citrate per 10 ml solution (Wade, 1977).

In Japan, phenacetin is available in 300 and 500 mg doses as a powder.

2. Production, Use, Occurrence and Analysis

2.1 Production and use

(a) Production

The original method used in 1887 to prepare phenacetin involved coupling of phenetole with a diazonium salt and reduction and acetylation to give phenacetin. The probable method for its commercial production is condensation of the sodium salt of *para*-nitrophenol with ethyl bromide to produce *para*-nitrophenetole, which, on reduction, is converted to *para*-phenetidine; this is acetylated to phenacetin (Swinyard, 1975).

Phenacetin has been produced commercially in the US for over 50 years. In 1978, two US companies produced an undisclosed amount (see preamble, p. 21). US imports of phenacetin through principal US customs districts were 67,000 mg in 1972. These increased to 282,000 kg in 1978 (US International Trade Commission, 1979).

Phenacetin is believed to be produced by one company in France, with an annual output of 100,000-500,000 kg, and by 3 producers in the Federal Republic of Germany, which produce over 500 thousand kg yearly. Most other countries in western Europe import 10,000-50,000 kg from these producers.

Phenacetin was first produced in Japan in 1935. In 1978, one company manufactured 290,000 kg, and 63,000 kg were imported; production and imports have been stable at about these levels in recent years.

(b) Use

Phenacetin is used as an analgesic and antipyretic drug. It is used alone, or in combination with aspirin and caffeine, for mild to moderate pain associated with the musculoskeletal system. The usual dose is 300 mg taken 4-6 times per day to a total of no more than 2.4 g per day (Goodman & Gilman, 1975; Swinyard, 1975). Since April 1964, the US Food & Drug Administration (1978) has required that all preparations containing phenacetin must bear a warning about possible kidney damage.

Phenacetin is used in human medicine in Japan and Europe as an analgesic and antipyretic, for treatment of such conditions as headache, neuritis, rheumatic pain and toothache. It is given either alone or in combination with aspirin, caffeine or codeine in tablets (Wade, 1977).

Phenacetin was withdrawn from use in Canada in 1978 (WHO, 1978) and will be banned in the UK in March 1980 (Anon., 1980) because of the reported association between long-term use of phenacetin and nephropathy. Several other countries are in the process of reviewing the status of phenacetin (WHO, 1979).

In Japan, the Ministry of Health and Welfare has issued a warning that prolonged use of large dosages of phenacetin may cause cancer (Anon., 1977; Iyakuhin Yoran, 1979).

Phenacetin is used in veterinary medicine as an analgesic and antipyretic agent (Windholz, 1976).

2.2 Occurrence

Phenacetin is not known to occur in nature.

2.3 Analysis

Typical methods for the analysis of phenacetin in various matrices are summarized in Table 1. Abbreviations used are: S, spectrometry; UV, ultra-violet spectrometry; GC/FID gas chromatography with flame-ionization detection.

Table 1. Analytical methods for phenacetin

Sample matrix	Sample preparation	Assay procedure	Sensitivity or limit of detection	Reference
Plasma	Mix with para-bromoacetanilide as internal standard; extract with diethyl ether; evaporate; dissolve in ethyl acetate; evaporate in rotary vacuum centrifuge; dissolve in trimethylanilinium hydroxide in methanol	GC/FID	0.1 mg/l	Evans & Harbison, 1977
Plasma and urine	Dilute with aqueous sodium hydroxide; add benzene and isoamyl alcohol; centrifuge; add hydrochloric acid; evaporate; dissolve in 1-propanol	UV	not given	Duggin & Mudge, 1976
Serum and urine	Extract with diethyl ether; wash with sodium hydroxide; filter; evaporate; add hydrochloric acid, n-hexane, tert-butanol and cobalt (III) oxide; reflux; extract solvent layer with sodium hydroxide	UV	not given	Wallace et al., 1973
Tissue	Homogenize; add sodium hydroxide; carry out the steps described above for serum and urine	UV	not given	Wallace et al., 1973
	Extract with isoamyl alcohol and benzene; evaporate; add hydrochloric acid; heat; diazotize with sodium nitrite; add α-naphthol in ethanol and sodium hydroxide; extract with isoamyl alcohol and benzene; add trichloroacetic acid and methylene chloride	S	not given	Maddock et al., 1977

3. Biological Data Relevant to the Evaluation of Carcinogenic Risk to Humans

3.1 Carcinogenicity studies in animals[1]

(a) Oral administration

Rat: A group of 30 BD I and BD III rats, 100 days of age (sex unspecified), received 40-50 mg/animal phenacetin daily in the diet (average total dose, 22 g). One rat died after a total dose of 10 g and was found to have an osteochondroma. The mean age at death was 770 days, compared with 750 days in an unspecified number of controls. No tumours related to treatment were observed (Schmähl & Reiter, 1954).

Female Sprague-Dawley rats were given 0 or 0.535% phenacetin in pelleted diet for 86 or 110 weeks. In the 86-week study, epithelial hyperplasia of renal papillae was found in 2/24 controls and in 21/38 treated animals (Johansson & Angervall, 1976a). In the 110-week study, the following changes were observed: urothelial hyperplasia of renal papillae in 26, dilatation of vasa recta in 28, and epithelial hyperplasia in 1. In addition, carcinomas of the mammary gland (5/30) and ear duct (4/30; P>0.05) were found in the treated group. In the control group, uroepithelial hyperplasia was found in 5 animals, dilatation of vasa recta in 8 and a mammary carcinoma in 1 animal (Johansson & Angervall, 1976b).

---

[1] Preliminary experiments have been reported in letters to the Editor of *Science* (Johansson & Angervall, 1979; Macklin et al., 1979). They are not quoted here, since insufficient details were given.

Subsequent to the meeting of the Working Group, the Secretariat was made aware of a study by Macklin & Szot (1980) in which 6 groups of 40 male and 40 female 4-week-old C57BL/6 mice were fed powder diets containing aspirin, phenacetin and caffeine, singly or in combination, for 75-80 weeks. Group 1 received 696 mg/kg bw/day aspirin-phenacetin-caffeine; Group 2, 693 mg/kg bw/day aspirin-phenacetin; Group 3, 321 mg/kg bw/day phenacetin-caffeine; Group 4, 754 mg/kg bw/day phenacetin; Group 5, 268 mg/kg bw/day phenacetin; and Group 6 received none of the compounds and served as controls. Intercurrent mortality in males and females combined was 18, 2, 10, 9, 5 and 17 in the 6 groups, respectively. Two males and 2 females from each group were killed after 6, 18, 33, 45 and 58 weeks of treatment, and all surviving animals were killed at the end of their treatment. Tissues from liver, kidney, spleen, heart, brain and urinary bladder and any abnormal lesions were removed at autopsy; only sections of bladder and kidney were examined histologically. One male mouse that received aspirin plus phenacetin developed a renal-cell carcinoma and one female on the same diet developed a hepatocellular carcinoma. No such tumours occurred in controls. [The limited duration of the experiment and the limited extent of histological examination were noted.]

The Working Group was also aware of a study in progress to assess the carcinogenicity of phenacetin in mice by oral administration (IARC, 1979).

Two groups of 50 male and 50 female 9-week-old Sprague-Dawley rats were fed, respectively, with 1.25% or 2.5% phenacetin (Japan Pharmacopeia grade) in pelleted diet for 18 months and fed thereafter with basal diet for 6 months; 65 male and 65 female control animals were fed basal diet. Among animals surviving for 24 months or dying within 24 months with tumour(s), neoplasms were detected in 26/27 males and 21/27 females fed 2.5%, in 20/22 males and 19/25 females fed 1.25% and in 1/19 males and 6/25 females of the control group. Tumours (benign and malignant) of the nasal cavity were found in 16/27 males and 7/27 females fed 2.5% and in 16/22 males and 6/25 females fed 1.25%. Malignant tumours of the urinary tract were detected in 13/27 males and 4/27 females fed the high dose and in 1/22 males and 0/25 females fed the low dose; 2 papillomas were found in females given the high dose. No nasal cavity or urinary-tract tumours were seen in controls (Isaka et al., 1979).

(b) Oral administration in a mixture

Mouse: A mixture of aspirin, phenacetin and caffeine (50:46:4) was incorporated into powdered diet at concentrations of 0, 0.7, or 1.4% and given to groups of 50 male and 50 female B6C3F1 mice (age not specified) for up to 78 weeks; observation continued for an additional 16 weeeks. Tumours were found in the lung, haematopoietic system and liver, with no significant difference between the treated and nontreated groups (National Cancer Institute, 1978).

Rat: A mixture of aspirin, phenacetin and caffeine (50:46:4) was incorporated into powdered diet at concentrations of 0, 0.7 or 1.4% and given to groups of 50 male and 50 female Fischer 344 rats (age not specified) for up to 78 weeks; observation continued for an additional 34-35 weeks. In male rats, adenomas and carcinomas of the pituitary gland were found in 18/47 (38%) fed 0.7% and in 12/44 (27%) fed 1.4%, *versus* 8/47 (17%) in the control group. In female rats, a transitional-cell carcinoma of the urinary bladder and a tubular-cell adenocarcinoma of the kidney were found in the low-dose group; and a transitional-cell carcinoma of the bladder and a transitional-cell papilloma of the kidney were observed in the high-dose group. In male rats fed the low dose, 1 tubular-cell adenocarcinoma of the kidney was observed. Three females treated with the high dose showed renal medullary necrosis, in 2 cases associated with hyperplasia of transitional-cell epithelium of the pelvis. Urinary bladder epithelial hyperplasia was seen in 1 male control and in 1 male treated with the high dose (National Cancer Institute, 1978).

(c) Other experimental systems

Administration in conjunction with a known carcinogen: Twenty male Wistar *rats* were given 2.5% phenacetin in stock diet for 30 weeks, followed by 6 weeks on control diet, at which point the experiment was terminated. Two groups of 30 and 28 male Wistar rats were given the phenacetin diet after they had received *N*-nitrosobutyl-*N*-(4-hydroxybutyl)amine (BBN) as a 0.05% or 0.01% solution in drinking-water for 4 weeks. Two further groups of 27 and 23 males were given only 0.05% or 0.01% BBN in drinking-water. Simple and papillary or nodular hyperplasia of the urinary bladder epithelium were found, respectively, in 11/20 (55%) and 4/20 (20%) rats given phenacetin only. Papillomas of the urinary bladder were observed in 26/30 rats fed 0.05% BBN plus phenacetin *versus* 8/27 in rats fed 0.05% BBN alone. Carcinomas of the urinary bladder occurred in 14/30 animals fed 0.05% BBN plus phenacetin *versus* 4/27 in rats fed 0.05% BBN alone. Both papillomas and carcinomas also developed in 7/28 and 1/28 rats fed 0.01% BBN plus phenacetin, while only papillomas developed in 3/23 fed 0.01% BBN alone (Nakanishi *et al.*, 1978). [Attention is drawn to the short duration of this experiment and the lack of untreated controls.]

(d) Carcinogenicity of metabolites

Rat: Groups of 20-24 male albino rats (strain unspecified) were fed synthetic *N*-hydroxyphenacetin, a metabolite of phenacetin, as a 0.05, 0.1 or 0.5% supplement in finely-ground diet. The animals were killed at between 30 and 73 weeks after the beginning of treatment. In the 3 groups, 9/20, 7/20 and 9/24 rats, respectively, died without tumours before the 45th, 45th and 38th week, when the first tumours were found at autopsy. Hepatocellular carcinomas were found in 8/11, 13/13 and 15/15 animals, respectively, that were alive when the first tumour was detected. Of rats fed 0.1%, 1/13 had a renal carcinoma with metastases to the liver, lung and bone marrow. No tumours were found in 15 control rats (Calder *et al.*, 1976).

3.2 Other relevant biological data

(a) Experimental systems

Toxic effects

The single oral LD_{50} of phenacetin in male Wistar rats is about 4 g/kg bw (Boyd & Hottenroth, 1968) and that in guinea-pigs 2.6 g/kg bw (Boyd & Carro-Ciampi, 1970).

Papillary necrosis of the kidney was produced in Wistar rats fed a mixture of aspirin (210 mg/kg bw/day), phenacetin (210 mg/kg bw/day) and caffeine (80 mg/kg bw/day), but not in rats receiving 500 mg/kg bw/day phenacetin alone (Saker & Kincaid-Smith, 1969). In homozygous Gunn rats genetically lacking glucuronyl transferase, a single oral dose of 6.4-12.54 mmol/kg bw phenacetin gave rise to renal papillary necrosis (Axelsen, 1976).

PHENACETIN

Phenacetin has only a weak nephrotoxic effect on its own, but readily induces renal papillary necrosis when given in mixtures with other analgesics (Molland, 1978). It potentiates the effect of caffeine on the central nervous system (Collins et al., 1977).

When an intragastric dose of 2 g/kg bw phenacetin was given in 5 divided doses per week to 25 male rats for up to 220 days, 80% of the rats were sterile at 176 days (Boyd, 1971).

N-Hydroxyphenacetin, a metabolite of phenacetin, was nephrotoxic in female Wistar rats following single i.v. injections of 1 mmol/kg bw of the synthetic compound (Calder et al., 1973).

Prenatal toxicity

When phenacetin-treated female rats were exposed to males, a decreased incidence of pregnancy was seen. Reduced fetal weight was found with oral doses of 600-1200 mg/kg bw per day phenacetin given from day 0 to day 20 of gestation. No increase in defect rate but some retardation in skeletal growth and an increase in supernumerary ribs occurred with doses of 150 mg/kg bw and over (Baethke & Muller, 1965).

Absorption, distribution, excretion and metabolism

The metabolism of phenacetin in rats has been compared with that of other structurally-related compounds (Smith & Griffiths, 1976a). Metabolic pathways for phenacetin involve de-ethylation, N-deacetylation and ring hydroxylation. The main route is oxidative de-ethylation, giving rise to N-acetyl-*para*-aminophenol, which is excreted in the urine as the sulphate or as the glucuronide (Dubach & Raaflaub, 1969). In rats, rabbits, guinea-pigs and ferrets given 125 mg/kg bw by oral intubation or mixed with food, 63, 57, 81 and 47% of the dose, respectively, were excreted as N-acetyl-*para*-aminophenol (free or conjugated). Metabolism by the second pathway, N-deacetylation, was greatest in rats (21% of the dose) and least in guinea-pigs and rabbits (7 and 4% of the dose) (Smith & Timbrell, 1974). The *para*-phenetidine resulting from N-deacetylation can be converted to 2-hydroxy-*para*-phenetidine, which in rats is excreted as the sulphate in increasing amounts with increasing doses of phenacetin (Dubach & Raaflaub, 1969).

Other metabolites that have been found in the urine of rats, guinea-pigs and rabbits are 2-hydroxyphenacetin and 3-[(5-acetamido-2-hydroxyphenyl)thio]alanine (Smith & Timbrell, 1974). Another thiomethyl metabolite, 3-methylthio-4-hydroxyacetanilide, representing 1-3% of the administered dose, has been identified in the urine of dogs (Klutch et al., 1978); the 2-hydroxyacetophenetidine glucuronide conjugate has been found in the urine of dogs and cats given phenacetin orally (Klutch et al., 1966). In rats and dogs given 200 mg/kg bw phenacetin, 1% of the total dose was excreted as 4-acetaminophenoxyacetic acid in the urine of rats, and 0.13% in dogs (Dittmann & Renner, 1977). Intestinal microflora in rats have been shown to deconjugate the metabolite N-acetyl-para-aminophenyl glucuronide, excreted partly in bile, to the N-acetyl-para-amino-phenol (Smith & Griffiths, 1976b).

It has been reported that a reactive metabolite of phenacetin is generated by cytochrome P-450 in hamster liver microsomes (Hinson et al., 1977). Evidence that phenacetin is N-hydroxylated by a cytochrome P-450 monooxygenase-catalysed reaction has been obtained in vitro with hamster and rabbit liver microsomes (Hinson & Mitchell, 1976; Fischbach et al., 1977). No N-hydroxyphenacetin was found when phenacetin metabolism was investigated in isolated rat hepatocytes (McLean, 1978). Following oral administration of 100 mg/kg bw phenacetin to dogs, 0.3-1.3% N-hydroxyphenacetin was found in the urine (Klutch & Bordun, 1968). N-Hydroxyphenacetin reacts with methionine under acid conditions or after esterification in vitro to give 4-hydroxy-3-methylthioacetanilide (Calder et al., 1974), which has also been found as a urinary metabolite of phenacetin in dogs (Focella et al., 1972; Klutch et al., 1978).

Using rat liver preparations, Mulder et al. (1977) demonstrated the formation of N-O-glucuronide and N-O-sulphate conjugates of N-hydroxyphenacetin. Both compounds led to products bound covalently to protein at pH 7.4, but the glucuronide conjugate did so at a slower rate than the sulphate.

In rats treated with 3-methylcholanthrene or benzo[a]pyrene or exposed to cigarette smoke, there was an increased rate of O-de-ethylation of phenacetin to N-acetyl-para-aminophenol in lung and intestine (Welch et al., 1972; Kuntzman et al., 1977). The stimulatory effects of other enzyme inducers and of dietary constituents on intestinal metabolism of phenacetin have been studied in rats (Pantuck et al., 1975, 1976).

Phenacetin can be N-nitrosated in vitro to form an unstable N-nitroso compound, N-nitroso-2-nitro-4-ethoxyacetanilide (Eisenbrand & Preussmann, 1975).

Mutagenicity and other, related short-term tests

Phenacetin was not mutagenic in several bacterial systems in the presence or absence of rat or mouse liver microsome preparations; the systems included a repair test in *Bacillus subtilis* (Tanooka, 1977) and reverse mutations in *Salmonella typhimurium* TA1535, TA1537, TA98 and TA100 (Shudo et al., 1978; King et al., 1979), *Escherichia coli* K 12/343/113 (King et al., 1979), and *B. subtilis* TKJ 5211 (Tanooka, 1977). Positive bacterial mutagenicity results have, however, been obtained by Bartsch et al. (1980) and by Matsushima et al. (1980) in *S. typhimurium* TA100 in the presence of hamster, but not rat, liver post-mitochondrial supernatant from Aroclor-treated animals.

Phenacetin was negative in an intrasanguineous host-mediated assay with *E. coli* K 12 in NMRI mice given 2 mmol/kg intraperitoneally. It induced neither an increased frequency of sex-linked recessive lethals in *Drosophila melanogaster* nor an enhanced number of micronucleated erythrocytes in the bone marrow of NMRI mice given 2x 5 mmol/kg bw intraperitoneally (King *et al.*, 1979).

Phenacetin produced a borderline positive result in an *in vitro* chromosome aberration test in Chinese hamster fibroblasts; gaps were observed in 8.8% of the metaphases of treated cells as compared with 1% in controls (Ishidate & Odashima, 1977). However, when combined with a rat liver metabolic activation system, the compound induced breaks, rings and translocations in up to 51% of the metaphases (Matsuoka *et al.*, 1979).

N-Hydroxyphenacetin, a metabolite of phenacetin, was mutagenic for *S. typhimurium* TA100 when activated by rat liver S-9 (Shudo *et al.*, 1978).

(b) Humans

Phenacetin is a mild analgesic and antipyretic (Goodman & Gilman, 1975).

Toxic effects

Prescott (1975) has reviewed the toxic effects of phenacetin in humans. Although phenacetin has been linked with nephrotoxicity in heavy users of analgesic mixtures containing it, there is no conclusive evidence that phenacetin itself is the causal agent (Prescott, 1979); there is, however, no evidence from long-term users of phenacetin alone. Acute hepatic necrosis has been reported after overdosage with *N*-acetyl-*para*-aminophenol (paracetamol), a major metabolite of phenacetin (Davidson & Eastham, 1966; Thomson & Prescott, 1966; Proudfoot & Wright, 1970; Prescott *et al.*, 1971; Clark *et al.*, 1973); this condition has become an increasing problem in many countries (Prescott, 1979).

A group of 623 women known to ingest phenacetin-containing analgesics regularly were compared over a 4-year period with a group of 621 controls. High intake of such analgesics was associated with increased serum creatinine levels and low urine specific gravity, suggesting renal damage (Dubach *et al.*, 1975).

Methaemoglobinaemia and haemolytic anaemia have occurred in subjects ingesting phenacetin. Methaemoglobinaemia has been associated with the formation of increased amounts of 2-hydroxyphenetidine (Shahidi, 1967; Shahidi & Hemaidan, 1969; Goodman & Gilman, 1975); this phenomenon has been associated with an impaired ability to *O*-de-ethylate phenacetin, a metabolic reaction known to exhibit genetic polymorphism (Evans, 1977; Sloan *et al.*, 1978).

Prenatal toxicity

In a survey of ingestion of phenacetin or paracetamol among approximately 10,000 pregnant women, 19 of the 911 mothers who delivered infants with congenital defects had taken these drugs; this was a reduction from the 31 expected on the basis of control data. No data on doses were available (Crombie *et al.*, 1970).

Heinonen *et al.* (1977) identified 5546 women who used phenacetin during the first 4 lunar months of pregnancy; no increase in the congenital malformation rate was observed in their children.

Absorption, distribution, excretion and metabolism

After 2 subjects were given an oral dose of 8.3 mg/kg bw (500 mg) ^{14}C-phenacetin, the major proportion of the dose (74 and 70%, respectively) was excreted in the urine within 24 hours as *N*-acetyl-*para*-aminophenol, either conjugated (~ 67%) or free (~ 3%). Small amounts of 2-hydroxyphenacetin, 3[(5-acetamido-2-hydroxyphenyl)thio]alanine and unchanged phenacetin were also found (Smith & Timbrell, 1974). In three male volunteers given 2 g phenacetin orally, about 2% of the dose was found to be excreted as *S*-(1-acetamido-4-hydroxyphenyl)cysteine in the urine (Jagenburg & Toczko, 1964).

Other metabolites have been detected in the urine in more recent studies. 3-Methylthio-4-hydroxyacetanilide represented 0.13-0.72% of an administered dose of 1000-1800 mg phenacetin (Klutch *et al.*, 1978). 4-Acetaminophenoxyacetic acid represented 0.04% of 3 ingested doses of 500 mg phenacetin (Dittmann & Renner, 1977). Following a single oral dose of 420 mg phenacetin, no *N*-hydroxyphenacetin could be detected in urine; however, after a dose of 1.8 g/day for 4 days to a different subject, 0.8% *N*-hydroxyphenacetin was found in urine after 24 hours and 0.7% after 96 hours (Klutch & Bordun, 1968). Excretion of *N*-hydroxyphenacetin was also reported by Belman *et al.* (1968) after doses of 900 mg. [The formation of *N*-hydroxyphenacetin thus appears to be a dose-dependent phenomenon.]

Urinary excretion of 2-hydroxyphenetidin and *N*-acetyl-*para*-aminophenol, and of their conjugates, was decreased when phenacetin was ingested in combination with aspirin, caffeine and codeine (Gault *et al.*, 1972).

In cigarette smokers, there is a higher ratio of *N*-acetyl-*para*-aminophenol:phenacetin in the plasma than in corresponding controls (Pantuck *et al.*, 1974).

The effect of dietary constituents on the metabolism of phenacetin was studied in 9 normal volunteers fed a diet containing charcoal-broiled beef for 4 days prior to the administration of phenacetin (900 mg). Plasma levels of phenacetin were markedly lower than in subjects given their customary home diet or a control hospital diet, and the ratio of N-acetyl-*para*-aminophenol:phenacetin was higher, suggesting enhancement of phenacetin metabolism in the gastrointestinal tract and/or during its first pass through the liver (Conney et al., 1976).

No data on the mutagenicity of phenacetin in humans were available.

3.3 Case reports and epidemiological studies of carcinogenicity in humans

Analgesic nephropathy is the term given to chronic interstitial nephritis (often with renal papillary necrosis) occurring in people consuming large amounts of analgesics, usually defined as at least 1 g of an analgesic per day for more than 1 year or at least 1 kg altogether. Although in some cases such levels are used appropriately for chronic pain, use of such amounts of analgesics is often termed 'analgesic abuse'. In some cases, patients have reported taking only one drug; but, more commonly, mixtures of analgesics have been taken. While the nephrotoxic effects were originally attributed to phenacetin, formerly a component common to the abused analgesic mixtures, there is now debate over which one or more of the components is mainly responsible (see, for example, Nanra et al., 1978).

Renal pelvic carcinoma was first associated with renal papillary necrosis in 6 patients, 5 of whom were abusers of analgesics containing phenacetin (Hultengren et al., 1965). Many further cases of this association have been reported (Adam et al., 1970; Grob, 1971; Høybye & Nielsen, 1971; Johansson et al., 1974; Liu et al., 1972; Nordenfelt, 1972; Güller & Dubach, 1973; Storey et al., 1977). The association of analgesic abuse and renal pelvic cancer without renal papillary necrosis has also been described, although these cases appear to be less common (Johansson et al., 1974; Landmann-Kolbert et al., 1975; Rathert et al., 1975; Moshakis & Hooper, 1978). In a series of 62 patients with renal pelvic cancer who abused mixtures of phenacetin, phenazone and caffeine, it was estimated that individuals had consumed from 1.5 to 27 kg (average, 9.1 kg) of phenacetin starting, on average, 22 years before appearance of the tumour (Johansson et al., 1974).

Tumours of the ureter and bladder have also been reported in patients with analgesic nephropathy and a history of analgesic abuse (Angervall et al., 1969; Begley et al., 1970; Mannion & Susmano, 1971; Taylor, 1972; Johansson et al., 1974; Rathert et al., 1975; Johansson & Wahlqvist, 1977; Güller & Dubach, 1973; Mahony et al., 1977; Storey et al., 1977; Tosi & Morin, 1977). In one series of 46 patients, it was estimated that, on average, patients had consumed 7.1 kg phenacetin and use had begun 30 years before appearance of the tumour (Johansson & Wahlqvist, 1977).

Several studies have documented the prevalence of analgesic abuse, with or without renal papillary necrosis, in series of patients with urinary tract tumours. Of all (28) patients admitted with renal pelvic carcinoma to a Swedish hospital between 1960 and 1967, 13 (46%) had been analgesic abusers. The mean age of the analgesic abusers was 56 years, compared with 67 years in the other patients ($P<0.001$) (Bengtsson et al., 1968). In another hospital series, of all (15) patients admitted with renal pelvic tumours between 1960 and 1968 in Jönköping, Sweden, 10 and possibly 2 more had abused phenacetin-containing analgesics; renal papillary necrosis was noted in 10. Nine had worked in a small-arms factory where, for many years, analgesic abuse had been common. Among workers in this factory the incidence of renal pelvic tumours [56/100,000 per year on the basis of the 9 cases] was over 100 times that in Sweden as a whole [0.5/100,000 per year] or in the remaining inhabitants of the same hospital catchment area [0.6/100,000 per year]. The authors noted that no other clusters of such tumours had been reported from similar factories (Angervall et al., 1969). [Nonetheless, the possible effect of occupational exposures cannot be excluded.]

Juusela (1973) identified all patients with renal pelvic carcinoma admitted to a Finnish hospital. Three (18%) of the 17 patients with such tumours had abused phenacetin-containing analgesics (more than 4 doses daily for more than 10 years), and 2 more (12%) had taken lesser amounts. In another hospital series, from Australia (Mahony et al., 1977), 14 (54%) of 26 consecutively admitted patients with renal pelvic carcinoma and 1 of 5 patients with ureteral tumours had abused analgesics (more than 2 kg total consumption). Twelve of the patients with carcinomas of the renal pelvis had renal papillary necrosis, 4 had renal papillary sclerosis and 11 (42%) also had tumours elsewhere in the urothelium. The patient with a ureteral tumour also had renal papillary necrosis and a bladder tumour. The cancer patients with renal papillary necrosis were, on average, 7 years younger than those without. In a Swiss autopsy study (Leistenschneider & Ehmann, 1973), 8 (47%) of 17 patients with renal pelvic cancer had been heavy abusers of analgesics. It was noted that, in comparison with earlier periods in which analgesic abuse had been less common, the prevalence of these tumours at autopsy had increased, the proportion of females with renal pelvic cancer had increased, and the mean age at onset had decreased.

[In all of these studies, it was presumed that the proportion of analgesic abusers among cancer patients was higher than would have been expected from the prevalence of analgesic abuse in the relevant general population. In none, however, was a control series available for comparison.]

In some series of patients with renal pelvic cancer, the prevalence of analgesic abuse has been compared with that in patients with other tumours of the urothelium. In an Australian series, Taylor (1972) reported a history of analgesic abuse in 7 (54%) of 13 patients with renal pelvic carcinoma, but in only 2 (7%) of 30 with carcinoma of the renal body, in none of 2 with carcinoma of the ureter and in 2 (1%) of 144 with carcinoma of the bladder. In a German autopsy study (Bock & Hogrefe, 1972), a history of analgesic abuse was noted in 1 (3%) of 31 cases of carcinoma of the renal pelvis, in none of 5 cases of carcinoma of the ureter and in 2 (2%) of 106 cases of carcinoma of the bladder. In a similar Swiss study (Küng, 1976), 4 (27%) of 15 patients with renal pelvic carcinoma were analgesic abusers compared with 5 (2%) of 269 with carcinoma of the renal body and 11 (5%) of 218 with bladder cancer.

In a case-control study of renal cancer in England, involving control subjects in the same hospital without urinary-tract tumours, 15 (14.2%) of 106 patients with cancer of the renal body had used analgesic tablets daily for 6 months or more, compared with 2 (1.9%, P<0.05) of 106 matched controls. There was no significant difference, however, in analgesic use between patients with renal pelvic cancer (none out of 33 cases had used analgesics daily for 6 months or more) and their controls (3 users out of 33) (Armstrong et al., 1976). None of the patients or controls had analgesic nephropathy, but this condition is rare in Britain, and the lowest rates are found in the areas in which this study was done (Murray, 1978). [An excess of analgesic abusers among patients with carcinoma of the renal body was not apparent in 2 other studies (Taylor, 1972; Küng, 1976), and this tumour has not been reported in follow-up studies of analgesic abusers (see below).]

Cancer of the bladder was the primary focus of 2 other case-control studies. In a Swiss study of 69 patients with epithelial tumours of the urinary tract (Landmann-Kolbert et al., 1975), history of analgesic abuse was investigated both by history and by testing the urine for a phenacetin metabolite. Twelve (17.4%; 1 with renal pelvic cancer and 11 with bladder cancer) had abused phenacetin-containing drugs, compared with 5 (7.2%) of 69 patients with nonurological tumours. This difference was not statistically significant. Among 1084 patients with bladder cancer in The Netherlands (Fokkens, 1979), 18 (1.7%) reported 'more than incidental' intake of phenacetin-containing analgesic mixtures, whereas 16 (1.5%) of 1094 age- and sex-matched controls gave a similar history (relative risk, 1.1; not statistically significant). When the groups were divided into those taking 2 kg or more of phenacetin and those taking less, cancer patients were more likely to have abused analgesics than controls (relative risk, 4; P = 0.02). [The division of the groups at 2 kg was chosen to maximize the difference. Division at the more conventional level of 1 kg gives a relative risk of 1.7, which is not statistically significant.]

Two series of patients who abused analgesics have been followed up for development of urinary-tract tumours. Of a group of 242 patients admitted to a Swedish hospital with chronic nonobstructive pyelonephritis, 104 analgesic abusers and 88 nonabusers were followed up for 1-11 years (average, 5.3 years). Eight (8%) abusers (7 with renal papillary necrosis) but no nonabusers developed renal pelvic tumours (Bengtsson et al., 1968; Bengtsson & Angervall, 1970). Of 110 patients with analgesic nephropathy identified in 2 Australian hospitals (Taylor, 1972), 7 (6.4%) developed renal pelvic cancer. Similar tumours occurred in 4 (0.7%) of 597 patients with 'chronic inflammatory damage of the kidneys not associated with analgesic abuse', a 9-fold difference in relative frequency. [The patients with 'nonanalgesic' chronic renal disease were not matched in any way to the patients with analgesic nephropathy, and possibly confounding variables were not documented or controlled in the analyses. It is doubtful, however, whether these deficiencies could account for effects of the magnitude observed.]

[All, or nearly all, of these studies involved analgesic mixtures containing phenacetin. In assigning responsibility for any putative carcinogenic effect, however, phenacetin cannot be separated from the other drugs (variously, aspirin or phenazone, caffeine or codeine and occasionally additional drugs) with which it was invariably associated. It may also be noted that most of the studies that suggested a carcinogenic effect were conducted in Sweden and Australia; studies from some other countries have been less suggestive of such an effect. These differences have been taken by some to indicate bias in the Swedish and Australian studies. While this is possible, the apparent inconsistencies might also be explained by differences in the prevalence of analgesic abuse, the composition of the analgesics used, or some other factor (Gault & Wilson, 1978; Murray, 1978; Murray & Goldberg, 1978).]

4. Summary of Data Reported and Evaluation

4.1 Experimental data

Phenacetin alone was tested in three studies in rats by oral administration and in combination with aspirin and caffeine in one study in mice and in one in rats by oral administration. In one study in rats, phenacetin alone induced benign and malignant tumours of the urinary tract and of the nasal cavity in males. When given in combination with aspirin and caffeine to rats or mice, no significant association was found between the administration of the mixture and the incidence of tumours. Phenacetin alone enhanced the urinary bladder carcinogenesis of N-nitrosobutyl-N-(4-hydroxybutyl)amine in rats.

Phenacetin is mutagenic to *Salmonella typhimurium* in the presence of a hamster liver microsome preparation, and it produces chromosome aberrations in Chinese hamster fibroblasts *in vitro*. No mutagenic effects were detected in *Drosophila melanogaster* or in mice *in vivo*, or in bacterial test systems when rat or mouse liver microsome preparations were used.

No teratogenic effects were found in rats, although embryotoxicity was observed.

N-Hydroxyphenacetin, a minor metabolite of phenacetin in humans, was tested by oral administration in male rats: it induced hepatocellular carcinomas.

N-Hydroxyphenacetin is mutagenic to *Salmonella typhimurium* in the presence of a rat liver microsome preparation.

4.2 Human data

Phenacetin is used extensively as a mild analgesic. Its use in certain countries has been restricted.

There are many case reports of renal pelvic cancer associated with abuse of analgesic mixtures containing phenacetin. In addition, an increased incidence of renal pelvic cancer has been reported in a population with a high prevalence of analgesic abuse; analgesic abuse has been reported to be more common in patients with renal pelvic cancer than in those with other urinary-tract neoplasms; and in one small follow-up study, renal pelvic cancer developed nine times more frequently in patients with analgesic nephropathy than in those with other chronic renal disease. One small case-control study showed no evidence of the association, although the prevalence of prior analgesic abuse was very low. Cases of other urinary-tract tumours have also been reported in association with analgesic abuse, but analytical studies have been inconclusive.

Two studies of pregnant women exposed to phenacetin alone or in combination with other drugs failed to find evidence of an increased rate of malformations in the offspring.

4.3 Evaluation

There is *limited evidence*[1] that phenacetin and *N*-hydroxyphenacetin, a metabolite, are carcinogenic in experimental animals.

There is *limited evidence*[1] that abuse of analgesic mixtures containing phenacetin causes cancer of the renal pelvis in humans. It is not possible to specify what component(s) of the analgesic mixtures may be responsible for this effect. There is insufficient evidence to link analgesic abuse with other tumours of the human urinary tract.

---

[1] See preamble, p. 18.

5. References

Adam, W.R., Dawborn, J.K., Price, C.G., Riddell, J. & Story, H. (1970) Anaplastic transitional-cell carcinoma of the renal pelvis in association with analgesic abuse. *Med. J. Aust., 1,* 1108-1109

Angervall, L., Bengtsson, U., Zetturlund, C.G. & Zsigmond, M. (1969) Renal pelvic carcinoma in a Swedish district with abuse of a phenacetin-containing drug. *Br. J. Urol., 41,* 401-405

Anon. (1977) *International Drug Regulatory Monitor, No. 51,* Washington DC, Monitor Publications, pp. 8-9

Anon. (1980) UK ban on phenacetin. *Pharm. Int., 1,* 270

Armstrong, B., Garrod, A. & Doll. R. (1976) A retrospective study of renal cancer with special reference to coffee and animal protein consumption. *Br. J. Cancer, 33,* 127-136

Axelsen, R.A. (1976) Analgesic-induced renal papillary necrosis in the Gunn rat: the comparative nephrotoxicity of aspirin and phenacetin. *J. Pathol., 120,* 145-150

Baethke, R. & Müller, B. (1965) Embryotoxic activity of phenacetin during chronic studies on rats (Ger.). *Klin. Wochenschr., 43,* 364-368

Bartsch, H., Malaveille, C., Camus, A.-M., Martel-Planche, G., Brun, G., Hautefeuille, A., Sabadie, N., Barbin, A., Kuroki, T., Drevon, C., Piccoli, C. & Montesano, R. (1980) Validation and comparative studies on 180 chemicals with *S. typhimurium* strains and V79 Chinese hamster cells in the presence of various metabolizing systems. *Mutat. Res., 76,* 1-50

Begley, M., Chadwick, J.M. & Jepson, R.P. (1970) A possible case of analgesic abuse associated with transitional-cell carcinoma of the bladder. *Med. J. Aust., 2,* 1133-1134

Belman, S., Troll, W., Teebor, G. & Mukai, F. (1968) The carcinogenic and mutagenic properties of *N*-hydroxy-aminonephthalenes. *Cancer Res., 28,* 535-542

Bengtsson, U. & Angervall, L. (1970) Analgesic abuse and tumours of renal pelvis. *Lancet, i,* 305

Bengtsson, U., Angervall, L., Ekman, H. & Lehmann, L. (1968) Transitional cell tumors of the renal pelvis in analgesic abusers. *Scand. J. Urol. Nephrol., 2,* 145-150

Bock, K.D. & Hogrefe, J. (1972) Analgesic abuse and malignant tumours of the efferent urinary tract. A retrospective study (Ger.). *Münch. med. Wschr., 114,* 645-652

Boyd, E.M. (1971) Sterility from phenacetin. *J. clin. Pharmacol., 11,* 96-102

Boyd, E.M. & Carro-Ciampi, G. (1970) The oral 100-day LD_{50} index of phenacetin in guinea pigs. *Toxicol. appl. Pharmacol., 16,* 232-238

Boyd, E.M. & Hottenroth, S.M.H. (1968) The toxicity of phenacetin at the range of the oral $LD_{50(100\ days)}$ in albino rats. *Toxicol. appl. Pharmacol., 12,* 80-93

Calder, I.C., Creek, M.J., Williams, P.J., Funder, C.C., Green, C.R., Ham, K.N. & Tange, J.D. (1973) N-Hydroxylation of p-acetophenetidide as a factor in nephrotoxicity. *J. med. Chem., 16,* 499-502

Calder, I.C., Creek, M.J. & Williams, P.J. (1974) N-Hydroxyphenacetin as a precursor of 3-substituted 4-hydroxyacetanilide metabolites of phenacetin. *Chem. - biol. Interactions, 8,* 87-90

Calder, I.C., Goss, D.E., Williams, P.J., Funder, C.C., Green, C.R., Ham, K.N. & Tange, J.D. (1976) Neoplasia in the rat induced by N-hydroxyphenacetin, a metabolite of phenacetin. *Pathology, 8,* 1-6

Clark, R., Thompson, R.P.H., Borirakchanyavat, V., Widdop, B., Davidson, A.R., Goulding, R. & Williams, R. (1973) Hepatic damage and death from overdose of paracetamol. *Lancet, i,* 66-70

Collins, C., Richards, P.T. & Starmer, G.A. (1977) Caffeine-phenacetin interaction in the rat: effects on absorption, metabolism and locomotor activity. *J. Pharm. Pharmacol., 29,* 217-221

Conney, A.H., Pantuck, E.J., Hsiao, K.-C., Garland, W.A., Anderson, K.E., Alvares, A.P. & Kappas, A. (1976) Enhanced phenacetin metabolism in human subjects fed charcoal-broiled beef. *Clin. Pharmacol. Ther., 20,* 633-642

Council of Europe (1969) *European Pharmacopoeia,* Vol. 1, Sainte-Ruffine, France, Maisonneuve, pp. 344-346

Crombie, D.L., Pinsent, R.J.F.H., Slater, B.C., Fleming, D. & Cross, K.W. (1970) Teratogenic drugs - R.C.G.P. survey. *Br. med. J., iv,* 178-179

Davidson, D.G.D. & Eastham, W.N. (1966) Acute liver necrosis following overdose of paracetamol. *Br. med. J., ii*, 497-499

Dittmann, B. & Renner, G. (1977) 4-Acetaminophenoxyacetic acid, a new urinary metabolite of phenacetin. *Naunyn-Schmiedeberg's Arch. Pharmacol., 296*, 87-89

Dubach, U.C. & Raaflaub, J. (1969) New aspect of the question of the nephrotoxicity of phenacetin (Ger.). *Experientia, 25*, 956-958

Dubach, U.C., Levy, P.S., Rosner, B., Baumeler, H.R., Müller, A., Peier, A. & Ehrensperger, T. (1975) Relation between regular intake of phenacetin-containing analgesics and laboratory evidence of urorenal disorders in a working female population of Switzerland. *Lancet, i*, 539-543

Duggin, G.G. & Mudge, G.H. (1976) Phenacetin: renal tubular transport and intrarenal distribution in the dog. *J. Pharmacol. exp. Ther., 199*, 10-16

Eisenbrand, G. & Preussmann, R. (1975) Nitrosation of phenacetin. Formation of *N*-nitroso-2-nitro-4-ethoxyacetanilide as an unstable product of the nitrosation in dilute aqueous-acidic solution. *Arzneimittel-Forsch., 25*, 1472-1475

Evans, D.A.P. (1977) *Human pharmacogenetics*. In: Parke, D.V. & Smith, R.L., eds, *Drug Metabolism - From Microbe to Man*, London, Taylor & Francis, pp. 369-391

Evans, M.A. & Harbison, R.D. (1977) GLC microanalysis of phenacetin and acetaminophen levels. *J. pharm. Sci., 66*, 1628-1629

Fischbach, T., Lenk, W. & Sackerer, D. (1977) *Additional routes in the metabolism of phenacetin.* In: Jollow, D.J., Kocsis, J.J., Snyder, R. & Vainio, H., eds, *Biological Reactive Intermediates,* New York, Plenum Press, pp. 380-386

Focella, A., Heslin, P. & Teitel, S. (1972) The synthesis of two phenacetin metabolites. *Can. J. Chem., 50*, 2025-2030

Fokkens, W. (1979) Phenacetin abuse related to bladder cancer. *Environ. Res., 20*, 192-198

Gault, M.H. & Wilson, D.R. (1978) Analgesic nephropathy in Canada : clinical syndrome, management, and outcome. *Kidney Int., 13*, 58-63

Gault, M.H., Shahidi, N.T. & Gabe, A. (1972) The effect of acetylsalicyclic acid, caffeine, and codeine on the excretion of phenacetin metabolites. *Can. J. Physiol. Pharmacol., 50,* 809-816

Goodman, L.S. & Gilman, A., eds (1975) *The Pharmacological Basis of Therapeutics,* 5th ed., New York, MacMillan, pp. 343-347, 368

Grob, H.U. (1971) Phenacetin abuse and renal pelvic carcinoma (Ger.). *Helv. chir. Acta, 38,* 537-539

Güller R. & Dubach, U.C. (1973) Tumours of the urinary tract after regular intake of analgesic containing phenacetin (Ger.). *Helv. med. Acta, 36,* 247-250

Heinonen, O.P., Slone, D. & Shapiro, S. (1977) *Birth Defects and Drugs in Pregnancy,* Littleton, MA, Publishing Sciences Group, Inc., pp. 286-295

Hinson, J.A. & Mitchell, J.R. (1976) N-Hydroxylation of phenacetin by hamster liver microsomes. *Drug. Metab. Disposition, 4,* 430-435

Hinson, J.A., Nelson, S.D. & Mitchell, J.R. (1977) Studies on the microsomal formation of arylating metabolites of acetaminophen and phenacetin. *Mol. Pharmacol., 13,* 625-633

Høybye, G. & Nielsen, O.E. (1971) Renal pelvic carcinoma in phenacetin abusers. *Scand. J. Urol. Nephrol., 5,* 190-192

Hultengren, N., Lagergren, C. & Ljungqvist, A. (1965) Carcinoma of the renal pelvis in renal papillary necrosis. *Acta chir. scand., 130,* 314-320

IARC (1977) *IARC Monographs on the Evaluation of Carcinogenic Risk of Chemicals to Man,* Vol. 13, *Some Miscellaneous Pharmaceutical Substances,* Lyon, pp. 141-155

IARC (1979) *Information Bulletin on the Survey of Chemicals Being Tested for Carcinogenicity,* No. 8, Lyon, p. 129

Isaka, H., Yoshii, H., Otsuji, A., Koike, M., Nagai, Y., Koura, M., Sugiyasu, K. & Kanabayashi, T. (1979) Tumors of Sprague-Dawley rats induced by long-term feeding of phenacetin. *Gann, 70,* 29-36

Ishidate, M., Jr & Odashima, S. (1977) Chromosome tests with 134 compounds on Chinese hamster cells *in vitro* - a screening for chemical carcinogens. *Mutat. Res., 48,* 337-354

Iyakuhin Yoran (1979) *Drug Index,* Osaka Prefecture, Association of Pharmacists, pp. 70-71

Jagenburg, O.R. & Toczko, K. (1964) The metabolism of acetophenetidine. Isolation and characterization of *S*-(1-acetamido-4-hydroxyphenyl)cysteine, a metabolite of acetophenetidine. *Biochem. J., 92,* 639-643

Johansson, S. & Angervall, L. (1976a) Urothelial hyperplasia of the renal papillae in female Sprague-Dawley rats induced by long term feeding of phenacetin. *Acta pathol. microbiol. scand., Sect. A, 84,* 353-354

Johansson, S. & Angervall, L. (1976b) Urothelial changes of the renal papillae in Sprague-Dawley rats induced by long term feeding of phenacetin. *Acta pathol. microbiol. scand., Sect. A, 84,* 375-383

Johansson, S. & Angervall, L. (1979) Carcinogenicity of phenacetin. *Science, 204,* 130

Johansson, S. & Wahlqvist, L. (1977) Tumours of urinary bladder and ureter associated with abuse of phenacetin-containing analgesics. *Acta pathol. microbiol. scand., Sect. A, 85,* 768-774

Johansson, S., Angervall, L., Bengtsson, U. & Wahlqvist L. (1974) Uroepithelial tumors of the renal pelvis associated with abuse of phenacetin-containing analgesics. *Cancer, 33,* 743-753

Juusela, H. (1973) Carcinoma of the renal pelvis and its relationship to analgesic abuse. *Ann. Chir. Gynaecol. Fenn., 62,* 386-390

King, M.-T., Beikirch, H., Eckhardt, K., Gocke, E. & Wild, D. (1979) Mutagenicity studies with X-ray-contrast media, analgesics, antipyretics, antirheumatics and some other pharmaceutical drugs in bacterial, *Drosophila* and mammalian test systems. *Mutat. Res., 66,* 33-43

Klutch, A. & Bordun, M. (1968) Chromatographic methods for analysis of the metabolites of acetophenetidin (phenacetin). *J. pharm. Sci., 57,* 524-526

Klutch, A., Harfenist, M. & Conney, A.H. (1966) 2-Hydroxyacetophenetidine, a new metabolite of acetophenetidine. *J. med. Chem., 9,* 63-66

Klutch, A., Levin, W., Chang, R.L., Vane, F. & Conney, A.H. (1978) Formation of a thiomethyl metabolite of phenacetin and acetaminophen in dogs and man. *Clin. Pharmacol. Ther., 24,* 287-293

Küng, L.G. (1976) Renal body carcinoma and carcinoma of the efferent urinary tract after phenacetin abuse (Ger.). *Schweiz. med. Wschr., 106,* 47-51

Kuntzman, R., Pantuck, E.J., Kaplan, S.A. & Conney, A.H. (1977) Phenacetin metabolism: effect of hydrocarbons and cigarette smoking. *Clin. Pharmacol. Ther., 22,* 757-764

Landmann-Kolbert, C., Rutishauser, G. & Dubach, U.C. (1975) Phenacetin-abuse and tumours of the urinary tract (Ger.). *Urologe, A/14,* 75-79

Leistenschneider, W. & Ehmann, R. (1973) Renal pelvic carcinoma after phenacetin abuse (Ger.). *Schweiz. med. Wschr., 103,* 433-439

Liu, T., Smith, G.W. & Rankin, J.T. (1972) Renal pelvic tumour associated with analgesic abuse. *Can. med. Assoc. J., 107,* 768, 771

Macklin, A.W. & Szot, R.J. (1980) Eighteen month oral study of aspirin, phenacetin and caffeine in C57BL/6 mice. *Drug Chem. Toxicol., 3,* 135-163

Macklin, A.W., Welch, R.M. & Cuatrecasas, P. (1979) Drug safety: phenacetin. *Science, 205,* 144, 146, 148

Maddock, J.T., Druck, K. & Neff, D. (1977) *Aspirin Substitutes,* Philadelphia, PA, Auerbach Associates, Inc. for US Consumer Product Safety Commission, Report No. AAI-2383/2384-200-TR-2, pp. 9-17

Mahony, J.F., Storey, B.G., Ibañez, R.C. & Stewart, J.H. (1977) Analgesic abuse, renal parenchymal disease and carcinoma of the kidney or ureter. *Aust. N.Z. J. Med., 7,* 463-469

Mannion, R.A. & Susmano, D. (1971) Phenacetin abuse causing bladder tumor. *J. Urol., 106,* 692

Matsuoka, A., Hayashi, M. & Ishidate, M., Jr (1979) Chromosomal aberration tests on 29 chemicals combined with S9 mix *in vitro*. *Mutat. Res., 66,* 277-290

Matsushima, T., Yahagi, T., Takamoto, Y., Nagao, M. & Sugimura, T. (1980) *Species differences in microsomal activation of mutagens and carcinogens, with special reference to new potent mutagens from pyrolysates of amino acids and proteins.* In: *Microsomes, Drug Oxidations and Chemical Carcinogenesis,* New York, Academic Press (in press)

McLean, S. (1978) Metabolism of phenacetin and N-hydroxyphenacetin in isolated rat hepatocytes. *Arch. Pharmacol., 305,* 173-180

Molland, E.A. (1978) Experimental renal papillary necrosis. *Kidney Int., 13,* 5-14

Moshakis, V. & Hooper, A.A. (1978) Analgesic nephropathy and transitional cell carcinoma. *Postgrad. med. J., 54,* 285-286

Mulder, G.J., Hinson, J.A. & Gillette, J.R. (1977) Generation of reactive metabolites of N-hydroxy-phenacetin by glucuronidation and sulfation. *Biochem. Pharmacol., 26,* 189-196

Murray, R.M. (1978) Genesis of analgesic nephropathy in the United Kingdom. *Kidney Int., 13,* 50-57

Murray, T.G. & Goldberg, M. (1978) Analgesic-associated nephropathy in the USA: epidemiologic, clinical and pathogenetic features. *Kidney Int., 13,* 64-71

Nakanishi, K., Fukushima, S., Shibata, M., Shirai, T., Ogiso, T. & Ito, N. (1978) Effect of phenacetin and caffeine on the urinary bladder of rats treated with N-butyl-N-(4-hydroxybutyl)nitrosamine. *Gann, 69,* 395-400

Nanra, R.S., Stuart-Taylor, J., de Leon, A.H. & White, K.H. (1978) Analgesic nephropathy: etiology, clinical syndrome and clinicopathologic correlations in Australia. *Kidney Int., 13,* 79-92

National Cancer Institute (1978) *Bioassay of a Mixture of Aspirin, Phenacetin, and Caffeine for Possible Carcinogenicity (Tech. Rep. Ser. No. 67),* DHEW Publication No. (NIH) 78-1317, Washington DC, US Government Printing Office

National Formulary Board (1970) *National Formulary,* 13th ed., Washington DC, American Pharmaceutical Association, pp. 66-68, 178-180

Nordenfelt, O. (1972) Deaths from renal failure in abusers of phenacetin-containing drugs. *Acta med. scand., 191,* 11-16

Pantuck, E.J., Hsiao, K.-C., Maggio, A., Nakamura, K., Kuntzman, R. & Conney, A.H. (1974) Effect of cigarette smoking on phenacetin metabolism. *Clin. Pharmacol. Ther., 15,* 9-17

Pantuck, E.J., Hsiao, K.-C., Kuntzman, R. & Conney, A.H. (1975) Intestinal metabolism of phenacetin in the rat: effect of charcoal-broiled beef and rat chow. *Science, 187,* 744-746

Pantuck, E.J., Hsiao, K.-C., Loub, W.D., Wattenberg, L.W., Kutzman, R. & Conney, A.H. (1976) Stimulatory effect of vegetables on intestinal drug metabolism in the rat. *J. Pharmacol. exp. Ther., 198,* 278-283

Prescott, L.F. (1975) *Antipyretic analgesics.* In: Dukes, M.N.G., ed., *Meyler's Side Effects of Drugs,* Vol. 8, Amsterdam, Excerpta Medica, pp. 176-186

Prescott, L.F. (1979) The nephrotoxicity and hepatotoxicity of antipyretic analgesics. *Br. J. clin. Pharmacol., 7,* 453-462

Prescott, L.F., Wright, N., Roscoe, P. & Brown, S.S. (1971) Plasma-paracetamol half-life and hepatic necrosis in patients with paracetamol overdosage. *Lancet, i,* 519-522

Proudfoot, A.T. & Wright, N. (1970) Acute paracetamol poisoning. *Br. med. J., iii,* 557-558

Rathert, P., Melchior, H. & Lutzeyer, W. (1975) Phenacetin: a carcinogen for the urinary tract? *J. Urol., 113,* 653-657

Saker, B.M. & Kincaid-Smith, P. (1969) Papillary necrosis in experimental analgesic nephropathy. *Br. med. J., i,* 161-162

Schmähl, D. & Reiter, A. (1954) Lack of a carcinogenic effect of phenacetin (Ger.). *Arzneimittel-forsch., 4,* 404-405

Shahidi, N.T. (1967) Acetophenetidin sensitivity. *Am. J. Dis. Child., 113,* 81-82

Shahidi, N.T. & Hemaidan, A. (1969) Acetophenetidin-induced methemoglobinemia and its relation to the excretion of diazotizable amines. *J. Lab. clin. Med., 74,* 581-585

Shudo, K., Ohta, T., Orihara, Y., Okamoto, T., Nagao, M., Takahashi, Y. & Sugimura, T. (1978) Mutagenicities of phenacetin and its metabolites. *Mutat. Res., 58,* 367-370

Sloan, T.P., Mahgour, A., Lancaster, R., Idle, J.R. & Smith, R.L. (1978) Polymorphism of carbon oxidation of drugs and clinical implications. *Br. med. J., ii,* 655-656

Smith, G.E. & Griffiths, L.A. (1976a) Comparative metabolic studies of phenacetin and structurally-related compounds in the rat. *Xenobiotica, 6,* 217-236

Smith, G.E. & Griffiths, L.A. (1976b) Metabolism of a biliary metabolite of phenacetin and other acetanilides by the intestinal microflora. *Experientia, 32,* 1556-1557

Smith, R.L. & Timbrell, J.A. (1974) Factors affecting the metabolism of phenacetin. I. Influence of dose, chronic dosage, route of administration and species on the metabolism of [1-^{14}C-acetyl] phenacetin. *Xenobiotica, 4,* 489-501

Storey, B.G., Mahony, J.F. & Stewart, J.H. (1977) Carcinoma of the upper urinary tract associated with analgesic nephropathy. *Br. J. Urol., 3,* 242

Swinyard, E.A. (1975) *Analgesics and antipyretics.* In: Osol, A., ed., *Remington's Pharmaceutical Sciences,* 15th ed., Easton, PA, Mack Publishing Co., p. 1051

Tanooka, H. (1977) Development and applications of *Bacillus subtilis* test systems for mutagens, involving DNA-repair deficiency and suppressible auxotrophic mutations. *Mutat. Res., 42,* 19-32

Taylor, J.S. (1972) Carcinoma of the urinary tract and analgesic abuse. *Med. J. Aust., 1,* 407-409

Thomson, J.S. & Prescott, L.F. (1966) Liver damage and impaired glucose tolerance after paracetamol overdosage. *Br. med. J., ii,* 506-507

Tosi, S.E. & Morin, L.J. (1977) Bladder tumor associated with phenacetin abuse. *Urology, 9,* 59-60

US Food & Drug Administration (1978) Food and drugs. *US Code Fed. Regul.,* Title 21, parts 200-299, pp. 38-39

US International Trade Commission (1979) *Imports of Benzenoid Chemicals and Products, 1978,* USITC Publication 990, Washington DC, US Government Printing Office, p. 86

US Pharmacopeial Convention, Inc. (1970) *The US Pharmacopeia,* 18th rev., Bethesda, MD, pp. 483-485

Wade, A., ed (1977) *Martindale, The Extra Pharmacopoeia,* 27th ed., London, The Pharmacuetical Press, pp. 205-206

Wallace, J.E., Biggs, J.D., Hamilton, H.E., Foster, L.L. & Blum, K. (1973) UV spectrophotometric method for determination of phenacetin in biological specimens. *J. pharm. Sci., 62,* 599-601

Welch, R.M., Cavallito, J. & Loh, A. (1972) Effect of exposure to cigarette smoke on the metabolism of benzo[a]pyrene and acetophenetidin by lung and intestine of rats. *Toxicol. appl. Pharmacol., 23,* 749-758

WHO (1978) *Drug Information - July-September 1978*, Geneva, p. 20

WHO (1979) *Drug Information Bulletin*, Geneva

Windholz, M. ed. (1976) *The Merck Index,* 9th ed., Rahway, NJ, Merck & Co., p. 9

PHENAZOPYRIDINE and PHENAZOPYRIDINE HYDROCHLORIDE

1. Chemical and Physical Data

PHENAZOPYRIDINE

1.1 Synonyms and trade names

Chem. Abstr. Services Reg. No.: 94-78-0

Chem. Abstr. Name: 2,6-Pyridinediamine, 3-(phenylazo)-

IUPAC Systematic Name: 2,6-Diamino-3-(phenylazo)pyridine

Synonym: 3-(Phenylazo)-2,6-pyridinediamine

Trade names: Gastracid; Gastrotest

1.2 Structural and molecular formulae and molecular weight

$C_{11}H_{11}N_5$ Mol. wt: 213.2

1.3 Chemical and physical properties of the pure substance

Melting-point: 139°C (Windholz, 1976)

1.4 Technical products and impurities

There are no technical products or pharmaceutical preparations containing the free base.

PHENAZOPYRIDINE HYDROCHLORIDE

1.1 Synonyms and trade names

Chem. Abstr. Services Reg. No.: 136-40-3

Chem. Abstr. Name: 2,6-Pyridinediamine, 3-(phenylazo)-, monohydrochloride

IUPAC Systematic Name: 2,6-Diamino-3-(phenylazo)pyridine monohydrochloride

Synonyms: 2,6-Diamino-3-phenylazopyridine hydrochloride; PAP; phenazopyridinium chloride; phenylazodiaminopyridine HCl; β-phenylazo-α,α'-diaminopyridine hydrochloride; 3-phenylazo-2,6-diaminopyridine hydrochloride; phenylazopyridine HCl

Trade names: Azodine; Azodium; Azodyne; Azo Gastanol; Azo Gantrisin; Azo-Mandelamine; Azo-Standard; Azo-Stat; Azotrex; Azodyne; Baridium; Bisteril; Cystamine 'McClung'; Cystopyrin; Cystural; Di-Azo; Diridone; Dolonil; Eucistin; Giracid; Mallophene; Mallofeen; NC 150; Nefrecil; Phenazo; Phenazodine; Phenylazo; Phenyl-Idium; Phenyl-Idium 200; Pirid; Piridacil; Pyrazodine; Pyrazofen; Pyredal; Pyridacil; Pyridenal; Pyridene; Pyridiate; Pyridium; Pyridivite; Pyripyridium; Pyrizin; Sedural; Sulodyne; Thiosulfil-A Forte; Urazium; Uridinal; Uriplex; Urobiotic - 250; Urodine; Urofeen; Uromide; Urophenyl; Uropyridin; Uropyrine; Utostan; Vestin; W 1655

1.2 Structural and molecular formulae and molecular weight

$C_{11}H_{12}ClN_5$ Mol. wt: 249.7

1.3 Chemical and physical properties of the pure substance

From Wade (1977) or Windholz (1976)

- (a) *Description:* Brick-red microcrystals with slight violet lustre
- (b) *Melting-point:* 235°C (dec.)
- (c) *Spectroscopy data:* λ_{max} (in methanol) 238 nm, A(1%, 1cm) = 437; 279 nm, A(1%, 1cm) = 188; and 402 nm, A (1%, 1cm) = 951 (Kráčmar & Kráčmarová, 1978)
- (d) *Solubility:* Slightly soluble in cold water (1 in 300) and ethanol; soluble in boiling-water (1 in 20), acetic acid, glycerol (1 in 100) and ethylene and propylene glycols; insoluble in acetone, benzene, chloroform, diethyl ether and toluene

1.4 Technical products and impurities

Commercial phenazopyridine hydrochloride may contain some β,β'-bis(phenylazo)-α,α'-diaminopyridine (Windholz, 1976). It is available in the US as a NF grade containing 99.0-101.0% active ingredient on a dried basis. Loss on drying should not exceed 1%; residue on ignition not exceed 0.2%; and water insoluble substances not exceed 0.1%. A test for heavy metals (not to exceed 0.002%) is also included. It is available in 100 and 200 mg doses as tablets containing 95.0-105.0% of the stated amount of phenazopyridine hydrochloride (National Formulary Board, 1975).

2. Production, Use, Occurrence and Analysis

2.1 Production and use

(a) *Production*

Phenazopyridine hydrochloride was first synthesized by Eisenberg and by Chichibabin and Zeide in 1914 (Wander & Pascoe, 1965; Windholz, 1976). The free base can be synthesized by diazotizing aniline with sodium nitrite and excess hydrochloric acid and coupling the product with 2,6-diaminopyridine (Shreve *et al.*, 1943). It is not known whether this is the method used for commercial production.

Although commercial production of the free base has not been reported in the US, it is undoubtedly produced as an unisolated intermediate in the production of the hydrochloride. The first commercial production of the hydrochloride in the US was reported in

1944 (US Tariff Commission, 1946). In 1979 only two US companies reported commercial production of an undisclosed amount (see preamble, p. 21). Annual production in the US and Canada is believed to be in the order of 10-50 thousand kg each. US imports through principal US customs districts in 1978 were 450 kg of the free base and 7000 kg of the hydrochloride (US International Trade Commission, 1979).

The only two major producers of phenazopyridine and phenazopyridine hydrochloride in western Europe are in Italy and Switzerland. Since 1948, Switzerland has produced less than 1000 kg of the free base and 10,000-50,000 kg of the hydrochloride yearly. Italy produces about 1000-10,000 kg of phenazopyridine hydrochloride yearly.

Phenazopyridine hydrochloride is not produced commercially in Japan. Small amounts are imported: 200 kg in 1976 and 300 kg in 1977.

(b) Use

Phenazopyridine hydrochloride is used as an analgesic and antiseptic in the management of genitourinary-tract infections. Its local effect may be an anaesthetic action. The usual oral dosage for adults is 200 mg, 3 times daily; the dosage for children is 12 mg/kg bw daily divided into 3 doses (Goodman & Gilman, 1975; Harvey, 1975; Wade, 1977). In Japan, phenazopyridine hydrochloride is used as a urinary antiseptic in a dose of 300 mg daily.

Phenazopyridine hydrochloride is most often given in combination with sulfonamides and antibiotics (Goodman & Gilman, 1975; Harvey, 1975).

2.2 Occurrence

Phenazopyridine and phenazopyridine hydrochloride are not known to occur in nature.

2.3 Analysis

Typical methods for the analysis of phenazopyridine hydrochloride are summarized in Table 1. Abbreviations used are: HPLC/UV, high-performance liquid chromatography with ultra-violet spectrometry; UV, ultra-violet spectrometry.

Table 1. Analytical methods for phenazopyridine hydrochloride

Sample matrix	Sample preparation	Assay procedure	Limit of detection	Reference
Solution	Dissolve in alcohol:sulphuric acid	UV	not given	National Formulary Board (1975)
Formulation	Dissolve in methanol	HPLC/UV	not given	Umagat et al. (1979)

3. Biological Data Relevant to the Evaluation of Carcinogenic Risk to Humans

3.1 Carcinogenicity studies in animals

(a) Oral administration

Mouse: Groups of 35 male and 35 female 7-week-old B6C3F1 mice received 0, 600 or 1200 mg/kg diet phenazopyridine hydrochloride (96.5% pure) for 80 weeks. The treated animals were fed test diets on 5 days per week and control diet on 2 days per week. A control group consisted of 15 female and 15 male mice. All surviving animals were killed at 105-107 weeks. The combined incidences of hepatocellular adenomas and carcinomas in control, low- and high-dose groups were as follows: males: 5/15, 15/35 and 15/33; females, 2/15, 11/34, 19/32 ($P = 0.003$ for females given the high dose). There were no significant differences in the incidences of tumours at other sites between treated and control mice (National Cancer Institute, 1978).

Rat: Groups of 35 male and 35 female 6-week-old Fischer 344 rats received 0, 3700 or 7500 mg/kg diet phenazopyridine hydrochloride (96.5% pure) for 78 weeks. The treated animals were fed test diets on 5 days per week and control diet on 2 days per week. A control group consisted of 15 female and 15 male rats. All surviving animals were killed at 104-105 weeks. The combined incidences of adenomas, adenocarcinomas and sarcomas of the colon and rectum in control, low- and high-dose groups were as follows: males, 0/14, 5/34 and 10/35; females, 0/14, 3/33 and 6/32. There were no significant differences in the incidences of tumours at other sites between treated and control rats (National Cancer Institute, 1978).

(b) Intraperitoneal administration

Mouse: Groups of 10 male and 10 female 6-8-week old A/He mice were given weekly i.p. injections of phenazopyridine hydrochloride for 24 weeks, at total doses of 0.310, 0.775 or 1.550 g/kg bw in steriod suspending vehicle. Survivors were killed at 24 weeks. The combined numbers of male and female mice that developed lung tumours were 6/20, 3/18 and 6/18 (0.40, 0.22 and 0.50 lung tumours per mouse) in the 3 groups, respectively. In a vehicle-control group, there were 14/58 lung-tumour bearing animals (0.24 lung tumours per mouse) (Stoner *et al.*, 1973). [Attention is drawn to the limitations of negative results obtained with this test system.]

3.2 Other relevant biological data

(a) Experimental systems

Toxic effects

In rats, the i.p. LD_{50} of phenazopyridine hydrochloride is about 270 mg/kg bw, while that of the base is 520 mg/kg bw (Walton & Lawson, 1934). In mice, the i.p. LD_{50} of phenazopyridine has been reported to be 600 mg/kg bw (Burba, 1967).

Absorption, distribution, excretion and metabolism

Following oral administration of 150 mg/kg bw phenazopyridine hydrochloride to rabbits, approximately 85% of the administered dose was eliminated in the urine during the first 12 hrs. Aniline, *para*-aminophenol (as 50% of the dose), *N*-acetyl-*para*-aminophenol, *ortho*-aminophenol (as traces), 2,3,6-triaminopyridine and phenazopyridine appeared in the urine (Johnson & Chartrand, 1976). 2,3,6-Triaminopyridine is more acutely toxic than is phenazopyridine (Burba, 1967).

In addition to reductive metabolism, phenazopyridine also undergoes oxidative metabolism: in the urine of rats treated with 50 mg/kg bw phenazopyridine, 2,6-diamino-3-[(4-hydroxyphenyl)azo]pyridine and 2,6-diamino-3-[(2-hydroxyphenyl)azo]pyridine have been detected (Pitrè & Maffei-Facino, 1977).

No data on the prenatal toxicity or mutagenicity of either compound were available.

(b) Humans

Phenazopyridine hydrochloride is an analgesic with a local anaesthetic action (Goodman & Gilman, 1975).

Toxic effects

Toxic signs which occur in humans given large doses of phenazopyridine hydrochloride include methaemoglobinaemia, Heinz-body formation, haemolytic anaemia, renal failure, hepatic enlargement, jaundice and hypersensitivity hepatitis (Crawford *et al.*, 1951; Sand & Edelmann, 1961; Gabor *et al.*, 1964; Greenberg & Wong, 1964; Wander & Pascoe, 1965; Hood & Toth, 1966; Bloch & Porter, 1969; Alano & Webster, 1970; Cohen & Bovasso, 1971; Goldfinger & Marx, 1972). Renal failure with acute tubular necrosis were reported in a 13-year-old girl following ingestion of 2 g in a suicide attempt (Feinfeld *et al.*, 1978).

Absorption, distribution, excretion and metabolism

After an oral dose of 600 mg phenazopyridine hydrochloride, about 80% is eliminated in the urine within 24 hours: 41-45% appears as conjugated phenazopyridine, 24-27% as *para*-aminophenol, 18-20% as conjugated *N*-acetyl-*para*-aminophenol, 7-8% as aniline and traces of *ortho*-aminophenol and 2,3,6-triaminopyridine (Johnson & Burba, 1965; Johnson & Chartrand, 1976).

No data on the prenatal toxicity or mutagenicity in humans of either compound were available.

3.3 Case reports and epidemiological studies of carcinogenicity in humans

In a hypothesis-seeking study involving determination of the incidence of all forms of cancer in relation to drug exposure in 143, 574 individuals, no significant excess of any cancer was observed in 2214 subjects who had received phenazopyridine hydrochloride. Follow-up was for a minimum of 3 years (Friedman & Ury, 1980). [About 10,000 person-years of follow-up would have been accumulated by subjects given phenazopyridine hydrochloride. Data on the age and sex distributions of the exposed subjects and the doses and durations of use of the drug were not given.]

4. Summary of Data Reported and Evaluation

4.1 Experimental data

Phenazopyridine hydrochloride was tested in mice and rats by oral administration and in mice by intraperitoneal administration. After its oral administration in female mice, it significantly increased the incidence of hepatocellular adenomas and carcinomas. In male and female rats, it induced tumours of the colon and rectum.

Attention is drawn to the absence of studies on the mutagenicity or teratogenicity of this compound.

4.2 Human data

Phenazopyridine hydrochloride is a weak urinary-tract analgesic and is possibly antiseptic.

In one epidemiological study, involving a limited period of observation, no association was observed between use of phenazopyridine hydrochloride and any cancer.

4.3 Evaluation

There is *sufficient evidence*[1] for the carcinogenicity of phenazopyridine hydrochloride in experimental animals. The available epidemiological data are insufficient to evaluate the carcinogenicity of phenazopyridine hydrochloride to humans. In the absence of adequate data in humans, phenazopyridine hydrochloride should be regarded, for practical purposes, as if it presented a carcinogenic risk to humans.

---

[1] See preamble, p. 18.

5. References

Alano, F.A., Jr & Webster, G.D., Jr (1970) Acute renal failure and pigmentation due to phenazopyridine (pyridium). *Ann. intern. Med., 72,* 89-91

Bloch, A. & Porter, B. (1969) Phenylazopyridine poisoning. *Am. J. Dis. Child., 117,* 369

Burba, J.V. (1967) The metabolism and toxicity of 2,3,6-triaminopyridine, a metabolite of pyridium. *Can. J. Biochem., 45,* 773-780

Cohen, B.L. & Bovasso, G.J., Jr (1971) Acquired methemoglobinemia and hemolytic anemia following excessive pyridium (phenazopyridine hydrochloride) ingestion. *Clin. Pediat., 10,* 537-540

Crawford, S.E., Moon, A.E., Jr, Panos, T.C. & Hooks, C.A. (1951) Methemoglobinemia associated with pyridium® administration. Report of a case. *J. Am. med. Assoc., 146,* 24-25

Feinfeld, D.A., Ranieri, R., Lipner, H.I. & Avram, M.M. (1978) Renal failure in phenazopyridine overdose. *J. Am. med. Assoc., 240,* 2661

Friedman, G.D. & Ury, H.K. (1980) Initial screening for carcinogenicity of commonly used drugs. *J. natl Cancer Inst.* (in press)

Gabor, E.P., Lowenstein, L. & de Leeuw, N.K.M. (1964) Hemolytic anemia induced by phenylazo-diamino-pyridine (pyridium). *Can. med. Assoc. J., 91,* 756-759

Goldfinger, S.E. & Marx, S. (1972) Hypersensitivity hepatitis due to phenazopyridine hydrochloride. *New Engl. J. Med., 286,* 1090-1091

Goodman, L.S. & Gilman, A., eds (1975) *The Pharmacological Basis of Therapeutics,* 5th ed., New York, Macmillan, p. 1009

Greenberg, M.S. & Wong, H. (1964) Methemoglobinemia and Heinz body hemolytic anemia due to phenazopyridine hydrochloride. *New Engl. J. Med., 271,* 431-435

Harvey, S.C. (1975) *Antimicrobial drugs.* In: Osol, A., ed., *Remington's Pharmaceutical Sciences,* 15th ed., Easton, PA, Mack Publishing Co., p. 1097

Hood, J.W. & Toth, W.N. (1966) Jaundice caused by phenazopyridine hydrochloride. *J. Am. med. Assoc., 198,* 1366-1367

Johnson, W.J. & Burba, J. (1965) Metabolic fate of diaminophenylazopyridine (DPP) (Abstract). *Fed. Proc., 25,* 734

Johnson, W.J. & Chartrand, A. (1976) The metabolism and excretion of phenazopyridine hydrochloride in animals and man. *Toxicol. appl. Pharmacol., 37,* 371-376

Kráčmar, J. & Kráčmarová, J. (1978) UV-spectrophotometry in drug control (Ger.). *Pharmazie, 33,* 27-32

National Cancer Institute (1978) *Bioassay of Phenazopyridine Hydrochloride for Possible Carcinogenicity (Tech. Rep. Ser. No. 99),* Department of Health, Education, & Welfare Publication No. (NIH) 78-1349, Washington DC, US Government Printing Office

National Formulary Board (1975) *National Formulary,* 14th ed., Washington DC, American Pharmaceutical Association, pp. 554-556

Pitrė, D. & Maffei-Facino, R. (1977) Isolation and identification of two hydroxylated metabolites of phenazopyridine in rat urine. *Farmaco-Ed. Sci., 32,* 453-460

Sand, R.E. & Edelmann, C.M., Jr (1961) Pyridium-induced methemoglobinemia. Report of a case. *J. Pediat., 58,* 845-848

Shreve, R.N., Swaney, M.W. & Riechers, E.H. (1943) Studies on azo dyes. I. Preparation and bacteriostatic properties of azo derivatives of 2,6-diaminopyridine. *J. Am. chem. Soc., 65,* 2241-2243

Stoner, G.D., Shimkin, M.B., Kniazeff, A.J., Weisburger, J.H., Weisburger, E.K. & Gori, G.B. (1973) Test for carcinogenicity of food additives and chemotherapeutic agents by the pulmonary tumor response in strain A mice. *Cancer Res., 13,* 3069-3085

Umagat, H., McGarry, P.F. & Tscherne, R.J. (1979) Stability-indicating sulfa drug analysis using high-performance liquid chromatography. *J. pharm. Sci., 68,* 922-924

US International Trade Commission (1979) *Imports of Benzenoid Chemicals and Products, 1978,* USITC Publication 990, Washington DC, US Government Printing Office, p. 86

US Tariff Commission (1946) *Synthetic Organic Chemicals, US Production and Sales, 1944,* Report No. 155, Second Series, Washington DC, US Government Printing Office, p. 95

Wade, A., ed. (1977) *Martindale, The Extra Pharmacopoeia,* 27th ed., London, The Pharmaceutical Press, p. 207

Walton, R.P. & Lawson, E.H. (1934) Pharmacology and toxicology of the azo dye, phenyl-azo-*alpha-alpha*-diaminopyridine (pyridium). *J. Pharmacol. exp. Ther., 51,* 200-216

Wander, H.J. & Pascoe, D.J. (1965) Phenylazopyridine hydrochloride poisoning. Report of case and review of literature. *Am. J. Dis. Child., 110,* 105-107

Windholz, M., ed. (1976) *The Merck Index,* 9th ed., Rahway, NJ, Merck & Co., pp. 935-936

PHENELZINE and PHENELZINE SULPHATE

1. Chemical and Physical Data

PHENELZINE

1.1 Synonyms and trade names

Chem. Abstr. Services Reg. No.: 51-71-8

Chem. Abstr. Name: Hydrazine, (2-phenylethyl)-

IUPAC Systematic Name: Phenethylhydrazine

Synonyms: 1-Hydrazino-2-phenylethane; phenalzine; phenylethylhydrazine; 2-phenylethylhydrazine; β-phenylethylhydrazine

Trade names: Phenodyn; W-1544-A; W1544

1.2 Structural and molecular formulae and molecular weight

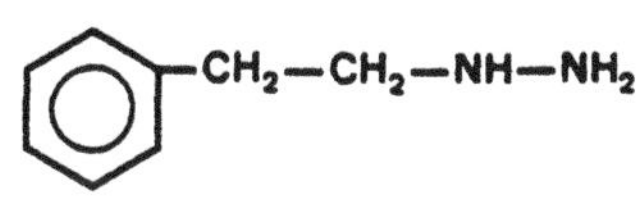

$$\text{C}_6\text{H}_5\text{-CH}_2\text{-CH}_2\text{-NH-NH}_2$$

$C_8H_{12}N_2$ Mol. wt: 136.2

1.3 Chemical and physical properties of the pure substance

From Windholz (1976)

(a) *Description:* Liquid
(b) *Boiling-point:* 74°C at 13 Pa
(c) *Refractive index:* $n_{20}^{D} = 1.5494$

1.4 Technical products and impurities

There are no technical products or pharmaceutical preparations containing the free base, which is used only in the preparation of the hydrochloride and sulphate salts.

PHENELZINE SULPHATE

1.1 Synonyms and trade names

Chem. Abstr. Services Reg. No.: 156-51-4

Chem. Abstr. Name: Hydrazine, (2-phenylethyl)-, sulfate (1:1)

IUPAC Systematic Name: Phenethylhydrazine sulfate (1:1)

Synonyms: 1-Hydrazino-2-phenylethane hydrogen sulphate; phenalzine dihydrogen sulphate; phenalzine hydrogen sulphate; phenethylhydrazine sulphate; phenylethylhydrazine dihydrogen sulphate; 2-phenylethylhydrazine dihydrogen sulphate; β-phenylethylhydrazine dihydrogen sulphate; 2-phenylethylhydrazine hydrogen sulphate; β-phenylethylhydrazine hydrogen sulphate; phenylethylhydrazine sulphate; 2-phenylethylhydrazine sulphate; β-phenylethylhydrazine sulphate

Trade names: Alazin; Estinerval; Fenelzin; Fenelzine; Kalgan; Mao-rem; Monofen; Nardelzine; Nardil; Phenelzine Bisulphate; Phenodyn; Stinerval

1.2 Structural and molecular formulae and molecular weight

$$\left[\bigcirc\!\!\!-CH_2CH_2-NHNH_2 \right] \cdot H_2SO_4$$

$C_8H_{12}N_2 \cdot H_2SO_4$ Mol. wt: 234.3

1.3 Chemical and physical properties of the pure substance

From Wade (1977) or Windholz (1976), unless otherwise specified

(a) Description: White powder with a pungent odour and a characteristic taste

(b) *Melting-point:* 164-168°C

(c) *Spectroscopy data:* λ_{max} (50% ethanol) 258 nm, A(1%, 1cm) = 8.0. Infrared, nuclear magnetic and mass spectral data have been tabulated (Daly, 1973).

(d) *Solubility:* Soluble in water (1 in 7); practically insoluble in ethanol; insoluble in chloroform and diethyl ether

(e) *Stability:* Sensitive to oxidation, light and temperature

1.4 Technical products and impurities

Various national and international pharmacopoeias give specifications for the purity of phenelzine in pharmaceutical products. For example, phenelzine sulphate is available in the US as a NF grade containing 97.0-100.5% active ingredient on a dried basis. The loss on drying should not exceed 1%; the limit for heavy metals is 0.002%; the melting-point range is 164-168°C; and the pH (1 in 100) should be between 1.4-1.9. It is available as tablets containing 95.0-105.0% of the stated amount as the free base, the equivalent of 15 mg phenelzine (National Formulary Board, 1975). Pharmaceutical preparations in the United Kingdom are the same as for the US (Wade, 1977).

2. Production, Use, Occurrence and Analysis

2.1 Production and use

(a) Production

The first synthesis of phenelzine was reported by Votocek and Leminger in 1932 (Windholz, 1976). It was synthezised by the reaction of hydrazine hydrate with phenethyl bromide, by Biel in 1961 (Daly, 1973). In another synthesis route, phenethyl alcohol is treated with thionyl chloride to give phenethyl chloride, which is then reacted with hydrazine hydrate in isopropanol to yield phenelzine hydrochloride. The hydrochloride is treated with alkali to liberate the free base, which is then neutralized with sulphuric acid to form phenelzine sulphate (Swinyard, 1975). It is not known whether this is the method used for commercial production.

One company in the US is believed to produce an undisclosed amount of this chemical (see preamble, p. 21). US imports of phenelzine sulphate through the principal US customs districts amounted to 450 kg in 1978 (US International Trade Commission, 1979); no data on its exports are available.

One company in Italy, which produced 700 kg in 1978, is believed to be the only producer of phenelzine sulphate in western Europe. There is no evidence that phenelzine sulphate has ever been produced in Japan.

(b) Use

Phenelzine sulphate is a monoamine oxidase inhibitor used, sometimes in combination with other drugs, in moderate to severe depressive states in adults and in certain phobic-anxiety states. It is given in a daily dose of 30-45 mg during the first week, adjusted to 15-75 mg after the first two weeks (Goodman & Gilman, 1975; Swinyard, 1975; Wade, 1977).

2.2 Occurrence

Phenelzine and phenelzine sulphate are not known to occur in nature.

2.3 Analysis

A review has been published giving several analytical methods for the determination of phenelzine sulphate in bulk or tablet form based on spectrophotometric methods, polarography, titrimetry, and gas and thin-layer chromatography (Daly, 1973).

Typical methods for the analysis of phenelzine or phenelzine sulphate in biological matrices are summarized in Table 1. Abbreviations used are: GC/FID, gas chromatography with flame-ionization detection; GC/ECD, gas-liquid chromatography with electron capture detection.

Table 1. Analytical methods for phenelzine sulphate

Sample matrix	Sample preparation	Assay procedure	Limit of detection	Reference
Plasma and whole blood (analysis of phenelzine in patients given phenelzine sulphate)	Extract with benzene-ethyl acetate mixture; back-extract with sulphuric acid; re-extract with benzene containing an internal standard and triethylamine; form heptafluorobutyric derivative; add water; neutralize with ammonium hydroxide	GC/ECD	0.1 µg/l	Cooper et al., 1978
Urine (oxidation of phenelzine sulphate to 2-phenylethanol)	Add 50% sulphuric acid and diethyl ether; add dodecan-1-ol, diethyl ether and potassium iodate solution; concentrate organic layer with stream of air	GC/FID	0.05 mg/l	Caddy & Stead, 1977

3. Biological Data Relevant to the Evaluation of Carcinogenic Risk to Humans

3.1 Carcinogenicity studies in animals

Oral administration

Mouse: A group of 50 male and 50 female random-bred Swiss mice, 6 weeks of age, were given 0.015% phenelzine sulphate in the drinking-water for lifetime. An untreated group of 100 females and 100 males served as controls. Of the treated females, 28/50 developed 69 lung tumours: 23 had 44 adenomas, 5 had 18 adenomas plus 7 adenocarcinomas. Their average age at death was 77 weeks; the first tumour was observed at the 48th week and the last at the 98th week of age. Of the untreated females, 21/100 developed 31 lung tumours: 17 had 23 adenomas, 3 had 5 adenocarcinomas, and 1 had an adenoma and 2 adenocarcinomas. Their average age at death was 95 weeks; the first tumour occurred at the 60th week and the last at the 122nd week of age. Of the treated males, 18/50 developed 30 neoplasms of the lung: 15 had 17 adenomas, 2 had 9 adenomas and 3 adenocarcinomas, and 1 mouse had an adenocarcinoma. Their average age at death was 78 weeks; the first tumour was found at the 42nd week and the last at the 101st week of age. Of the untreated males, 23/100 developed 35 lung tumours: 10 had 12 adenomas, 8 had 11 adenocarcinomas, and 5 had 6 adenomas and 6 adenocarcinomas. Their average age at death was 92 weeks; the first tumour was found at the 53rd week and the last at the 125th week of age. Blood vessel tumours developed at various sites in 22 of the treated females: 4 mice had angiomas and 18 had angiosarcomas. The average age at death was 83 weeks; the first tumour was found at 69 weeks and the last at 98 weeks of age. Of untreated females, 5 developed vascular tumours. Of the treated males, 4 developed angiosarcomas. The average age at death was 50 weeks; the first tumour was observed at the 14th week and the last at the 91st week of age. Of untreated males, 6 developed blood vessel tumours (Toth & Shimizu, 1974; Toth, 1976; Toth & Nagel, 1976).

3.2 Other relevant biological data

(a) Experimental systems

Toxic effects

The oral, i.v. and i.p. LD_{50}'s of phenelzine in mice are 160, 160 and 135 mg/kg bw, respectively (Barnes & Eltherington, 1964; Lapin & Samsonova, 1969). The oral LD_{50} in rats is 210 mg/kg bw (Barnes & Eltherington, 1964).

Prenatal toxicity

When mice were given 25 mg/kg bw per day phenelzine sulphate by s.c. injection during the first 6 days of gestation, implantation was partially suppressed (Poulson & Robson, 1964).

Absorption, distribution, excretion and metabolism

Following i.p. injection of 2.5 mg/kg bw phenelzine-1-^{14}C sulphate to rats, 62% of the dose was recovered in the urine within 24 hours. The major excretion product was phenylacetic acid (Clineschmidt & Horita, 1969), which is also a metabolite of phenelzine in mice (Leverett *et al.*, 1960). The first enzyme involved in this elimination process is monoamine oxidase (Clineschmidt & Horita, 1969).

Mutagenicity and other, related short-term tests

Phenelzine sulphate was mutagenic for *Salmonella typhimurium* TA100 in the absence of metabolic activation by rat liver homogenate (Shimizu *et al.*, 1978). Phenelzine sulphate exhibits reactivity towards DNA, as evidenced by positive results in the *pol A$^+$/A$^-$* test in *Escherichia coli* (Rosenkranz & Carr, 1971) and by the inactivation of *Bacillus subtilis* transforming DNA (Freese *et al.*, 1968).

(b) Humans

Phenelzine sulphate is a monoamine oxidase inhibitor (Goodman & Gilman, 1975).

Toxic effects

Numerous acute toxic reactions to phenelzine sulphate can occur, including agitation, hallucinations, hyperreflexia, hyperpyrexia and convulsions. Both hypotension and hypertension have been reported. Chronic toxicity may involve the liver, central nervous system and cardiovascular system (orthostatic hypotension) (Goodman & Gilman, 1975).

Absorption, distribution, excretion and metabolism

Phenelzine is readily absorbed from the gastrointestinal tract. There is little excretion in the urine (Wade, 1977). The mean apparent half-life, estimated from urinary excretion data in patients who received oral doses of 30 mg thrice daily, was 0.87 hours following the initial dose and 3.11 hours after 13 days of treatment (Caddy *et al.*, 1978).

No data on the prenatal toxicity or mutagenicity in humans of either compound were available.

3.3 Case reports and epidemiological studies of carcinogenicity in humans

A 64-year old woman who developed angiosarcoma of the liver had taken phenelzine sulphate (15 to 45 mg daily) for at least 6 years before onset of the disease. Diazepam (5 to 10 mg occasionally) was the only other medication reported. There was no history of exposure to thorium dioxide, arsenic or vinyl chloride, which are known or suspected to cause angiosarcoma of the liver in humans. The patient also had multiple angiosarcomas in the peritoneum and an osteolytic lesion in the right humerus (Daneshmend et al., 1979).

4. Summary of Data Reported and Evaluation

4.1 Experimental data

Phenelzine sulphate was tested in mice by oral administration: it significantly increased the incidence of lung and blood vessel tumours in females.

Phenelzine sulphate is mutagenic in bacteria.

Phenelzine sulphate has been shown to be embryotoxic in mice.

4.2 Human data

Phenelzine sulphate is a monoamine oxidase inhibitor with limited use in the treatment of depressive states.

The single case report of angiosarcoma in a woman taking phenelzine sulphate provides insufficient evidence to assess the carcinogenicity of this compound in humans.

4.3 Evaluation

There is *limited evidence*[1] that phenelzine sulphate is carcinogenic in experimental animals. In view of the evidence in experimental animals, the mutagenicity of phenelzine sulphate and a single case report of angiosarcoma of the liver in a patient taking phenelzine sulphate, further studies on the carcinogenicity of this compound are warranted.

---

[1] See preamble, p. 18.

5. References

Barnes, C.D. & Eltherington, L.G. (1964) *Drug Dosage in Laboratory Animals, a Handbook*, Berkeley, CA, University of California Press, p. 176

Caddy, B. & Stead, A.H. (1977) Indirect determination of phenelzine in urine. *Analyst, 102*, 42-49

Caddy, B., Stead, A.H. & Johnstone, E.C. (1978) The urinary excretion of phenelzine. *Br. J. clin. Pharmacol., 6*, 185-188

Clineschmidt, B.V. & Horita, A. (1969) The monoamine oxidase catalysed degradation of phenelzine-1-^{14}C, an irreversible inhibitor of monoamine oxidase-II. *Biochem. Pharmacol., 18*, 1021-1028

Cooper, T.B., Robinsin, D.S. & Nies, A. (1978) Phenelzine measurement in human plasma: a sensitive GLC-ECD procedure. *Commun. Psychopharmacol., 2*, 505-512

Daly, R.E. (1973) *Phenelzine sulfate*. In: Florey, K., ed., *Analytical Profiles of Drug Substances*, Vol. 2, New York, Academic Press, pp. 383-407

Daneshmend, T.K., Scott, G.L. & Bradfield, J.W.B. (1979) Angiosarcoma of liver associated with phenelzine. *Br. med. J., i*, 1679

Freese, E., Sklarow, S. & Bautz Freese, E. (1968) DNA damage caused by antidepressant hydrazines and related drugs. *Mutat. Res., 5*, 343-348

Goodman, L.S. & Gilman, A., eds (1975) *The Pharmacological Basis of Therapeutics*, 5th ed., New York, Macmillan, pp. 177-188

Lapin, I.P. & Samsonova, M.L. (1969) Comparison of pharmacological activity and toxicity of the antidepressants - nialamid, phenelzine and iproniazid (Russ.). *Farmakol. Toksikol., 32*, 526-530

Leverett, R., Leeson, G.A. & Dubnick, B. (1960) Metabolism of β-phenylethylhydrazine (Abstract no. 172). *Abstr. Am. chem. Soc.*, p. 65C

National Formulary Board (1975) *National Formulary*, 14th ed., Washington DC, American Pharmaceutical Association, pp. 556-557

Poulson, E. & Robson, J.M. (1964) Effect of phenelzine and some related compounds on pregnancy and on sexual development. *J. Endocrinol., 30*, 205-215

Rosenkranz, H.S. & Carr, H.S. (1971) Hydrazine antidepressants and isoniazid: potential carcinogens. *Lancet, i*, 1354-1355

Shimizu, H., Hayashi, K. & Takemura, N. (1978) Relationships between the mutagenic and carcinogenic effects of hydrazine derivatives (Jpn.). *Jpn. J. Hyg., 33*, 474-485

Swinyard, E.A. (1975) *Psychopharmacologic agents*. In: Osol, A., ed., *Remington's Pharmaceutical Sciences*, 15th ed., Easton, PA, Mack Publishing Co., pp. 1032-1033

Toth, B. (1976) Tumorigenicity of β-phenylethylhydrazine sulfate in mice. *Cancer Res., 36*, 917-921

Toth, B. & Nagel, D. (1976) Tumorigenesis investigations with β-phenylethylhydrazine sulfate, phenylhydrazine hydrochloride, and ethylhydrazine hydrochloride in mice (Abstract no. 41). *Am. J. Pathol., 82*, 40a-41a

Toth, B. & Shimizu, H. (1974) 1-Carbamyl-2-phenylhydrazine tumorigenesis in Swiss mice. Morphology of lung adenomas. *J. natl Cancer Inst., 52*, 241-251

US International Trade Commission (1979) *Imports of Benzenoid Chemicals and Products, 1978*, USITC Publication 990, Washington DC, US Government Printing Office, p. 86

Wade, A., ed. (1977) *Martindale, The Extra Pharmacopoeia*, 27th ed., London, The Pharmaceutical Press, pp. 1203-1207

Windholz, M., ed. (1976) *The Merck Index*, 9th ed., Rahway, NJ, Merck & Co., p. 936

PHENOXYBENZAMINE and PHENOXYBENZAMINE HYDROCHLORIDE

These substances were considered by a previous working group, in April, 1975 (IARC, 1975). Since that time new data have become available, and these have been incorporated into the monograph and taken into account in the present evaluation.

1. Chemical and Physical Data

PHENOXYBENZAMINE

1.1 Synonyms and trade names

Chem. Abstr. Services Reg. No.: 59-96-1

Chem. Abstr. Name: Benzenemethanamine, *N*-(2-chloroethyl)-*N*-(1-methyl-2-phenoxyethyl)-

IUPAC Systematic Name: *N*-(2-Chloroethyl)-*N*-(1-methyl-2-phenoxyethyl)-benzylamine

Synonyms: 2-(*N*-Benzyl-2-chloroethylamino)-1-phenoxypropane; benzyl(2-chloroethyl)-(1-methyl-2-phenoxyethyl)amine; *N*-phenoxyisopropyl-*N*-benzyl-β-chloroethylamine

Trade name: Bensylyte

1.2 Structural and molecular formulae and molecular weight

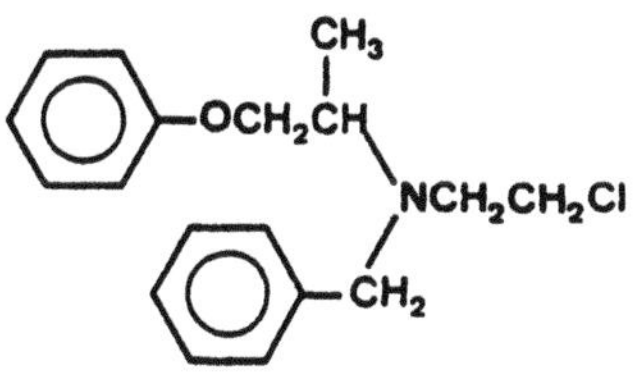

$C_{18}H_{22}ClNO$ Mol. wt: 303.8

1.3 Chemical and physical properties of the pure substance

From Windholz (1976)

- (a) *Description:* Crystals (from petroleum ether)
- (b) *Melting-point:* 38-40°C
- (c) *Solubility:* Soluble in benzene

1.4 Technical products and impurities

Phenoxybenzamine is available only as the hydrochloride.

PHENOXYBENZAMINE HYDROCHLORIDE

1.1 Synonyms and trade names

Chem. Abstr. Services Reg. No.: 63-92-3

Chem. Abstr. Name: Benzenemethanamine, *N*-(2-chloroethyl)-*N*-(1-methyl-2-phenoxyethyl)-, hydrochloride

IUPAC Systematic Name: *N*-(2-Chloroethyl)-*N*-(1-methyl-2-phenoxyethyl)benzylamine hydrochloride

Synonyms: 2-(*N*-Benzyl-2-chloroethylamino)-1-phenoxypropane hydrochloride; benzyl(2-chloroethyl) (1-methyl-2-phenoxyethyl)amine hydrochloride; phenoxybenzamine HCl; *N*-phenoxyisopropyl-*N*-benzyl-β-chloroethylamine hydrochloride

Trade names: Bensylyt NEN; Benzylyt; Blocadren; Dibenylin; Dibenyline; Dibenzylene; Dibenzyline; Dibenzyran; Fenoxybenzamin; SKF 688A

1.2 Structural and molecular formulae and molecular weight

$C_{18}H_{23}Cl_2NO$ Mol. wt: 340.3

1.3 Chemical and physical properties of the pure substance

From Wade (1977)

(a) *Description:* White, odourless, almost tasteless crystalline powder
(b) *Melting-point:* 137.5-140°C
(c) *Spectroscopy data:* λ_{max} (in chloroform) 272 nm, A(1%, 1cm) = 56.3; 279 nm, A(1%, 1cm) = 46.1
(d) *Solubility:* Sparingly soluble in water; soluble in ethanol (1 in 9), chloroform (1 in 9) and propylene glycol; insoluble in diethyl ether
(e) *Stability:* Neutral and alkaline solutions are unstable; sensitive to oxidation and photodegradation

1.4 Technical products and impurities

Phenoxybenzamine hydrochloride is available in the US as a NF grade containing 98.0-101.0% active ingredient calculated on the dried basis. It is also available in 10 mg capsules containing 90.0-110.0% of the labelled amount of phenoxybenzamine hydrochloride (National Formulary Board, 1975).

The *British Pharmacopoeia* specifies a purity of not less than 98.5% and gives a thin-layer chromatography test to limit the presence of related substances. The loss on drying should not exceed 0.5% and the sulphated ash not more than 0.1% (British Pharmacopoeia Commission, 1973).

2. Production, Use, Occurrence and Analysis

2.1 Production and use

(a) Production

Phenoxybenzamine can be prepared by the treatment of 2-phenoxy-1-methyl ethanol with thionyl chloride to yield 2-phenoxy-1-methyl-1-chloroethane, which is treated with ethanolamine. The reaction product is then alkylated with benzyl chloride to produce the N-benzyl derivative. Subsequent treatment with thionyl chloride yields phenoxybenzamine hydrochloride, which can be neutralized to produce the free base (Kerwin & Ullyot, 1954).

Phenoxybenzamine hydrochloride has been produced by a single company in the US since 1953, in an undisclosed amount (see preamble, p. 21). Phenoxybenzamine hydrochloride is believed to be produced by a single company in Italy. It is not produced in Japan.

(b) Use

Phenoxybenzamine hydrochloride is an α-adrenergic receptor blocking agent with prolonged action. It is used in the treatment of peripheral vascular disorders such as Raynaud's disease, acrocyanosis, frostbite sequelae, acute arterial occlusion and other conditions with vasospasm, and in phlebitis, phlebothrombosis, diabetic gangrene, causalgia and chronic skin ulcers. It is also used to control hypertension caused by phaeochromocytoma and has been given intravenously in the treatment of shock. In chronic treatment, dosage may vary from 10 to 200 mg/day (Goodman & Gilman, 1975; Harvey, 1975).

2.2 Occurrence

Phenoxybenzamine and phenoxybenzamine hydrochloride are not known to occur in nature.

2.3 Analysis

Phenoxybenzamine can be determined by thin-layer chromatography using a solvent system of heptane, chloroform and methanol (Masuoka *et al.*, 1967). The phenoxybenzamine hydrochloride content of a chloroform solution can be determined by ultraviolet spectrometry (US Pharmacopeial Convention, Inc., 1975).

3. Biological Data Relevant to the Evaluation of Carcinogenic Risk to Humans

3.1 Carcinogenicity studies in animals

Intraperitoneal administration

Mouse: Three groups of 10 male and 10 female A/He mice, 6-8 weeks old, were given 4 i.p. injections (injection interval not specified) of phenoxybenzamine (free base) dissolved in tricaprylin to give total doses of 40, 100 or 200 mg/kg bw. Twenty-four weeks after the first injection, the 20, 14 and 7 survivors in the 3 groups, respectively, were killed, and 9, 9 and 3 had lung tumours, with averages of 0.45, 0.79 and 0.71 tumours per mouse. As controls, 80 mice of each sex received 24 weekly injections of tricaprylin; of the 77 male and 77 female survivors in each group, lung tumours were found in 28% of males (average, 0.24 tumours/mouse) and 20% of females (average, 0.20 tumours/mouse) (Stoner *et al.*, 1973). [The difference in incidence of lung tumours between treated and control mice was statistically significant at the low ($P<0.05$) and medium ($P<0.01$) dose levels. The short duration of the test may have precluded the observation of tumours at sites other than the lung.]

Groups of 35 male and 35 female $B6C3F_1$ mice, 6-8 weeks old at the start of the experiment, received 12.5 or 25 mg/kg bw phenoxybenzamine hydrochloride 3 times a week, in phosphate-buffered saline containing 0.05% polysorbate 80 for the first 10 weeks and then in 6% propylene glycol in saline for an additional 42 weeks (1 ml/100 g bw). Due to the death of all high-dose male mice, treatment lasted only 50 weeks in this group. A group of 14 male and 16 female mice and one of 15 males and 15 females were kept as untreated and vehicle-treated controls, respectively. All surviving mice were killed at 83-85 weeks. In the high-dose group, 17/21 males ($P<0.001$) and 16/20 females ($P<0.001$) developed abdominal cavity (peritoneal) sarcomas. No such tumours were found in the low-dose group (0/30 males, 0/33 females) or in the controls. There was no significant difference in the incidence of other types of tumours among treated and control mice (National Cancer Institute, 1978).

Rat: Groups of 35 male and 35 female Sprague-Dawley rats, 5-6 weeks old at the start of treatment, received 5 or 10 mg/kg bw phenoxybenzamine hydrochloride 3 times a week, in phosphate-buffered saline for the first week, in phosphate-buffered saline containing 0.05% polysorbate 80 for 13 weeks and then in 6% propylene glycol in saline for an additional 37 weeks (0.25 ml/100 g bw). Two groups of 10 male and 10 female rats each were kept as untreated and vehicle-treated controls. The experiment was terminated at 82-85 weeks. The incidence of abdominal cavity (peritoneal) sarcomas was 16/20 in males and 16/30 in females in the high-dose group (P<0.001 and 0.004), and 11/31 in males (P = 0.027) and 0/35 in females in the low-dose group. No such tumours were found in the control groups. There was no significant difference in the incidence of other types of tumours among treated and control rats (National Cancer Institute, 1978).

3.2 Other relevant biological data

(a) Experimental systems

Toxic effects

The oral LD_{50} of phenoxybenzamine hydrochloride in rats is 2500 mg/kg bw and that for guinea-pigs 500 mg/kg bw (Barnes & Eltherington, 1965).

Prenatal toxicity

No decrease in implantation rate was found in rats fed 10 mg/kg bw daily on the first 5 days of gestation (Saksena & Gokhale, 1972) or given an i.p. dose of 20 mg/kg bw phenoxybenzamine hydrochloride on days 2-5 (Sethi & Chaudhury, 1970).

Absorption, distribution, excretion and metabolism

After i.v. injection into mice of 0.54 mg, ^{14}C-phenoxybenzamine hydrochloride remained in blood for 40 minutes. Radioactive material was widely distributed in the tissues (notably the heart and central nervous system), and persisted for 4 days. Biliary excretion was an important route of elimination (Masuoka *et al.*, 1967).

After oral or i.p. administration of ^{15}N-labelled phenoxybenzamine hydrochloride to rats (20 mg/kg bw) and after oral administration to dogs (10 mg/kg bw), the following urinary metabolites were identified: *N*-benzyl-*N*-(*para*-hydroxyphenoxyisopropyl)amine was found to be the major metabolite in both species; *N*-benzyl-*N*-phenoxyisopropylamine was a minor metabolite in dogs and was also observed in small amounts in rats, only after i.p. injection; and phenoxyisopropylamine was found to be a metabolite in dogs. 2-Benzylamino-1-propanol was found in rat urine after i.p. but not after oral dosing (Knapp *et al.*, 1976).

Mutagenicity and other, related short-term tests

It was reported in an abstract that phenoxybenzamine increased the number of micronucleated erythrocytes in mouse bone marrow (Molina *et al.*, 1978).

(b) Humans

Phenoxybenzamine hydrochloride blocks α-adrenergic receptors with actions on the peripheral vascular system (Goodman & Gilman, 1975).

Toxic effects

Side effects reported in persons taking phenoxybenzamine include postural hypotension with dizziness, compensatory tachycardia, nasal stuffiness, inhibition of ejaculation, nausea and vomiting, miosis and lassitude (Goodman & Gilman, 1975; Roberts & Breckenridge, 1975).

Metabolism

N-Benzyl-*N*-(*para*-hydroxyphenoxyisopropyl)amine was identified in the urine of two patients treated orally with 10 mg/day phenoxybenzamine hydrochloride (Knapp *et al.*, 1976).

No data on the prenatal toxicity or mutagenicity of phenoxybenzamine in humans were available.

3.3 Case reports and epidemiological studies of carcinogenicity in humans

No data were available to the Working Group.

4. Summary of Data Reported and Evaluation

4.1 Experimental data

Phenoxybenzamine was tested intraperitoneally in mice; it produced an increased incidence of lung tumours.

Phenoxybenzamine hydrochloride was tested intraperitoneally in mice and rats; it produced local peritoneal sarcomas in animals of both sexes.

Attention is drawn to the absence of adequate studies on the mutagenicity or teratogenicity of phenoxybenzamine or its hydrochloride.

4.2 Human data

Phenoxybenzamine hydrochloride has limited use as an α-adrenergic receptor blocking agent.

No case reports or epidemiological studies were available to the Working Group.

4.3 Evaluation

There is *sufficient evidence*[1] that phenoxybenzamine hydrochloride is carcinogenic in experimental animals by intraperitoneal administration. No data on humans were available.

---

[1] See preamble, p. 18.

5. References

Barnes, C.D. & Eltherington, L.G. (1965) *Drug Dosages in Laboratory Animals, a Handbook*, Berkeley, CA, University of California Press, p. 176

British Pharmacopoeia Commission (1973) *British Pharmacopoeia*, London, Her Majesty's Stationery Office, p. 361

Goodman, L.S. & Gilman, A., eds (1975) *The Pharmacological Basis of Therapeutics*, 5th ed., New York, Macmillan, pp. 533-540

Harvey, S.C. (1975) *Adrenergic blocking drugs*. In: Osol, A., ed., *Remington's Pharmaceutical Sciences*, 15th ed., Easton, PA, Mack Publishing Co., p. 834

IARC (1975) *IARC Monographs on the Evaluation of Carcinogenic Risk of Chemicals to Man*, Vol. 9, *Some aziridines, N- S- and O-mustards and selenium*, Lyon, pp. 223-228

Kerwin, J.F. & Ullyot, G.E. (1954) *N-(2-Phenoxyisopropyl)ethanolamines*. US Patent 2,683,719, 13 July to Smith, Kline & French Laboratories [*Chem. Abstr.*, 49, 11011-11012]

Knapp, D.R., Holcombe, N.H., Krueger, S.A. & Privitera, P.J. (1976) Qualitative metabolic fate of phenoxybenzamine in rat, dog, and man. Use of ^{15}N-labeling. *Drug Metab. Disposition, 4*, 164-168

Masuoka, D., Appelgren, L.-E. & Hansson, E. (1967) Autoradiographic distribution studies of adrenergic blocking agents. I. Phenoxybenzamine-^{14}C (Bensylyt NFN), an α-receptor-type blocking agent. *Acta pharmacol. toxicol. (Kbh), 25*, 113-122

Molina, L., Rinkus, S. & Legator, M.S. (1978) Evaluation of the micronucleus procedure over a 2-year period (Abstract). *Mutat. Res., 53*, 125

National Cancer Institute (1978) *Bioassay of Phenoxybenzamine Hydrochloride for Possible Carcinogenicity (Tech. Rep. Ser. No. 72)*, US Department of Health, Education, & Welfare Publication No. (NIH) 78-1322, Washington DC, US Government Printing Office

National Formulary Board (1975) *National Formulary*, 14th ed., Washington DC, American Pharmaceutical Association, pp. 556-557

Roberts, J.B. & Breckenridge, A.M. (1975) *Drugs affecting autonomic functions.* In: Dukes, M.N.G., ed., *Meyler's Side Effects of Drugs,* Vol. 8, Amsterdam, Excerpta Medica, p. 310

Saksena, S.K. & Gokhale, S.V. (1972) Effect of some adrenergic receptor blocking drugs on early pregnancy in rats. *Indian J. med. Res., 60,* 281-283

Sethi, A. & Chaudhury, R.R. (1970) Effect of adrenergic receptor-blocking drugs in pregnancy in rats. *J. Reprod. Fertil., 21,* 551-554

Stoner, G.D., Shimkin, M.B., Kniazeff, A.J., Weisburger, J.H., Weisburger, E.K. & Gori, G.B. (1973) Test for carcinogenicity of food additives and chemotherapeutic agents by the pulmonary tumor response in strain A mice. *Cancer Res., 13,* 3069-3085

US Pharmacopeial Convention, Inc. (1975) *The US Pharmacopeia,* 19th rev., Rockville, MD, p. 746

Wade, A., ed. (1977) *Martindale, The Extra Pharmacopoeia,* 27th ed., London, The Pharmaceutical Press, pp. 1655-1657

Windholz, M., ed. (1976) *The Merck Index,* 9th ed., Rahway, NJ, Merck & Co., pp. 943-944

PROFLAVINE, PROFLAVINE DIHYDROCHLORIDE, PROFLAVINE HEMISULPHATE and PROFLAVINE MONOHYDROCHLORIDE

1. Chemical and Physical Data

PROFLAVINE

1.1 Synonyms and trade names

Chem. Abstr. Services Reg. No.: 92-62-6

Chem. Abstr. and IUPAC Systematic Name: 3,6-Acridinediamine

Synonyms: 2,8-Diaminoacridinium; 3,6-diaminoacridinium; 3,7-diamino-5-aza-anthracene; proflavin

Trade names: Isoflav base; Profoliol; Profoliol-B; Proformiphen; Profundol; Profura; Progarmed; Pro-Gen; Progesic

1.2 Structural and molecular formulae and molecular weight

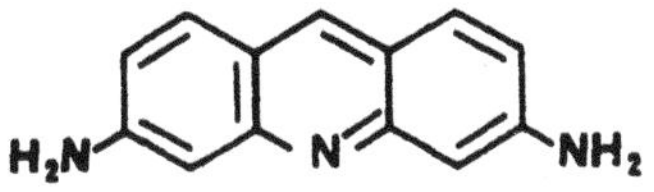

$C_{13}H_{11}N_3$ Mol. wt: 209.3

1.3 Chemical and physical properties of the pure substance

From Weast (1977)

(a) *Description*: Yellow needles from water or ethanol
(b) *Melting-point*: 284-286°C
(c) *Solubility*: Soluble in boiling-water and ethanol

1.4 Technical products and impurities

There are no technical products or pharmaceutical preparations containing the free base, which is used as an intermediate in the preparation of the dihydrochloride, hemisulphate and monohydrochloride salts.

PROFLAVINE DIHYDROCHLORIDE

1.1 Synonyms and trade names

Chem. Abstr. Services Reg. No.: 531-73-7

Chem. Abstr. and IUPAC Systematic Name: 3,6-Acridinediamine, dihydrochloride

Synonyms: 3,6-Diaminoacridine dihydrochloride; 2,8-diaminoacridinium chloride hydrochloride; 3,6-diaminoacridinium chloride hydrochloride; proflavin dihydrochloride

1.2 Structural and molecular formulae and molecular weight

$C_{13}H_{11}N_3 \cdot 2HCl$ Mol. wt: 282.2

1.3 Chemical and physical properties of the pure substance

From Windholz (1976)

(a) *Description:* The dihydrate is an orange-red to brown-red crystalline powder
(b) *Solubility:* Soluble in water (1 in 10 w/v); very slightly soluble in diethyl ether, chloroform and liquid petroleum
(c) *Stability:* Sensitive to oxidation and light

1.4 Technical products and impurities

There are no technical products or pharmaceutical preparations containing proflavine dihydrochloride.

PROFLAVINE HEMISULPHATE

1.1 Synonyms and trade names

Chem. Abstr. Services Reg. No.: 1811-28-5

Chem. Abstr. Name: 3,6-Acridinediamine, sulfate (2:1)

IUPAC Systematic Name: 3,6-Acridinediamine sulfate

Synonyms: 3,6-Acridinediamine sulphate; 3,6-diaminoacridine bisulphate; 3,6-diaminoacridine sulphate (1:1); 3,6-diaminoacridinium monohydrogen sulphate; 2,8-diaminoacridinium sulphate; neutral proflavine sulphate; proflavin hemisulphate; flavin sulphate; proflavine sulphate

Trade names: Flavine; Isoflav; Pancridine; Sanoflavin

1.2 Structural and molecular formulae and molecular weight

$[H_2N\text{-acridine-}NH_2]_2 \cdot H_2SO_4$

$C_{26}H_{22}N_6 \cdot H_2SO_4$ Mol. wt: 516.6

1.3 Chemical and physical properties of the pure substance

From Wade (1977)

(a) Description: Orange-to-red, odourless, hygroscopic, crystalline powder with a bitter taste

(b) Solubility: Soluble in cold water (1 in 300 w/v), boiling-water (1 in 1 w/v) and glycerol (1 in 35 w/v); very slightly soluble in ethanol; insoluble in chloroform and diethyl ether

(c) Stability: Sensitive to oxidation and light

1.4 Technical products and impurities

Published specifications for proflavine hemisulphate are included in the *Belgian Pharmacopoeia* (Anon., 1962) (monohydrate) and in the *British Pharmaceutical Codex* (Pharmaceutical Society of Great Britain, 1973) (dihydrate). The latter requires a purity, expressed as the anhydrous substance, of not less than 98% and imposes a test for certain other acridine derivatives that may be present as impurities. Proflavine is used for local application only and is available in the form of a lotion (containing from 0.1-1% of the hemisulphate), as pessaries (0.2% of the hemisulphate in a glycerol base) and as a cream (containing 0.1% of the hemisulphate in an emulsified base) (Wade, 1977).

PROFLAVINE MONOHYDROCHLORIDE

1.1 Synonyms and trade names

Chem. Abstr. Services Reg. No.: 952-23-8

Chem. Abstr. and IUPAC Systematic Name: 3,6-Acridinediamine monohydrochloride

Synonyms: 3,6-Diaminoacridine monohydrochloride; 3,6-diaminoacridinium chloride hydrochloride; 2,8-diaminoacridinium chloride monohydrochloride; proflavin monohydrochloride

1.2 Structural and molecular formulae and molecular weight

$C_{13}H_{11}N_3 \cdot HCl$ Mol. wt: 246.5

1.3 Chemical and physical properties of the pure substance

From Windholz (1976)

(a) Stability: Sensitive to oxidation and light

1.4 Technical products and impurities

At present there are no technical products or pharmaceutical preparations containing proflavine monohydrochloride.

2. Production, Use, Occurrence and Analysis

2.1 Production and use

(a) Production

Proflavine was first synthesized by the condensation of *meta*-phenylenediamine and formic acid in 1919 (Windholz, 1976). In 1941, methods were described for the preparation of proflavine as the result of a single condensation, starting from *meta*-phenylenediamine (with oxalic or formic acid), from *meta*-amino-oxanilic acid, or from mono(or di)-formyl-*meta*-phenylenediamine (Albert, 1941). It is not known whether any of these methods are used for commercial production of proflavine.

No evidence was found that proflavine or its salts have ever been produced in commercial quantities in the US. US imports of proflavine hemisulphate through the principal US customs districts amounted to 10 kg in 1977 (US International Trade Commission, 1978).

(b) Use

The different salts of proflavine are slow-acting disinfectants. They are bacteriostatic against many gram-positive bacteria, but less effective against gram-negative organisms, and not effective against *Proteus vulgaris, Pseudomonas aeruginosa*, some strains of *Escherichia coli* or acid-fast bacteria. They also inactivate or inhibit some viruses (Wade, 1977).

The proflavine salts are used as topical antiseptics for treatment of contaminated or suppurative wounds and for disinfection of the skin. For the treatment of infected wounds and burns, they are used once or twice daily, usually as a 0.1% solution, but strengths ranging from 0.1-1% have been used for the treatment of local infections of the ear, mouth and throat. In preliminary studies, proflavine (0.1% solution) has been painted on ulcers caused by herpes virus followed by exposure to incandescent or fluorescent light (Wade, 1977), and it has been considered for reintroduction for use against psoriasis in conjuction with ultra-violet light (National Cancer Institute, 1977).

Proflavine dihydrochloride is a component (along with the hydrochloride of 3,6-diamino-10-methylacridinium chloride) of acriflavinium chloride (see IARC, 1977), a topical antiseptic. Acridine derivatives were reported to have been withdrawn from use in Sweden in 1979.

Proflavine salts are reportedly used as topical antiseptics in veterinary medicine (Windholz, 1976).

2.2 Occurrence

Proflavine and its salts are not known to occur in nature.

2.3 Analysis

No data were available to the Working Group.

3. Biological Data Relevant to the Evaluation of Carcinogenic Risk to Man

3.1 Carcinogenicity studies in animals

(a) Oral administration

Mouse: Groups of 50 male and 50 female B6C3F1 mice, 5-6 weeks of age, were fed diets containing 200 or 400 mg/kg diet proflavine monohydrochloride, as the hemihydrate[1], for up to 104 weeks. (The percentage of amine was 103.4 ± 0.3% of the theoretical amount; minor unidentified impurities were present.) Of the treated mice, 20/49 females (P<0.001) and 28/49 males in the low-dose group, and 22/50 females (P<0.001) and 30/50 males (P = 0.04) in the high-dose group developed hepatocellular carcinomas, compared with 4/50 and 20/49, respectively, in the controls. Haemangiosarcomas of the liver developed in 0/49 females and 6/49 males in the low-dose group and in 2/50 females and 3/50 males in the high-dose group, compared with 1/50 and 6/49, respectively, in the controls. The overall incidence of malignant lymphomas was high: 16/50 females and 11/50 males in the low-dose group, and 20/50 females and 13/50 males in the high-dose group, compared with 23/50 and 11/50, respectively, in the controls. Because a positive control carcinogen, *N*-2-fluorenylacetamide, was tested in the same room with these animals, the authors questioned the validity of these bioassay results; the statistical inference was made, however, that in female mice there was a strong association of development of hepatocellular carcinomas with the dose of proflavine monohydrochloride hemihydrate administered (National Cancer Institute, 1977). [The Working Group could not assess the significance of these results, given the possibility that the experimental animals were exposed to a known carcinogen.]

Rat: Proflavine monochloride, as the hemihydrate (percentage of amine, 103.4 ± 0.3% of the theoretical amount; minor unidentified impurities present), was administered in the diet at concentrations of 300 or 600 mg/kg diet to groups of 50 male and 50 female Fischer 344/ CR rats, 5-6 weeks of age, for 109 weeks. In male rats in the high-dose group, 3/48 leiomyosarcomas of the small intestine, 1/48 adenocarcinoma of the small intestine, 1/48 sarcoma of the large intestine and 1/49 hepatocellular carcinoma occurred; 1/50 females in the high-dose group developed a hepatocellular carcinoma. Hepatocellular carcinomas occurred in 1/50 males and 2/50 females in the low-dose group. None of these tumours occurred in the control group. The incidences of other neoplasms in treated animals were approximately the same or lower than those reported for controls (National Cancer Institute, 1977).

---

[1] $C_{12}H_{11}N_3 \cdot HCl \cdot \frac{1}{2}H_2O$

(b) Skin application

Mouse: In a study in which the tumour-promoting effect of sclerosing agents was investigated on skin initiated with 9,10-dimethyl-1,2-benzanthracene, a control group of 20 male albino 's' strain mice were given weekly skin applications of 0.3 ml of a 1% solution of proflavine hemisulphate (B.P.) alone in 1:2 water:carbowax 300 for 24 weeks. No tumours were found in this group within 31 weeks. In addition, no tumour-promoting effect of proflavine hemisulphate was noted in this experiment (Salaman & Glendenning, 1957). [Attention was drawn to the short duration of treatment.]

(c) Other experimental systems

Intradermal administration: In a study in which the tumour-promoting effect of sclerosing agents was investigated on skin initiated with 9,10-dimethyl-1,2-benzanthracene, a control group of 20 male albino 's' strain *mice* were given weekly intradermal injections in 4 areas of 0.1 ml of a 0.1% solution of proflavine hemisulphate (B.P.) in water for 24 weeks. No tumours were found in this group within 46 weeks. However, the intradermal injections of proflavine hemisulphate enhanced the development of skin tumours which occurred in 12/27 animals after 33 weeks following the initiation (Salaman & Glendenning, 1957). [Attention was drawn to the short duration of treatment.]

Subcutaneous implantation: In a study in which the tumour-promoting effect of sclerosing agents was investigated on skin initiated with 9,10-dimethyl-1,2-benzanthracene, two solid pellets of proflavine hemisulphate (B.P.) suspended in paraffin wax were implanted subcutaneously in the backs of a control group of 20 male albino 's' *mice*. No tumours were found within 47 weeks. No tumour-promoting effect of proflavine hemisulphate was noted in this experiment (Salaman & Glendenning, 1957). [Attention was drawn to the short duration of treatment.]

3.2 Other relevant biological data

(a) *Experimental systems*

Toxic effects

The s.c. LD_{50} of proflavine in mice is 140 mg/kg bw (Rubbo, 1947).

The incorporation of ^{3}H-thymidine into mouse testicular DNA *in vivo* was reduced by an i.p. injection of 100 mg/kg bw proflavine (Seiler, 1977). Proflavine also inhibited the incorporation of radioactive precursors into DNA, RNA and protein of HeLa cells *in vitro;* RNA was the most and protein the least sensitive target (Watts & Davis, 1966).

No data were available on the prenatal toxicity, absorption, distribution, excretion or metabolism of proflavine.

Mutagenicity and other, related short-term tests

The mutagenicity of proflavine and other acridines has been reviewed (Nasim & Brychcy, 1979); in most studies, the salt of proflavine used was not specified.

Proflavine binds to DNA and RNA by intercalation (Lerman, 1961; Scholtissek & Rott, 1964; Georghiou, 1977). Thus, it induces frameshift mutations in various bacteriophages and viruses (DeMars, 1953; Orgel & Brenner, 1961; Gendon, 1963; Drake, 1970; Kadohama et al., 1972; Pervikov et al., 1973; Haspel & Rapp, 1975). In the presence of proflavine or its hemisulphate, visible light has an inactivating (lethal) effect on DNA, phage and bacteria (Kaufman & Hiatt, 1959; Ritchie, 1965; Janíková, 1966; Piette et al., 1978) as well as a mutagenic effect (Ritchie, 1964; Brendel, 1973; Piette et al., 1978). However, no prophage induction could be obtained (Speck et al., 1978).

Proflavine and its hemisulphate are mutagenic for *Escherichia coli* (DeMars, 1953; Zampieri & Greenberg, 1965; Maillet, 1969). It has been found to induce forward mutations to 8-azaguanine-resistance in *Salmonella typhimurium* TM35 and TM677 (Skopek et al., 1978) as well as reverse mutations in TA1537, TA1538, TA98 and TA100 (McCann et al., 1975; Gatehouse, 1978; Skopek et al., 1978).

Exposure of *Salmonella* strains to proflavine in the dark resulted in frameshift mutagenesis (i.e., reversion of TA1537 and TA98), whereas, in the light, base substitution (TA1535) as well as frameshift mutations (TA1537, TA1538, TA98) occurred. In the presence of a liver microsome activating system, mutagenic activity could also be observed with TA1538 (Speck & Rosenkranz, 1980).

Proflavine did not induce reverse mutations in *Saccharomyces cerevisiae* (Brusick & Zeiger, 1972), but it induced mitotic gene conversion (Fahrig, 1970).

Feeding *Drosophila melanogaster* larvae on proflavine dihydrochloride produced no mutations and only a slight increase in nondisjunction (Ostertag & Haake, 1966). Feeding of adult *Drosophila* with proflavine (salt unspecified) had no effect on chromosome loss or nondisjunction (Mittler, 1976).

Treatment of HeLa cells with proflavine hemisulphate hemihydrate resulted in a large increase of chromatid breakage (Ostertag & Kersten, 1965). Chromatid breaks were also observed in conjunction with sister chromatid exchange in Chinese hamster Don-D6 and V79-4 cells with proflavine (salt unspecified) (Kato, 1974; Popescu et al., 1977). Sister chromatid exchanges were also obtained by treatment of human lymphocytes *in vitro* with proflavine hemisulphate (Crossen, 1979).

Sister chromatid exchanges were also induced by proflavine in a V79 Chinese hamster cell line in the dark and (in enhanced numbers) in the presence of visible light (Speit & Vogel, 1979).

Exposure to proflavine and visible light inactivated *Herpes simplex* virus type 2; when hamster embryo cells were treated with such inactivated virus they underwent morphological transformation *in vitro* and produced undifferentiated fibrosarcomas (with no detectable virus) when inoculated into newborn hamsters (Li & Rapp, 1976).

(b) Humans

Dermatitis has been reported to be associated with topical application of proflavine dihydrochloride (Mitchell, 1972). Skin sensitivity to proflavine hemisulphate, confirmed by patch tests, was observed in 3 subjects (Morgan, 1968).

No data on the prenatal toxicity, absorption, distribution, metabolism or mutagenicity of proflavine in humans were available.

3.3 Case reports and epidemiological studies of carcinogenicity in humans

No data were available to the Working Group.

4. Summary of Data Reported and Evaluation

4.1 Experimental data

Proflavine monohydrochloride, as the hemihydrate, was tested in mice and rats by oral administration. Proflavine hemisulphate was tested in mice by skin application, intradermal administration and subcutaneous implantation. All tests were inadequate for evaluation.

Proflavine is mutagenic in viral and bacterial systems. It increased the number of chromatid breaks and induced sister chromatid exchanges in mammalian cells.

Attention is drawn to the absence of studies on the teratogenicity of this compound.

4.2 Human data

Proflavine and its salts have limited use as topical disinfectants.

No case reports or epidemiological studies were available to the Working Group.

4.3 Evaluation

The available experimental results were inadequate for an evaluation of the carcinogenicity of proflavine in experimental animals, and no data were available from human studies. However, in view of its mutagenicity, confirmed in several experimental systems, further studies on the carcinogenicity of this compound are warranted.

5. References

Albert, A. (1941) Acridine syntheses and reactions. Part I. Synthesis of proflavine from *m*-phenylenediamine and its derivatives. *J. chem. Soc.*, 121-125

Anon. (1962) *Pharmacopée Belge*, Vol. 2, 5th ed., Strée (Hainaut), F. & N. Dantinne, pp. 485-486

Brendel, M. (1973) Different photodynamic action of proflavine and methylene blue on bacteriophage. II. Mutation induction in extracellularly treated *Serratiaphage* kappa. *Molec. gen. Genet.*, *120*, 171-180

Brusick, D.J. & Zeiger, E. (1972) A comparison of chemically induced reversion patterns of *Salmonella typhimurium* and *Saccharomyces cerevisiae* mutants, using *in vitro* plate tests. *Mutat. Res.*, *14*, 271-275

Crossen, P.E. (1979) The effect of acridine compounds on sister-chromatid exchange formation in cultured human lymphocytes. *Mutat. Res.*, *68*, 295-299

DeMars, R.I. (1953) Chemical mutagenesis in bacteriophage T2. *Nature*, *172*, 964

Drake, J.W. (1970) *The Molecular Basis of Mutation*, San Francisco, CA, Holden-Day, pp. 123-145

Fahrig, R. (1970) Acridine-induced mitotic gene conversion (paramutation) in *Saccharomyces cerevisiae*. The effect of two different modes of binding to DNA. *Mutat. Res.*, *10*, 509-514

Gatehouse, D. (1978) Detection of mutagenic derivatives of cyclophosphamide and a variety of other mutagens in a 'microtrite'® fluctuation test, without microsomal activation. *Mutat. Res.*, *53*, 289-296

Gendon, Y.Z. (1963) Induction of mutations in poliomyelitis virus by direct action of proflavine on virus RNA. *Vopr. virusol.*, *8*, 542-544

Georghiou, S. (1977) Interaction of acridine drugs with DNA and nucleotides. *Photochem. Photobiol.*, *26*, 59-68

Haspel, M.V. & Rapp, F. (1975) Measles virus: an unwanted variant causing hydrocephalus. *Science*, *187*, 450-451

IARC (1977) *IARC Monographs on the Evaluation of the Carcinogenic Risk of Chemicals to Man*, Vol. 13, *Some miscellaneous pharmaceutical substances*, Lyon, pp. 31-37

Janíková, A. (1966) The photodynamic action of acridine orange and proflavine on the survival of *Escherichia coli* B and its capacity for phage T3. *Folia Biol. (Praha), 12*, 132-136

Kadohama, N., Muhlstock, B. & McCarter, J.A. (1972) Mutagenicity of 10-methylated acridines for bacteriophage T4. *Mutat. Res., 15*, 227-228

Kato, H. (1974) Induction of sister chromatid exchanges by chemical mutagens and its possible relevance to DNA repair. *Exp. Cell Res., 85*, 239-247

Kaufman, E. & Hiatt, C.W. (1959) Photodynamic action of proflavine on T2 coliphage. *Virology, 9*, 478-479

Lerman, L.S. (1961) Structural considerations in the interaction of DNA and acridines. *J. mol. Biol., 3*, 18-30

Li, J.-L.H. & Rapp, F. (1976) Oncogenic transformation of mammalian cells *in vitro* by proflavine-photoinactivated *Herpes simplex* virus type 2. *Cancer Lett., 1*, 319-326

Maillet, S. (1969) Specific mutagenic action of three dyes on the reverse mutation of a gene Pro^-_A in *E. coli* K12 (Fr.). *C.R. Acad. Sci. Paris, 269*, 1708-1711

McCann, J., Choi, E., Yamasaki, E. & Ames, B.N. (1975) Detection of carcinogens as mutagens in the *Salmonella*/microsome test: assay of 300 chemicals. *Proc. natl Acad. Sci. USA, 72*, 5135-5139

Mitchell, J.C. (1972) Contact dermatitis from proflavine dihydrochloride. *Arch. Dermatol., 106*, 924

Mittler, S. (1976) Screening for induced chromosome loss and nondisjunction in *Drosophila melanogaster* (Abstract no. 58). *Mutat. Res., 38*, 406-407

Morgan, J.K. (1968) Iatrogenic epidermal sensitivity. *Br. J. clin. Pract., 22*, 261-264

Nasim, A. & Brychcy, T. (1979) Genetic effects of acridine compounds. *Mutat. Res., 65*, 261-288

National Cancer Institute (1977) *Bioassay of Proflavine for Possible Carcinogenicity (Tech. Rep. Ser. No. 5)*, Department of Health, Education, & Welfare Publication No. (NIH) 77-805, Washington DC, US Government Printing Office

Orgel, A. & Brenner, S. (1961) Mutagenesis of bacteriophage T4 by acridines. *J. mol. Biol., 3*, 762-768

Ostertag, W. & Haake, J. (1966) The mutagenicity in *Drosophila melanogaster* of caffeine and of other compounds which produce chromosome breakage in human cells in culture. *Z. Vererbungsl., 98*, 299-308

Ostertag, W. & Kersten, W. (1965) The action of proflavin and actinomycin D in causing chromatid breakage in human cells. *Exp. Cell Res., 39*, 296-301

Pervikov, Y.V., Vorohsilova, M.K., Chumakov, M.P., Savinov, A.P. & Yurovetskaya, A.L. (1973) Studies on the mutagenic action of proflavine on type 3 poliovirus. *Acta virol., 17*, 365

Pharmaceutical Society of Great Britain (1973) *British Pharmaceutical Codex*, London, The Pharmaceutical Press, p. 407

Piette, J., Calberg-Bacq, C.M. & Van de Vorst, A. (1978) Photodynamic effect of proflavine on ϕX174 bacteriophage, its DNA replicative form and its isolated single-stranded DNA: inactivation, mutagenesis and repair. *Molec. gen. Genet., 167*, 95-103

Popescu, N.C., Turnbull, D. & DiPaolo, J.A. (1977) Sister chromatid exchange and chromosome aberration analysis with the use of several carcinogens and noncarcinogens: brief communication. *J. natl Cancer Inst., 59*, 289-292

Ritchie, D.A. (1964) Mutagenesis with light and proflavine in phage T4. *Genet. Res., Camb., 5*, 168-169

Ritchie, D.A. (1965) The photodynamic action of proflavine on phage T4. *Biochem. biophys. Res. Commun., 20*, 720-726

Rubbo, S.D. (1947) The influence of chemical constitution on toxicity. Part I: A general survey of the acridine series. *Br. J. exp. Pathol., 28*, 1-11

Salaman, M.H. & Glendenning, O.M. (1957) Tumour promotion in mouse skin by sclerosing agents. *Br. J. Cancer, 11*, 434-444

Scholtissek, C. & Rott, R. (1964) Binding of proflavine to deoxyribonucleic acid and ribonucleic acid and its biological significance. *Nature, 204*, 39-43

Seiler, J.P. (1977) Inhibition of testicular DNA synthesis by chemical mutagens and carcinogens. Preliminary results in the validation of a novel short term test. *Mutat. Res., 46*, 305-310

Skopek, T.R., Liber, H.L., Kaden, D.A. & Thilly, W.G. (1978) Relative sensitivities of forward and reverse mutation assays in *Salmonella typhimurium. Proc. natl Acad. Sci. USA, 75*, 4465-4469

Speck, W.T. & Rosenkranz, H.S. (1980) Proflavine: an unusual mutagen. *Mutat. Res., 77*, 37-43

Speck, W.T., Santella, R.M. & Rosenkranz, H.S. (1978) An evaluation of the prophage λ induction (inductest) for the detection of potential carcinogens. *Mutat. Res., 54*, 101-104

Speit, G. & Vogel, W. (1979) The effect on sister-chromatid exchanges of drugs and dyes by intercalation and photoactivation. *Mutat. Res., 59*, 223-229

US International Trade Commission (1978) *Imports of Benzenoid Chemical and Products, 1977*, USITC Publication 900, Washington DC, US Government Printing Office, p. 87

Wade, A., ed. (1977) *Martindale, The Extra Pharmacopoeia*, 27th ed., London, The Pharmaceutical Press, pp. 531-532

Watts, J.W. & Davis, M.A.F. (1966) The effect of proflavine on HeLa cells. *Biochem. J., 100*, 467-472

Weast, R.C. (1977) *CRC Handbook of Chemistry and Physics*, 56th ed., Cleveland, OH, Chemical Rubber Co., p. C-96

Windholz, M., ed. (1976) *The Merck Index*, 9th ed., Rahway, NJ, Merck & Co., p. 1007

Zampieri, A. & Greenberg, J. (1965) Mutagenesis by acridine orange and proflavine in *Escherichia coli* strain S. *Mutat. Res., 2*, 552-556

RESERPINE

This substance was considered by a previous working group, in October 1975 (IARC, 1976). Since that time new data have become available, and these have been incorporated into the monograph and taken into account in the present evaluation.

1. Chemical and Physical Data

1.1 Synonyms and trade names

Chem. Abstr. Services Reg. No.: 50-55-5

Chem. Abstr. Name: Yohimban-16-carboxylic acid, 11,17-dimethoxy-18-[(3,4,5-trimethoxybenzoyl)oxy]-, methyl ester, (3β,16β,17α,18β,20α)-

IUPAC Systematic Name: Methyl 11, 17α-dimethoxy-18β (3,4,5-trimethoxybenzoyloxy)-3β, 20α-yohimbane-16β-carboxylate

Synonyms: 11,17α-Dimethoxy-18β[(3,4,5-trimethoxybenzoyl)oxy]-3β, 20α-yohimban-16β-carboxylic acid methyl ester; 18β-hydroxy-11,17α-dimethoxy-3β, 20α-yohimban-16β-carboxylic acid methyl ester 3,4,5-trimethoxybenzoate (ester); methyl-1α,2β,3α,4,4aα,5,7,8,13,13bβ,14,14aβ-dodecahydro-2α,11-dimethoxy-3β-(3,4,5-trimethoxybenzoyloxy)benz[g]indolo(2,3α)quinolizine-1β-carboxylate; methyl reserpate 3,4,5-trimethoxybenzoic acid ester; 3,4,5-trimethoxybenzoic acid ester with methyl 18β-hydroxy-11,17α-dimethoxy-3β,20α-yohimban-16β-carboxylate; 3,4,5-trimethoxybenzoyl methyl reserpate; yohimban-16-carboxylic acid derivative of benz[g]indolo(2,3α)quinolizine; 3β,16β,17α,18β,20α-yohimban-16-carboxylic acid-11,17-dimethoxy-18-[(3,4,5-trimethoxybenzoyl)oxy] methyl ester

Trade names: Abesta; Abicol; Adelfan; Adelphane; Adelphin; Adelphin-Esidrex-K; Alkarau; Alkaserp; Alserin; Anquil; Apoplon; Apsical; Arcum R-S; Ascoserp; Austrapine; Banasil; Banisil; Bendigon; Bioserpine; Brinderdin; Briserine; Broserpine; Butiserpazide-25; Butiserpazide-50; Butiserpine; Cardioserpin; Carditivo; Carrserp; Crystoserpine; Darebon; Deserpine; Diupres; Diutensen-R; Drenusil-R; Dypertane Compound; Ebserpine; Elfanex; Elserpine; ENT-50146; Eserpine; Eskaserp; Gamaserpin; Gilucard; Hexaplin; Hiposerpil; Hiserpia; Hydromox R; Hydropres; Hydropres KA; Hygroton-Reserpine; Hypercal B; Hypertane Forte;

Hypertensan; Idoserp; Interpina; Key-Serpine; Kitine; Klimanosid; Lemiserp; Loweserp; Marnitension simple; Maviserpin; Mayserpine; Mephaserpin; Metatensin; Mio-pressin; Modenol; Naquival; Nembu-Serpin; Neo-antitersol; Neo-serfin; Neo-Serp; Neoslowten; Ondasil; Orthoserpina; Perskleran; Pressimedin; Purserpine; Quiescin; Raucap; Raudixin; Raudixoid; Raugal; Raulen; Rauloycin; Rauloydin; Raunervil; Raunormin 'Orzan'; Raupasil; Raurine; Rausan; Rau-Sed; Rausedan; Rausedil; Rausedyl; Rauserpen-Alk; Rauserpin; Rausingle; Rautrin; Rauvilid; Rauwasedin; Rauwilid; Rauwiloid; Rauwiloid +; Rauwipur; Rauwita; Rauwoleaf; Rauwopur 'Byk'; Recipin; Regroton; Renese R; Resaltex; Resedrex; Resedril; Rese-Lar; Reser-Ar; Reserbal; Resercaps; Resercen; Resercrine; Reserfia; Reserjen; Reserlor; Reserpamed; Reserpanca; Reserpene; Reserpex; Reserpidefe; Reserpil; Reserpin; Reserpka; Reserpoid; Reserpur; Reserp 'Wander'; Resersana; Reserutin; Resiatric; Resine; Resocalm; Resomine; Respital; Restran; Rezerpin; Riserpa; Rivased; Rivasin; Rolserp; Roxel; Roxinoid; Salupres; Salutensin; Sandril; Sarpagen; Sedaraupin; Seda-Recipin; Seda-Salurepin; Sedserp; Seominal; Serfin; Serolfia; Serp; Serp-AFD; Serpalan; Serpaloid; Serpanray; Serpasil; Serpasil Apresoline; Serpasil-Esidrex; Serpasil-Esidrex No. 1; Serpasil-Esidrex No. 2; Serpasil-Esidrex K; Serpasil premix; Serpasol; Serpate; Serpatone; Serpax; Serpedin; Serpen; Serpena; Serpentil; Serpentina; Serpentine 'Pharbil'; Serpicon; Serpiloid; Serpilum; Serpine; Serpipur; Serpivite; Serplex K; Serpoid; Serpone; Serpresan; Serpyrit; Sertabs; Sertens; Sertensin; Sertina; Sinesalin composition; Solfo Serpine; Supergan; Temposerpine; Tendoscen-Compr.; Tensanyl; Tenserlix; Tenserp; Tenserpine 'Assia'; Tensional; Tensionorme; Terbolan; Transerpin; Triserpin; T-Serp; Tylandril; Unilord; Unitensen; Vio-Serpine; Vioserpine; Veriloid; V-Serp

1.2 Structural and molecular formulae and molecular weight

$C_{33}H_{40}N_2O_9$ Mol. wt: 608.7

1.3 Chemical and physical properties of the pure substance

From Wade (1977) or Windholz (1976), unless otherwise specified

(a) *Description:* White or slightly yellow crystals or crystalline powder
(b) *Melting-point:* 264-265°C (dec.); 277-277.5°C (dec.) in evacuated tube
(c) *Spectroscopy data:* λ_{max} (in chloroform): 216 nm, A (1%, 1 cm) = 101; 267 nm, A(1%, 1 cm) = 28; 295 nm, A(1%, 1 cm) = 17. Infrared and nuclear magnetic spectral data have been tabulated (Schirmer, 1975).
(d) *Optical rotation:* $[\alpha]_D^{23}$ − 118° (in chloroform);

$[\alpha]_D^{26}$ − 164° (0.96% in pyridine):

$[\alpha]_D^{26}$ − 168° (0.624% in dimethylformamide)
(e) *Solubility:* Practically insoluble in water; soluble in chloroform (1 in 6), dichloromethane, glacial acetic acid, benzene and ethyl acetate; slightly soluble in acetate, methanol, ethanol (1 in 1800), diethyl ether and aqueous solutions of acetic and citric acids
(f) *Stability:* Sensitive to oxidation and hydrolysis. It acquires a yellow colour with pronounced fluorescence, especially after addition of acid or exposure to light.
(g) *Reactivity:* A weak base (pK_a 6.6); forms salts with strong acids

1.4 Technical products and impurities

Various national and international pharmacopoeias give specifications for the purity of reserpine in pharmaceutical products. For example, reserpine is available in the US as a USP grade containing 97.0-101.0% active ingredient on a dried basis. The loss on drying at temperatures below 60°C should not exceed 0.5%, and the residue on ignition should not exceed 0.1%. It is available in injections containing 2.5 and 5 mg/ml reserpine; and in tablets as 0.1, 0.25, 0.5, 1, and 2 mg doses containing 90.0-110.0% of the stated amount of reserpine (US Pharmacopeial Convention, Inc., 1975). In the UK, reserpine is available as 2.5 and 5 mg/ml injections and in 0.1, 0.15, 0.25, 0.5, 1, and 2 mg doses as tablets by itself or in combination with bendrofluazide, phenobarbitone, theobromine hydrochlorothiazide or potassium chloride (Wade, 1977). Perhaps the most exacting specification presently published is that of the *European Pharmacopoeia* (Council of Europe, 1975), which requires a total alkaloid content of not less than 99% and a content of reserpine (by a specific method) of not less than 98%. There is also a test to limit (by light absorption measurements) the presence of oxidation products of reserpine; related alkaloids that may contaminate it include, for example, rescinnamine which may co-exist with reserpine in

Rauwolfia species (AMA Department of Drugs, 1977). Reserpine is available in Japan in 0.03 and 0.25 mg/ml doses as injections and in 0.1, 0.2, and 0.5 mg doses as tablets by itself or in combination with hydralazine hydrochloride.

2. Production, Use, Occurrence and Analysis

2.1 Production and use

(a) Production

Reserpine was isolated from the roots of *Rauwolfia serpentina* L. and its structure determined by Dorfman and coworkers in 1954 (Windholz, 1976). It was first synthesized by the now legendary method of Woodward and co-workers (Woodward *et al.*, 1956). Synthetic reserpine has been marketed, but has at no time been able to compete with the natural product. Natural reserpine is extracted from the roots of various *Rauwolfia* species with alcohols or aqueous acid and then further purified by extraction at pH 3.4-3.6 and crystallization.

There are several suppliers (Sittig, 1979) of reserpine in the US; however, only one company reports production of an undisclosed amount (see preamble, p. 21). According to trade and industry sources, 4 or 5 pharmaceutical companies based in the Federal Republic of Germany, France, Italy, Switzerland and the US account for the bulk of world consumption of *Rauwolfia* root and bark.

Reserpine was first marketed in Japan in 1954. The annual production rate of the two producers remained remarkably stable at approximately 65 kg in 1976-1978.

The major producing countries of *Rauwolfia* are Thailand, India, Nepal, Malaysia, Indonesia and Zaire.

(b) Use

Extracts of *Rauwolfia serpentina* have been used medicinally in India for centuries. They were used in primitive Hindu medicine for a variety of conditions, including snakebite, hypertension, insomnia and insanity. Reserpine is now used primarily as a peripheral antihypertensive and as a central depressant and sedative. It is used alone or in combination with thiazide diuretics for the management of mild labile hypertension and in conjunction with potent hypotensive agents for the management of essential hypertension and hypertension associated with toxaemia of pregnancy. For control of mild or moderate hypertension, the usual dosage for adults is 0.25 mg, 3-4 times daily for 2 weeks; the dosage is then reduced to the lowest dose necessary to maintain the response. Children may be given 20 µg/kg bw daily in divided doses. For hypertensive crises, an i.m. dose of 0.5-1 mg is used; if there is little or no fall in blood pressure within 3 hours, 2-4 mg are given at 3- to 12-hour intervals until the pressure falls to the desired level. Reserpine has also been used as a sedative in mild anxiety states and chronic psychoses in daily doses of 0.1 to 1 mg but is now rarely used for this purpose (Goodman & Gilman, 1975; Harvey, 1975; AMA Department of Drugs, 1977; Wade, 1977; Office de Vulgarisation Pharmaceutique, 1979).

Reserpine is used in veterinary practice as a tranquilizer and sedative for horses, cattle, dogs and cats (Harvey, 1975). It has also been used in feeds for chicken and turkeys as a sedative and to prevent aortic rupture in turkeys (Windholz, 1976).

2.2 Occurrence

Reserpine is a naturally occurring alkaloid produced by several members of the genus *Rauwolfia*, a climbing shrub of the *Apocynaceae* family, indigenous to India, Burma, Malaysia, Thailand, Nepal and Indonesia (Harvey, 1975).

2.3 Analysis

Analytical methods for the determination of reserpine based on chromatography, titration, electrochemistry and spectrometry have been reviewed by Schirmer (1975). Typical methods for the analysis of reserpine in various matrices are summarized in Table 1. Abbreviations used are: CC/F, column chromatography with fluorescence spectrometry; TLC/F, thin-layer chromatography with fluorescence spectrometry; UV, ultra-violet spectrometry; HPLC/F, high-performance liquid chromatography with fluorescence spectrometry.

Table 1. Analytical methods for reserpine

Sample matrix	Sample preparation	Assay procedure	Limit of detection	Reference
Formulations (injections and tablets)	Dissolve in chloroform; add citric acid solution; separate chloroform layer; add sodium bicarbonate; filter into methanol; extract bicarbonate layer with chloroform; collect in two flasks; add hydrochloric acid in methanol; add sodium nitrite to one and add methanol to the other; to both add ammonium sulphamate solution and methanol; measure absorbances from each flask	UV	not given	US Pharmacopeial Convention, Inc., 1975
Rauwolfia serpentina root powder and tablets	Powder; add ethanol; reflux; add chloroform; filter; treat with sulphuric acid; elute organic phase on chromatographic column with methanol and chloroform; add hydrochloric and sulphamic acids	CC/F	not given	Clark, 1970
Plasma	Extract with benzene; oxidize to fluorophor with vanadium pentoxide in phosphoric acid; separate on octadecylsilane column; determine fluorescence	HPLC/F	0.1 µg/l	Sams, 1978
	Add saturated sodium tetraborate solution and benzene; centrifuge; evaporate benzene; dissolve in dichloromethane; spot on TLC plates; develop with glacial acetic acid	TLC/F	10 ng	Sams & Huffman, 1978

3. Biological Data Relevant to the Evaluation of Carcinogenic Risk to Humans

3.1 Carcinogenicity studies in animals[1]

(a) Oral administration

Mouse: A group of 24 female C3H mice 45-50 days of age and a further group of 11 female XV11nc mice of the same age received an average of 0.24 µg reserpine (purity not specified) per day in the food, while 22 C3H controls received the basal diet only. Of the treated C3H females, 15/24 developed mammary carcinomas, the earliest by 216 days and the latest by 15 months; of the controls, 12/12 animals developed mammary tumours, the earliest appearing at 320 days and the latest at 17 months. No mammary tumours occurred in treated XV11nc mice that lived for 200 days to 32 months (Lacassagne & Duplan, 1959). [Attention is drawn to the low dose used.]

Two groups, each of 50 male and 50 female B6C3F1 mice, 5 weeks old, were fed diets containing 5 or 10 mg/kg diet reserpine (USP grade) for 103 weeks and observed for an additional 2 weeks. A third group of 50 mice of each sex were used as matched controls. All surviving animals were killed at the end of 104-105 weeks. Of the 50 high-dose females, 48 were examined; 7 had developed malignant tumours of the mammary glands ($P = 0.005$), while in the low dose-treated females the corresponding figure was 7/49 ($P = 0.006$). No such tumours were found in 50 control females. Of the high-dose males, 5/49 developed carcinomas of the seminal vesicles ($P = 0.027$); while in the low-dose males, the corresponding figure was 1/50. No such tumours were found in 50 control males. The incidences of tumours at other sites were no higher in treated mice than in controls (National Cancer Institute, 1980).

Rat: A group of 92 female and 43 male Wistar rats received 100 µg/kg diet reserpine (purity not specified) daily in a semi-liquid diet. A group of 30 female and 20 male controls received a solid, dry, basal diet only. The experiment lasted 18 months, at which time both test and control animals were sacrificed. The first tumours (lymphosarcomas and hepatomas) appeared in females after 8-8½ months and in males 2 months later; 16% of the test animals, but no controls, developed tumours. In a later experiment, in which 80 female and 50 male Wistar controls received a semi-liquid diet and were killed at 18 months, 13% of the animals developed lymphosarcomas and hepatomas from about the 9th month onwards (Tuchmann-Duplessis & Mercier-Parot, 1962). [Attention is drawn to the short duration of the experiment.]

---

[1] The Working Group was aware of a study in progress to assess the carcinogenicity of reserpine to mice by oral administration (IARC, 1979).

Two groups, each of 50 male and 50 female 5-week-old Fischer 344 rats, were fed diets containing 5 or 10 mg/kg diet reserpine (USP grade) for 103 weeks and observed for an additional 2 weeks. A third group of 50 rats of each sex were used as matched controls. All surviving animals were killed at the end of 104-105 weeks. In the high-dose males the combined incidence of adrenal medullary pheochromocytomas was 24/48 ($P<0.001$) (15 benign and 9 malignant tumours); while in the low-dose males, the corresponding figure was 18/49 ($P<0.001$) (14 benign and 4 malignant neoplasms). In the matched controls, only 3 benign and 1 malignant pheochromocytoma developed in 3/48 males. In the high-dose females, the combined incidence of pheochromocytomas was 4/49 (3 benign and 1 malignant); while in the low-dose females, the corresponding figure was 3/48 (all benign). Of the matched controls, only 1/49 females developed a benign pheochromocytoma. Tumours at other sites occurred in similar incidences in test and control animals (National Cancer Institute, 1980).

Groups of 25 male and 25 female Wistar rats received 0, 30 or 60 mg/kg of diet reserpine (purity not specified) for 75 weeks, at which time all surviving rats (22 males and 22 females, 18 males and 18 females, 15 males and 24 females, in the 3 groups, respectively) were killed. A few pituitary adenomas, fibroadenomas of the mammary gland and lymphosarcomas were found in both treated and control rats; however, the differences in incidence were not statistically significant (Tatematsu et al., 1978). [Attention is drawn to the short duration of observation.]

(b) *Other experimental systems*

Administration in conjunction with known carcinogens: The number of mammary tumours per animal in 16 Sprague-Dawley female *rats* given a single i.v. injection of 5 mg 9,10-dimethylbenz[a]anthracene (DMBA) at 55 days of age was increased in all animals by subsequent daily s.c. administration of 100 µg/kg bw reserpine for 50 days after the appearance of the first tumour over that observed in controls treated with DMBA only (Welsch & Meites, 1970).

Nine male Wistar *rats* given 16 mg/kg of diet reserpine were protected against the carcinogenic effects of administration of 50 mg/l of drinking-water N-nitrosodiethylamine (Lacassagne et al., 1968).

3.2 Other relevant biological data

(a) Experimental systems

Toxic effects

In rats, the i.v. LD_{50} is 18 mg/kg bw (Usdin & Efron, 1972); in mice, the oral LD_{50} is 500 mg/kg bw and the i.p. LD_{50} 70 mg/kg bw (National Cancer Institute, 1980).

Reserpine given at a s.c. dose of 2.5 or 10 mg/kg bw induces gastric erosion and haemorrhage in mice (Blackman *et al.*, 1959). An i.p. dose of 0.25 mg/kg bw or an s.c. dose of 1 mg/kg bw suppresses the immune response of lymph-node cells in C57Bl/6 and CBA mice (Devoino & Yeliseyeva, 1971).

Administration of 2.5 mg/kg bw reserpine inhibited thymidine incorporation into rat brain DNA by 50-70% (Lewis *et al.*, 1977).

Prenatal toxicity

The extensive literature on the effect of prenatal administration of reserpine can be divided roughly into three spheres: 1) reproductive effects, 2) abnormal organogenesis, and 3) postnatal effects on the central nervous and endocrine systems.

Reserpine inhibits the pituitary ovarian axis in the rat (Tuchmann-Duplessis *et al.*, 1957), rabbit (Kehl *et al.*, 1956) and guinea-pig (Deanesly, 1966). The studies in the rabbit showed interruption of pregnancy when doses of as little as 0.125 mg (0.04 mg/kg bw) were administered intramuscularly either early or late in gestation (Kehl *et al.*, 1956). When given at 14-15 days of gestation to guinea-pigs, reserpine caused death and resorption of fetuses (Deanesly, 1966). Pregnancy was interrupted in rats given 250 µg/kg bw per day subcutaneously starting on the 1st, 3rd or 6th day of gestation (Tuchmann-Duplessis *et al.*, 1957).

Eye defects and spina bifida were reported in rats when 0.8-1.5 mg/kg bw reserpine was given on the 9th day, or 1.5-2 mg/kg bw on the 10th day, of gestation (Goldman & Yakovac, 1965). Hydronephrosis and deformities of the brain ventricles were found when 1 mg/kg bw was injected to rats daily for 3 days in the last third of gestation (Kanoh & Moriyama, 1977). Doses up to 0.5 mg per day (0.16 mg/kg bw) injected intramuscularly during mid-gestation in rabbits caused no fetotoxicity (Kehl *et al.*, 1956).

In rats, some form of intrauterine growth retardation has commonly been observed postnatally. In pair-fed animals, starved controls did not have an equivalent amount of fetal weight reduction (Moriyama & Kanoh, 1976).

Werboff & Kesner (1963) reported a reduction in the ability to learn a maze after administration of 0.1 mg/kg bw reserpine prenatally to rats; however, in another report, Werboff *et al.* (1961) reported increased emotionality and susceptibility to audiogenic seizures but no decrease in maze-learning. Hoffeld & Webster (1965) detected no maze-learning defects in the offspring of rats that received the same dose. Murai (1966) found no reduction in either postnatal activity or intelligence as measured by enclosed field testing in rats given reserpine. Hoffeld *et al.* (1967) found a prolongation of conditioned avoidance extinction in the offspring of rats after prenatal treatment on days 5-8 of gestation. Studies of postnatal neuroendocrine function indicate a permanent increase in sympathoadrenal tone in the offspring of rats exposed early in gestation and chemical changes in brain transmitters in the offspring of rats treated subcutaneously with 1 mg/kg bw reserpine 6, 5 and 4 days before delivery (Bartolomé *et al.*, 1976). A decreased cold stress response was found in 70-80-day-old rats whose mothers had been given 0.1 mg/kg bw reserpine daily from day 8 of pregnancy (Dailey, 1978).

In chicks treated with reserpine *in ovo*, various permanent alterations in postnatal function, including behavioural changes, and in biochemical maturation were observed (Sparber, 1972).

Absorption, distribution, excretion and metabolism

In rats, after an i.v. injection of 400 μg ^{14}C-reserpine, peak radioactivity occurred in most tissues within 60 minutes, with a rapid decline for up to 6 hours (Sheppard *et al.*, 1955). In male guinea-pigs, radioactivity in the brain after i.v. injection of 2 mg ^{3}H-reserpine reached a maximum within 20-30 minutes and then declined rapidly, whereas radioactivity in the liver reached similar levels but fell more slowly (Sheppard *et al.*, 1958).

Essentially no unchanged reserpine is excreted in the urine of rats, dogs, rhesus monkeys (Glazko *et al.*, 1956) or mice (Numerof *et al.*, 1955); but 35% of an i.v. dose was excreted in mouse faeces (Numerof *et al.*, 1955).

In rats, orally administered reserpine is rapidly hydrolysed to methyl reserpate (Glazko *et al.*, 1956); and in mice, orally or intravenously administered reserpine is metabolized to trimethoxybenzoic acid (Numerof *et al.*, 1955). In rats, methyl reserpate appears to be formed in the intestinal mucosa (Glazko *et al.*, 1956). Trimethoxybenzoic acid is rapidly eliminated in the urine of mice (Numerof *et al.*, 1955).

Mutagenicity and other, related short-term tests

Reserpine has no mutagenic activity in *Salmonella typhimurium* TA1950 or TA1538, either with or without metabolic activation by a rat liver homogenate (Fonstein *et al.*, 1978). Reserpine (in the form of the pharmaceutical preparations Adelfan and Serpasil) had no effect in a diploid *Aspergillus nidulans* system for the detection of induced non-disjunction and crossing over (Bignami *et al.*, 1974).

In mouse bone-marrow cells, reserpine was reported to stimulate mitosis and induce an increased number of chromosome aberrations (Jameela & Subramanyam, 1979). An increase in mitotic activity was also observed in cultured human peripheral leucocytes exposed to reserpine; no chromosome aberrations were noted (Bishun *et al.*, 1975).

I.p. doses of 0.92 and 4.6 mg/kg reserpine did not induce dominant lethality in mice (Epstein *et al.*, 1972). Zolotareva *et al.* (1978) reported a dominant lethal effect in mice in the 2nd and 3rd week after treatment with 0.2 - 8 mg/kg reserpine in the form of the pharmaceutical preparation Rausedil. They also reported that chromosome aberrations are induced in mouse bone-marrow cells at doses up to 10 mg/kg. [Attention is drawn to the inadequate reporting of the latter experiment.]

Effects on intermediary metabolism

Reserpine blocks the release of prolactin-inhibiting factor and thus raises serum prolactin levels (Welsch & Meites, 1970).

Other effects

Reserpine (30 mg/kg bw) has been reported to inhibit the growth of L1210 leukaemic cells in male mice (Goldin *et al.*, 1957) and to suppress the growth of sarcoma 37 in mice (50 mg/kg bw) (Belkin & Hardy, 1957). In contrast, reserpine did not affect the growth of transplanted mammary adenocarcinomas in C3H mice (Cranston, 1958).

(b) Humans

The primary therapeutic effect of reserpine is its peripheral antihypertensive action; it is also used as a central depressant and sedative (Goodman & Gilman, 1975).

Toxic effects

Death has been reported after ingestion of 50 mg/kg bw reserpine (Gleason et al., 1969).

Prenatal toxicity

In 475 women treated with reserpine and other *Rauwolfia* drugs at different times during pregnancy, there was no overall evidence of an association with malformations. This association was, however, found in the course of multiple comparisons; the data were only partially controlled in the context of a hypothesis-seeking study (Heinonen et al., 1977). Sobel (1960) reported one stillborn and congenital lung cysts in one of a pair of twins in the pregnancy outcomes of 15 treated women. Nasal congestion with cyanosis, costal retraction and lethargy were found in 12 newborn babies whose mothers were treated with reserpine shortly before delivery (Budnick et al., 1955).

Absorption, distribution, excretion and metabolism

After oral administration of 0.25 mg ^{3}H-reserpine, tritium was rapidly absorbed into the blood, reaching a peak within 1-2 hours. Radioactivity was tightly bound to red blood cells and remained constant over a 96-hour period. Disappearance of radioactivity in plasma was biphasic: the first component had a half-life of 4.5 hours, and the second, 271 hours. Six percent of the dose was excreted in the urine by 24 hours, mainly as trimethoxybenzoic acid; but radioactivity was still detectable in plasma, urine and faeces 11-12 days after drug administration (Maass et al., 1969).

Hypertensive patients who received reserpine had significantly greater ($P<0.005$) serum prolactin levels than those measured 6 weeks after treatment had been discontinued (Lee et al., 1976).

No data were available on the mutagenicity of reserpine in humans.

3.3 Case reports and epidemiological studies of carcinogenicity in humans

The relationship of reserpine use to breast cancer was reviewed previously (IARC, 1976). On the basis of information from the 6 studies available, it was concluded at that time that the results, taken together, were 'not consistent in indicating an increased risk of cancer in patients exposed to *Rauwolfia* derivatives', and that further evidence was needed.

A number of studies have since been published. In addition, the topic has been reviewed by Henderson (1977), Labarthe (1979) and Shapiro & Slone (1979).

Thirteen case-control studies (including the 6 already reviewed in IARC, 1976) available to the Working Group are summarized: in Table 1: some aspects of selection of cases and controls; Table 2: methods of ascertainment of the history of reserpine use; Table 3: definitions and criteria of exposure to reserpine; and Table 4: estimates of association between reserpine exposure and breast cancer. These studies will be discussed in the order that they appear in the tables, and then data from two cohort studies will be considered. Estimates of association for the cohort studies are included in Table 4.

Boston study: the first report (Boston Collaborative Drug Surveillance Program, 1974) was based upon the screening of multiple associations between drugs and diseases. The relative risk for breast cancer associated with reserpine use was 3.5 with 95% confidence limits of 1.6-8.0. [Since it was a hypothesis-generating study, however, information on possible confounding and other relevant factors was not available.]

Bristol and Helsinki studies: the Boston study eliminated two other studies. An association was found in the Bristol study (Armstrong et al., 1974), but the low prevalence of reserpine use resulted in wide confidence limits (0.7-5.5) about the relative risk (2.0). An association was also found in the Helsinki study (relative risk, 2.0; confidence limits, 1.2-3.4) (Heinonen et al., 1974), but it has been suggested by one of the original investigators that inconsistency in the relative risk estimates over three calendar periods could suggest one or more undetected sources of bias (Shapiro & Slone, 1979). [On the other hand, this variation might have been due simply to chance.]

[The three initial studies reported associations between recent reserpine use and breast cancer. Little information was available concerning earlier use.]

Los Angeles study: Mack et al. (1975) reported a modest association for 'ever-use' of reserpine (relative risk, 1.2; confidence limits, 0.7-2.2) and a slightly stronger one for recent use (1.6; 0.7-3.4), but drug use in general was associated with breast cancer, thus casting doubt on the relation to reserpine per se.

Rochester study: O'Fallon et al. (1975) found no evidence of an association (relative risk, 1.0; one-sided upper 95% confidence limit, 1.6). [This study, however, used different exposure criteria (past exposure) from those in the initial three studies. In addition, the selection of controls with only one condition, such as gallbladder disease (as in this study) can obscure an association if that condition is itself positively related to the exposure.]

Rockland study: the relative risk estimates in the Rockland study (Laska et al., 1975) were based on small numbers (55 case-control pairs), and the confidence intervals were wide (1.1; 0.5-2.3).

Baltimore study: Lilienfeld et al. (1975) found no statistically significant increase in the risk of breast cancer associated with reserpine use. The relative risks were 1.6 (95% confidence limits, 0.9-2.9) using hospital controls, 0.9 (95% confidence limits, 0.4-1.7) using neighbourhood controls, and 1.1 (95% confidence limits, 0.5-2.2) using hospital and neighbourhood controls. The hospital controls were of lower socio-economic status than the cases, whereas the neighbourhood controls were not; the slightly higher risk seen when using hospital controls may thus have been due to confounding by socio-economic status.

England and Wales study: to control for possible confounding due to hypertension Armstrong et al. (1976) limited their study to women whose death certificates mentioned hypertension. The subjects were selected from random samples of death certificates of women who died in England and Wales in 1972 or 1973. Fifteen of 33 patients with breast cancer (45%) and 30 of 97 matched controls without cancer (31%) were found ever to have used *Rauwolfia* derivatives; a relative risk of 2.1 (95% confidence limits, 0.9-4.9). When controls with selected cancers other than breast were used, 15 of 35 breast cancer patients (43%) and 27 of 76 matched controls (36%) were identified as users (relative risk, 1.4; 95% confidence limits, 0.6-3.4). Breast cancer risk did not increase with increasing duration of *Rauwolfia* use.

Finland study: Aromaa et al. (1976), in a matched-pairs analysis using hypertensive cases and controls, found a relative risk for breast cancer of 1.0, with 95% confidence limits of 0.5-1.9, when *Rauwolfia* was the main compound used. For 'any' use of *Rauwolfia*, the relative risk was 1.2, with 95% confidence limits of 0.6-2.3. Information on reserpine use in both cases and controls was obtained from hypertension registers, and cases were limited to those entered independently in a population-based cancer registry after their date of enrollment in the hypertension registry. [The possibility of certain biases would thereby be reduced.]

Berlin study: in this study (Kewitz et al., 1977), cases of breast cancer and controls with benign breast disease were all interviewed before the diagnosis had been made [thus limiting the possibility of interviewer bias]. The relative risk estimate of 0.6 (95% confidence limits: 0.4-1.1) was interpreted as strong evidence against a causal relationship. To test the possibility that reserpine use may be related to the risk of both benign breast disease and breast cancer, the cases were compared with a second control group of women subjected to surgery for other benign conditions. For this control group the interviewers were aware of the diagnosis. The relative risk was 0.9, with 95% confidence limits of 0.4-1.7. [In this study the exact timing of reserpine use was not specified.]

Scotland and England study: Christopher et al. (1977) used a matched-sets design to evaluate the use of reserpine at various times in relation to breast cancer. For 'ever-use', when comparing cases with controls who did not have cancer, the relative risks in Aberdeen and Dundee were 1.0 and 1.2, respectively. [No confidence limits were given. The estimate for 116 matched sets studied in London was also not given.] Timing of reserpine use was examined in detail: rates of use - whether at the time of diagnosis, within 1 year of diagnosis, more than 1 year before diagnosis or ever (including 'unknowns') - were similar when cases and controls were compared.

Oakland study: Kodlin & McCarthy (1978) reported conflicting results, with relative risk for breast cancer estimates varying from 1.3 to 4.7. When hypertensive cases were compared with matched controls who had had diagnosed hypertension for the same length of time (their preferred comparison), the relative risk estimate was 1.3 [approximate 95% confidence limits, 0.6-2.9, calculated by the Working Group].

United States study: in this study (Williams et al., 1978), women with breast cancer and controls were enrolled from among 80,000 women who volunteered for screening in the nationwide Breast Cancer Detection Demonstration Project; and 481 cases were compared with 1268 randomly selected controls. Although the women were said to be asymptomatic, it was estimated that two-thirds of the cancers were large enough to be detected on physical examination. The use of reserpine in the year before admission was not associated with breast cancer (relative risk estimate, 1.1); but earlier use for 5 or more years was (relative risk adjusted for several potentially confounding factors, 2.0; $P<0.05$). A similar association was evident when 359 women who were biopsied and found not to have breast cancer were compared with 1071 controls (adjusted relative risk, 2.1; $P<0.1$). [The biopsy-negative women presumably had benign breast disease.] The use of thiazide diuretics for 5 or more years, either alone or in combination with other drugs, was also associated with benign breast disease. The use, especially for 5 or more years, of other antihypertensive drugs such as methyldopa, chlorthalidone and hydralazine, was also associated with breast cancer, benign breast disease or both. Moreover, the relative risks tended to rise progressively, both among the breast cancer subjects and among those with benign breast disease, as the number of antihypertensive agents used increased. This applied particularly to women who had taken multiple agents for 5 or more years. The authors felt that the combined data suggested that causality (of breast cancer by reserpine) was a serious possibility. [The multiple associations reported in this study may be explicable in terms of the unique population selected for study. To illustrate this, consider 2 women who have a breast lump, one of whom takes reserpine or another antihypertensive drug. It is plausible that the user of antihypertensives would, in general, be more 'health conscious' than the nonuser. The health-conscious woman might be more likely to find a lump and volunteer for screening as soon as she suspected that she had cancer. The nonuser with a breast lump might be less health conscious, less likely to find the lump and consequently not volunteer for screening and instead have her cancer diagnosed in the usual way. She would thus be less likely to appear in the population of screened women but would appear in a hospital or population series. This preferential inclusion of reserpine users in a screened population would probably be less pronounced in women without breast lumps. Even if this were not true, the question would still arise as to whether these data confirm the original reports in which recent reserpine use was associated with breast cancer. In the study of Williams *et al.*, recent use was not associated with breast cancer. This is not coherent with the first three original reports.]

Two cohort studies have also been reported. In the first, Labarthe & O'Fallon (1980) describe the experience of 450 women who used reserpine, 250 of whom took the drug for 1 year or more. All the women were residents of Olmstead County, Minnesota; expected numbers of cases of breast cancer were estimated from data from the same county and from the Connecticut Tumor Registry. Among all 450 users, 11 breast cancers were observed during 6 months to 26 years of follow-up (10.8 and 10.0 expected); and in the 250 longterm users, 4 were observed (5.6 and 5.1 expected). The relative risks were close to unity for each comparison, with an upper 95% confidence limit of about 1.8. The use of thiazide diuretics alone or in combination with reserpine was not associated with breast cancer. This study also suggested that hypertension *per se* is not a risk factor for breast cancer and therefore not of concern as a confounding factor in other studies.

The second study was based upon screening data from a medical care programme (Friedman & Ury, 1980). Among 4270 *Rauwolfia* recipients followed for 3-7 years (number of women unspecified), there were 30 cases of breast cancer (31.2 expected) and 211 cases of all cancers (226.5 expected). [Since these data were generated in the course of routine screening for the presence or absence of associations, and since no specific relationship was evaluated in detail, they must be interpreted with caution.]

Table 1. Some aspects of selection of cases and controls in 13 case-control studies of reserpine use in relation to breast cancer[a]

Boston:	Cases, 25,000 hospitalized patients in Boston area, 1972; 159 new cases, less 9 with inadequate drug history; n = 150 Controls, surgical - 6500 candidates; less 309 with other cancers; less 180 with inadequate drug history; remainder sampled for 4:1 match by decade of age, hospital; n = 600 Controls, medical - 5200 candidates: less 1686 with cardiovascular diseases or other cancer; less 171 with inadequate drug history; remainder sampled for 4:1 match; n = 600
Bristol:	Cases, 750 newly registered cases, 1971-1973; less 32 with inadequate history; n = 708 Controls, all other cancers sampled to provide 3:1 match by 5-year age range, year of registration; removed matched subjects not newly diagnosed and treated in Bristol area hospitals; removed 121 with inadequate history; final matching ratio variable; n = 1430 Controls, selected other cancers - subset of above after exclusion of subjects with cancers of pancreas, skin, corpus uteri, kidney, nervous system; n = 963
Helsinki:	Cases, subjects with mastectomy for breast cancer in a Helsinki hospital, 1960-1972; less those with any other cancer; less those with inadequate history in case or paired controls; n = 438 Controls, surgical - subjects with elective surgery and no cancer, less those with surgery for gall-bladder, thyroid or kidney disease, cardiac or vascular surgery or sympathectomy; less those with inadequate history; matched by 5-year age interval and year of surgery, 1:1; n = 438
Los Angeles:	Cases, 120 notifications of breast cancer, 1971-1975; less 2 with metastases to breast, 7 lacking records; including those with prior breast cancer and other cancers; n = 111. In most analyses the latter are excluded; n = 99 Controls, community residents - roster searched for age and community-entry matches within 6 months; excluding subjects without charts and subjects with benign breast disease; n = 444 or 396
Rochester:	Cases, 453 breast cancer cases; from defined population, diagnosed 1955-1973; less 3 with inadequate history; n = 450; 167 hypertensive Controls, gall-bladder disease - from 2000 subjects, 475 diagnosed 1955-1970, drawn at random within age strata to match age distribution of cases; no exclusions; n = 475; 225 hypertensive
Rockland:	Cases, 55 cases with breast cancer diagnosed while resident in institution, 1965-1974, on average 18 years before diagnosis; no exclusions; n = 55 Controls, 55 controls matched on age, psychiatric diagnosis, admission date, (sometimes) race and religion; all resident in hospital April 1, 1969; no exclusions; n = 55

Table 1 (contd)

Baltimore:	Cases, 273 newly diagnosed patients in Breast Tumor Collaborative Study, July 1973-January 1975; less 38 without interview; less 39 with inadequate history in the case or the match; less 32 not matched with hospital control; n = 164 matched to hospital control; less 57 not matched with neighbourhood control; n = 139 matched to neighbourhood control Controls, hospital - 242 subjects matched by sex, age (within 5 years), Baltimore residence, race, hospital service, date of admission; free of prior breast cancer; less 30 with no interview; less 48 with inadequate history; n = 164 Controls, neighbourhood - 201 subjects with similar demographic matching; less 35 without interviews; less 27 with inadequate history; n = 139
England & Wales:	Cases, 58 subjects with death certificates in special analysis samples (10% of 1972, 25% of 1973), with all diagnoses coded, having breast cancer and hypertension coded; less 11 with inadequate history; n = 47 (33, 35) Controls, other cancers - 105 subjects with other cancers and hypertension found when seeking match on year of death, 5-year interval of age at death, position of hypertension on death certificate and rubric coded; less 14 with inadequate history; n = 91 (76) Controls, no cancer - 254 subjects identified as above; less 70 with inadequate history; n = 184 (97)
Finland:	Cases - 126 subjects linked in Finnish Cancer Registry and Social Insurance Institution as having breast cancer reported in 1973, antihypertensive medications reimbursed by 1972; less 7 pairs in which case or control lacked adequate history; n = 109 Controls, other hypertensives - selected from among 3 tentative controls per case after matching by geographic area, age (within 1 year) and duration of hypertension; n = 109
Berlin:	Cases, 526 women admitted to any of 20 hospitals for breast biopsy, with no other cancer; less 336 without breast cancer on biopsy; less persons over 80 years old; n = 181 Controls, benign breast disease - remainder of cancer-free biopsy series; less persons under 30 years old; n = 307 Controls, other surgery - other surgical patients, excluding those with gallbladder disease or any cancer; n = 101
Scotland & England:	Cases, all cases with discharge diagnosis of breast cancer in 1969-1974 or a shorter interval in participating hospitals; Aberdeen, 1000 cases less 354 with inadequate history or match yielded 646 matched sets with 2 controls, 1 case; Dundee, 233 matched sets with 2 controls, 1 case; Hammersmith, 177 cases less 61 exclusions yielded 116 matched sets (or 107); total n = 986

Table 1 (contd)

Scotland & England (contd)	Controls, other cancer - combined Aberdeen and Dundee controls; age-matched; total n = 879 Controls, other - combined Aberdeen, Dundee and Hammersmith controls; age-matched; total n = 986 Controls, cardiac rematch - combined Aberdeen and Dundee 'controls, other' after replacement of all with cardiac diagnosis (n = 102) gives total n = 879
Oakland:	Cases, breast cancer diagnosed between 1974 and April 1975; selected from 789 breast cancer cases because hypertension diagnosed in multiphasic screening 1964-1973; n = 108 Controls, selected from a pool of sets of 20 potential controls matched to each case by race, year of multiphasic screening examination, age (within 1 year) and hypertension diagnosed during screening; n = 324
United States:	All subjects selected from the nationwide Breast Cancer Detection Demonstration Project Cases, 543 with biopsy-proven breast cancer; 62 nonrespondents; n = 481 Controls, 1422 subjects screened negative; 154 nonrespondents; n = 1268

[a] Adapted from Labarthe (1979) and supplemented by the Working Group

Table 2. Methods of ascertainment of the history of reserpine use in 13 case-control studies of reserpine use in relation to breast cancer[a]

Boston:	In-hospital interview responses to items on use of medications during the 3 months prior to admission; if response positive for treatment of high blood pressure, identity, frequency and duration of use of antihypertensive medications sought
Bristol:	Medical record sources of several types searched in sequence until exhausted or adequate data obtained, the first 3 types relating to drugs in use at time of admission: (1) General practitioner (GP) admission form; (2) admission medical history; (3) project-initiated inquiry similar to GP admission form; and (4) GP practice notes; if *Rauwolfia* derivatives identified, GP notes sought for dose and duration
Helsinki:	Medical record sources linked to current hospitalization; prior use information limited to referral letters, outpatient notes, current and previous admission histories, inpatient drug records, anaesthetic records and consultants' notes

Table 2 (contd)

Los Angeles:	Outpatient clinic records, including general medical history recorded at entry to community, possibly including pre-entry drug use
Rochester:	Outpatient and inpatient medical records
Rockland:	Inpatient medical records
Baltimore:	Interview response whether ever hypertensive; if yes, when and by whom treated; letters to physicians named plus search of clinic records when a participating hospital involved; interview response linked to hospital admission for cases and hospital controls, not neighbourhood controls; but only approximately two-thirds of interviews actually completed in hospital
England & Wales:	GP records sought when subjects were attended at the time of death, or from local family-practitioner committee, if returned there following death
Finland:	Social Insurance Institution records of reimbursement for medications purchased during 1972, giving name, amount purchased and dosage for all purchases; physicians contacted to determine duration of hypertension, but evidently not for drug information
Berlin:	In-hospital response positive for long-term medication, if 'regular use for at least three months'; then dosages, duration of treatment and between-treatment intervals sought. If history positive for hypertension, physican contact sought and questionnaire sent for similar data on antihypertensive and other cardiovascular drugs
Scotland & England:	Hospital records at admission for diagnosis of breast cancer or other conditions, plus request for supplemental information from GP (or committee); except at Hammersmith, with no corresponding hospital history for controls
Oakland:	Inpatient and outpatient records from a medical care programme
United States:	Questionnaire mailed to all subjects; patients asked to record all drugs taken for 1 year or more; supplementary questionnaires mailed to each physician listed by patient as prescribing therapy for hypertension or oedema

[a] Adapted from Labarthe (1979) and supplemented by the Working Group

Table 3. Definitions and criteria of exposure to reserpine in 13 case-control studies of reserpine use in relation to breast cancer[a]

Boston:	Use within past 3 months = user (recent) Also analysed by duration of use (1, 1-3, 4-5, 5+ years)
Bristol:	Use at time of admission to hospital = user (recent)
Helsinki:	Any positive history = user (ever)
Los Angeles:	Any positive history = user (ever) Separate analysis for users at least 5 years prior to diagnosis
Rochester:	Positive history occurring at least 6 months prior to diagnosis = user (ever) Also analysed by interval from first use to diagnosis (more than 1, 2, 3... 8, 9, 10+ years)
Rockland:	Any positive history before 6 months from diagnosis = user (ever) Also analysed by years of use in which 25 mg+ used, relative to year of diagnosis; cumulative years: mean number of days and mean dosage of reserpine
Baltimore:	Any positive history = user (ever) Also analysed by average dose per user and average duration of use per user
England & Wales:	Any positive history = user (ever) Also analysed by use before cancer diagnosis, before and after, after only, any period of 3+ months before diagnosis, and any period of 5+ years before diagnosis
Finland:	Any positive history = user (recent) Also analysed as 'main' antihypertensive agent (use on same number or more days than other agents)
Berlin:	Any positive history = user (ever) Also analysed by duration of use 1+ years, by proximity of use to date of diagnosis (within the same year), and use for 1+ years up to the time of diagnosis
Scotland & England:	Any positive history = user (ever) Also analysed by use at time of diagnosis of cancer, within 1 year, and more than 1 year from diagnosis; Aberdeen also grouped at more than 6 months before diagnosis
Oakland:	Any positive history = user (ever)
United States:	Any positive history of use for 1+ years = user (ever) Also analysed by use for 5+ years

[a] Adapted from Labarthe (1979) and supplemented by the Working Group

Table 4. Estimates of association between reserpine and breast cancer in 13 case-control and 2 cohort studies[a]

Study	Relative risk[b] (95% confidence intervals)	Reserpine exposure recorded[c]
Case-control studies		
Boston	3.5 (1.6-8.0)	Recent
Bristol	2.0 (0.7-5.5)	Recent
Helsinki	2.0 (1.2-3.4)	Recent
Los Angeles	1.2 (0.7-2.2)	Ever
	1.6 (0.7-3.4)	Recent
Rochester	1.0 (one-sided upper confidence limit: 1.6)	Recent
Rockland	1.1 (0.5-2.3)	Ever
Baltimore	1.6 (0.9-2.9)[d]	Ever
	0.9 (0.4-1.7)	Ever
	1.1 (0.5-2.2)	Ever
England & Wales	2.1 (0.9-4.9)[d]	Ever
	1.4 (0.6-3.4)	Ever
Finland	1.0 (0.5-1.9)	Recent (main drug)
	1.2 (0.6-2.3)	Recent (any use)
Berlin	0.6 (0.4-1.1)[d]	Ever
	0.9 (0.4-1.7)	Ever
Scotland & England	1.0 (no confidence limits given) (Aberdeen)	Ever
	1.2 (no confidence limits given) (Dundee)	Ever
Oakland	1.3 (0.6-2.9)[e]	Ever
United States	1.2	Ever
	2.0 (P<0.05)[f]	
	1.1	Recent

Table 4 (contd)

Study	Relative risk[b] (95% confidence intervals)	Reserpine exposure recorded[c]
Cohort studies		
Olmstead County	1.0 (0.5-1.8)[e]	Any[g]
Medical care programme (Kaiser-Permanente)	1.0 (0.6-1.4)[e]	Any[h]

[a] Prepared from data supplied by Labarthe (1979) and supplemented by the Working Group

[b] Relative risks shown were selected as those most representative of the data

[c] Recent = last use, usually within 6 months of diagnosis of breast cancer
Ever = ever exposed (including unknown timing)

[d] Different relative risks associated with different control goups (see text)

[e] Approximate interval estimated by the Working Group

[f] Use for 5 or more years

[g] Any use occurring 6 months to 26 years before end of follow-up

[h] Any use occurring 3-7 years before end of follow-up

4. Summary of Data Reported and Evaluation

4.1 Experimental data

Reserpine was tested in two experiments in mice by oral administration; in one experiment it induced malignant mammary tumours in females and carcinomas of the seminal vesicles in males. It was tested in three experiments in rats by oral administration; in one experiment it increased the incidence of pheochromocytomas in males. The other study in mice and the other two studies in rats were inadequate for evaluation.

Reserpine is embryotoxic and has effects on reproduction. There is limited evidence that it is teratogenic in experimental animals. It was not mutagenic in *Salmonella typhimurium*.

4.2 Human data

Reserpine is used mainly for the treatment of mild or moderate hypertension.

Thirteen case-control and two cohort studies on the relationship of reserpine to breast cancer were available to the Working Group. Between and within studies, estimates of relative risk for different measures of reserpine use varied from as low as 0.6 to over 3. Many of the positive findings were not coherent with one another; and the studies considered to be the most satisfactory, methodologically, showed little or no evidence of an increased risk.

Two studies of pregnant women receiving reserpine failed to find clear evidence of teratogenicity.

4.3 Evaluation

There is *limited evidence*[1] that reserpine is carcinogenic in experimental animals.

The studies in humans are not consistent in showing an increase in risk of breast cancer associated with reserpine use; and, considering all studies together and the methodological problems of some, such an increase appears unlikely. Because of sampling variation, however, a small increase in risk (of the order of 50% or less) cannot be ruled out.

---

[1] See preamble, p. 18.

5. References

AMA Department of Drugs (1977) *AMA Drug Evaluations,* 3rd ed., Littleton, MA, Publishing Sciences Group, Inc., pp. 62-63

Armstrong, B., Stevens, N. & Doll, R. (1974) Retrospective study of the association between use of *Rauwolfia* derivatives and breast cancer in English women. *Lancet, ii,* 672-675

Armstrong, B., Skegg, D., White, G. & Doll, R. (1976) *Rauwolfia* derivatives and breast cancer in hypertensive women. *Lancet, ii,* 8-12

Aromaa, A., Hakama, M., Hakulinen, T., Saxén, E., Teppo, L. & Indänpään-Heikkilä, J. (1976) Breast cancer and use of *Rauwolfia* and other antihypertensive agents in hypertensive patients: a nationwide case-control study in Finland. *Int. J. Cancer, 18,* 727-738

Bartolomé, J., Seidler, F.J., Anderson, T.R. & Slotkin, T.A. (1976) Effects of prenatal reserpine administration on development of the rat adrenal medulla and central nervous system. *J. Pharmacol. exp. Ther., 197,* 293-302

Belkin, M. & Hardy, W.G. (1957) Effect of reserpine and chlorpromazine on sarcoma 37. *Science, 125,* 233-234

Bignami, M., Morpurgo, G., Pagliani, R., Carere, A., Conti, G. & Di Giuseppe, G. (1974) Non-disjunction and crossing-over induced by pharmaceutical drugs in *Aspergillus nidulans. Mutat. Res., 26,* 159-170

Bishun, N., Smith, N. & Williams, D. (1975) Chromosomes, mitosis, and reserpine. *Lancet, i,* 926

Blackman, J.G., Campion, D.S. & Fastier, F.N. (1959) Mechanism of action of reserpine in producing gastric haemorrhage and erosion in the mouse. *Br. J. Pharmacol., 14,* 112-116

Boston Collaborative Drug Surveillance Program (1974) Reserpine and breast cancer. *Lancet, ii,* 669-671

Budnick, I.S., Leikin, S. & Hoeck, L.E. (1955) Effect in the newborn infant of reserpine administered *ante partum. Am. J. Dis. Child., 90,* 286-289

Christopher, L.J., Crooks, J., Davidson, J.F., Erskine, Z.G., Gallon, S.C., Moir, D.C. & Weir, R.D. (1977) A multicentre study of *Rauwolfia* derivatives and breast cancer. *Eur. J. clin. Pharmacol., 11,* 409-417

Clark, C.C. (1970) Spectrofluorometric determination of *Rauwolfia serpentina* tablets and whole root. *Interbureau By-Lines, 6,* 288-293

Council of Europe (1975) *European Pharmacopoeia (European Treaty Series No. 50),* Vol. 3, Paris, Maisonneuve, pp. 339-341

Cranston, E.M. (1958) Effects of some tranquilizers on a mammary adenocarcinoma in mice. *Cancer Res., 18,* 897-899

Dailey, J.W. (1978) Effects of maternally administered reserpine on the development of the cold stress response and its possible relation to adrenergic nervous system function. *Res. Commun. chem. Pathol. Pharmacol., 19,* 389-402

Deanesly, R. (1966) The effects of reserpine on ovulation and on the corpus luteum of the guinea-pig. *J. Reprod. Fertil., 11,* 429-438

Devoino, L.V. & Yeliseyeva, L.S. (1971) Influence of some drugs on the immune respone. III. Effect of serotonin, 5-hydroxytryptophan, reserpine, monoamine oxidase inhibitors, and DOPA on the involvement of lymph node cells in the immune response. *Eur. J. Pharmacol., 14,* 71-76

Epstein, S.S., Arnold, E., Andrea, J., Bass, W. & Bishop, Y. (1972) Detection of chemical mutagens by the dominant lethal assay in the mouse. *Toxicol. appl. Pharmacol., 23,* 288-325

Fonstein, L.M., Revazova, Y.A., Zolotareva, G.N., Abilev, S.K., Akinjshina, L.P., Brazlavsky, V.A., Iskhakova, E.N., Meksin, V.A., Radchenko, L.U. & Shapiro, A.A. (1978) Studies of mutagenic activity of dioxydine (Russ.). *Genetika, 14,* 900-908

Friedman, G.D. & Ury, H.K. (1980) Initial screening for carcinogenicity of commonly used drugs. *J. natl Cancer Inst., 65* (in press)

Glazko, A.J., Dill, W.A., Wolf, L.M. & Kazenko, A. (1956) Studies on the metabolism of reserpine. *J. Pharmacol. exp. Ther., 118,* 377-387

Gleason, M.N., Gosselin, R.E., Hodge, H.C. & Smith, R.P. (1969) *Clinical Toxicology of Commercial Products,* 3rd ed., Baltimore, Williams & Wilkins, p. 123

Goldin, A., Burton, R.M., Humphreys, S.R. & Venditti, J.M. (1957) Antileukemic action of reserpine. *Science, 125,* 156-157

Goldman, A.S. & Yakovac, W.C. (1965) Teratogenic action in rats of reserpine alone and in combination with salicylate and immobilization. *Proc. Soc. exp. Biol. Med., 118,* 857-862

Goodman, L.S. & Gilman, A., eds (1975) *The Pharmacological Basis of Therapeutics,* 5th ed., New York, Macmillan, pp. 167-169, 557-559

Harvey, S.C. (1975) *Adrenergic blocking drugs.* In: Osol, A., ed., *Remington's Pharmaceutical Sciences,* 15th ed., Easton, PA, Mack Publishing Co., p. 837-838

Heinonen, O.P., Shapiro, S., Tuominen, L. & Turunen, M.I. (1974) Reserpine use in relation to breast cancer. *Lancet, ii,* 675-677

Heinonen, O.P., Slone, D. & Shapiro, S. (1977) *Birth Defects and Drugs in Pregnancy,* Littleton, MA, Publishing Sciences Group, Inc., pp. 372-373, 441

Henderson, M. (1977) *Reserpine and breast cancer. A review.* In: Colombo, F., Shapiro, S., Slone, D. & Tognoni, G., eds, *Epidemiological Evaluation of Drugs,* Amsterdam, Elsevier, pp. 211-227

Hoffeld, D.R. & Webster, R.L. (1965) Effect of injection of tranquillizing drugs during pregnancy on offspring. *Nature, 205,* 1070-1072

Hoffeld, D.R., Webster, R.L. & McNew, J. (1967) Adverse effects on offspring of tranquillizing drugs during pregnancy. *Nature, 215,* 182-183

IARC (1976) *IARC Monographs on the Evaluation of Carcinogenic Risk of Chemicals to Man,* Vol. 10, *Some Naturally Occurring Substances,* Lyon, pp. 217-229

IARC (1979) *Information Bulletin on the Survey of Chemicals Being Tested for Carcinogenicity, No. 8,* Lyon, p. 70

Jameela, Miss & Subramanyam, S. (1979) Cytogenetic action of the antihypertensive agent adelphane on meiotic cells of *Poekilocerus pictus. Mutat. Res., 67,* 295-299

Kanoh, S. & Moriyama, I.S. (1977) Effect of reserpine on the pregnant rat: 2nd report (Abstract). *Teratology., 16,* 110

Kehl, R., Audibert, A., Gage, C. & Amarger, J. (1956) Action of reserpine at different periods of gestation in rabbits (Fr.). *C.R. Soc. Biol. (Alger), 150,* 2196-2199

Kewitz, H., Jeskinsky, H.J., Schröter, P.-M. & Lindtner, E. (1977) Reserpine and breast cancer in women in Germany. *Eur. J. clin. Pharmacol., 11,* 79-83

Kodlin, D. & McCarthy, N. (1978) Reserpine and breast cancer. *Cancer, 41,* 761-768

Labarthe, D.R. (1979) Methodologic variation in case-control studies of reserpine and breast cancer. *J. chronic Dis., 32,* 95-104

Labarthe, D.R. & O'Fallon, W.M. (1980) Reserpine and breast cancer: a community-based longitudinal study of 2000 hypertensive women. *J. Am. med. Assoc.* (in press)

Lacassagne, A. & Duplan, J.-F. (1959) The mechanism of cancer production in the mammary gland in mice, considered on the basis of the results of experiments with reserpine (Fr.). *C.R. Acad. Sci. (Paris), 249,* 810-812

Lacassagne, A., Buu-Hoi, N.P., Giao, N.B. & Ferrando, R. (1968) Retarding action of reserpine on the production of liver cancer in rats by diethylnitrosamine (Fr.). *Bull. Cancer., 55,* 87-90

Laska, E.M., Siegel, C., Meisner, M., Fischer, S. & Wanderling, J. (1975) Matched-pairs study of reserpine use and breast cancer. *Lancet, ii,* 296-300

Lee, P.A., Kelly, M.R. & Wallin, J.D. (1976) Increased prolactin-levels during reserpine treatment of hypertensive patients. *J. Am. med. Assoc., 235,* 2316-2317

Lewis, P.D., Patel, A.J., Béndek, G. & Balázs, R. (1977) Effect of reserpine on cell proliferation in the developing rat brain: a quantitative histological study. *Brain Res., 129,* 299-308

Lilienfeld, A.M., Chang, L., Thomas, D.B. & Levin, M.L. (1975) *Rauwolfia* derivatives and breast cancer. *Johns Hopkins med. J., 139,* 41-50

Maass, A.R., Jenkins, B., Shen, Y. & Tannenbaum, P. (1969) Studies on absorption, excretion and metabolism of ^{3}H-reserpine in man. *Clin. Pharmacol. Ther., 10,* 366-371

Mack, T.M., Henderson, B.E., Gerkins, V.R., Arthur, M., Baptista, J. & Pike, M.C.. (1975) Reserpine and breast cancer in a retirement community. *New Engl. J. Med., 292,* 1366-1371

Moriyama, I.S. & Kanoh, S. (1976) Effect of reserpine on the pregnant rat (Abstract). *Teratology, 14,* 247

Murai, N. (1966) Effect of maternal medication during pregnancy upon behavioral development of offspring. *Tohoku J. exp. Med., 89,* 265-272

National Cancer Institute (1980) *Bioassay of Reserpine for Possible Carcinogenicity,* Department of Health, Education, & Welfare Publication No. (NIH) 80-1749, Washington DC, US Government Printing Office

Numerof, P., Gordon, M. & Kelly, J.M. (1955) The metabolism of reserpine. I. Studies in the mouse with C-14 labeled reserpine. *J. Pharmacol. exp. Ther., 115,* 427-431

O'Fallon, W.M., Labarthe, D.R. & Kurland, L.T. (1975) *Rauwolfia* derivatives and breast cancer. *Lancet, ii,* 292-296

Office de Vulgarisation Pharmaceutique (1979) *Dictionnaire Vidal,* 55th ed., Paris, pp. 9-10, 1022, 1746-1747, 1848-1849, 2029, 2032

Sams, R. (1978) Determination of reserpine in plasma using high-performance liquid chromatography with fluorescence detection. *Anal. Letter., B11,* 697-707

Sams, R.A. & Huffman, R. (1978) Thin-layer chromatographic test for reserpine in plasma. *J. Chromatogr., 161,* 410-414

Schirmer, R.E. (1975) *Reserpine.* In: Florety, K., ed., *Analytical Profiles of Drug Substances,* Vol. 4, New York, Academic Press, pp. 384-430

Shapiro, S. & Slone, D. (1979) Comment. *J. chronic Dis., 32,* 105-113

Sheppard, H., Lucas, R.C. & Tsien, W.H. (1955) The metabolism of reserpine-C^{14}. *Arch. int. Pharmacodyn., 103,* 256-269

Sheppard, H., Tsien, W.H., Plummer, A.J., Peets, E.A., Giletti, B.J. & Schulert, A.R. (1958) Brain reserpine levels following large and small doses of reserpine-H^3. *Proc. Soc. exp. Biol. Med., 97,* 717-721

Sittig, M. (1979) *Pharmaceutical Manufacturing Encyclopedia,* Park Ridge, NJ, Noyes Data Corporation, p. 556

Sobel, D.E. (1960) Fetal damage due to ECT, insulin coma, chlorpromazine, or reserpine. *AMA Arch. gen. Psychiatry, 2,* 606-611

Sparber, S.B. (1972) Effects of drugs on the biochemical and behavioral responses of developing organisms. *Fed. Proc., 31,* 74-80

Tatematsu, M., Takahashi, M., Tsuda, H., Ogiso, T. & Ito, N. (1978) The administration of reserpine to rats for 75 weeks. *Toxicol. Lett., 1,* 201-205

Tuchman-Duplessis, H. & Mercier-Parot, L. (1962) Occurrence of malignant tumours in a strain of Wistar rats (Fr.). *C.R. Acad. Sci. (Paris), 254,* 1535-1537

Tuchmann-Duplessis, H., Gershon, R. & Mercier-Parot, L. (1957) Disturbances of gestation in rats caused by reserpine and tests of compensatory hormone therapy (Fr.). *J. Physiol., 49,* 1007-1019

Usdin, E. & Efron, D.H. (1972) *Psychotropic Drugs and Related Compounds,* 2nd ed., Washington DC, US Department of Health, Education, & Welfare, p. 80

US Pharmacopeial Convention, Inc. (1975) *The US Pharmacopeia,* 19th rev., Rockville, MD, pp. 438-440

Wade, A., ed. (1977) *Martindale, The Extra Pharmacopoeia,* 27th ed., London, The Pharmaceutical Press, pp. 674-677

Welsch, C.W. & Meites, J. (1970) Effects of reserpine on development of 7,12-dimethylbenzanthracene induced mammary tumors in female rats. *Experientia, 26,* 1133-1134

Werboff, J. & Kesner, R. (1963) Learning deficits of offspring after administration of tranquillizing drugs to the mothers. *Nature, 197,* 106-107

Werboff, J., Gottlieb, J.S., Havlena, J. & Word, T.J. (1961) Behavioral effects of prenatal drug administration in the white rat. *Pediatrics, 27,* 318-324

Williams, R.R., Feinleib, M., Connor, R.J. & Stegens, N.L. (1978) Case-control study of antihypertensive and diuretic use by women with malignant and benign breast lesions detected in a mammography screening program. *J. natl Cancer Inst., 61,* 327-335

Windholz, M., ed. (1976) *The Merck Index,* 9th ed., Rahway, NJ, Merck & Co., p. 1057

Woodward, R.B., Bader, F.E., Bickel, H., Frey, A.J. & Kierstead, R.W. (1956) The total synthesis of reserpine. *J. Am. chem. Soc., 78,* 2023-2025

Zolotareva, G.N., Akaeva, E.A., Iskhakova, E.N., Oblapenko, N.G., Kotelyanskaya, A.E. & Epshtein, S.I. (1978) Comparative study of the mutagenic activity of a series of hypotensive agents in mice (Russ.). *Khim. -Farm. Zh., 12,* 19-22

RIFAMPICIN

1. Chemical and Physical Data

1.1 Synonyms and trade names

Chem. Abstr. Services Reg. No.: 13292-46-1

Chem. Abstr. Name: Rifamycin, 3-{[(4-methyl-1-piperazinyl)imino]methyl}-

IUPAC Systematic Name: (12Z,14E,24E)-(2S,16S,17S,18R,19R,20R,21S,22R,-23S)-1,2-Dihydro-5,6,9,17,19-pentahydroxy-23-methoxy-2,14,12,16,18,20,22-heptamethyl-8-(4-methylpiperazin-1-yliminomethyl)-1,11-dioxo-2,7-epoxypentadeca-1,11,13-trienoimino)naphtho[2,1-6]furan-21-yl acetate

Synonyms: 5,6,9,17,19,21-Hexahydroxy-23-methoxy-2,4,12,16,18,20,22-heptamethyl-8-[N-(4-methyl-1-piperazinyl)formimidoyl]-2,7-[epoxypentadeca(1,11,13)trienimino]-naphtho(2,1-b)furan-1,11(2H)-dione-21-acetate; 3-(4-methylpiperazinyliminomethyl)-rifamycin SV; 3-{[(4-methyl-1-piperazinyl)imino]methyl} rifamycin SV; rifaldazin; rifaldazine; rifampicin SV; rifampicinum; rifamycin AMP

Trade names: Archidyn; Arficin; NSC 113926; R/AMP; Rifa; Rifadin; Rifadine; Rifagen; Rifaldin; Rifamate; Rifampin; Rifaprodin; Rifinah; Rifobac; Rifoldin; Rifoldine; Riforal; Rimactan; Rimactane; Rimactazid; Rimactizid; Tubocin

1.2 Structural and molecular formulae and molecular weight

$C_{43}H_{58}N_4O_{12}$ Mol. wt: 823.0

1.3 Chemical and physical properties of the pure substance

From Wade (1977) or Windholz (1976), unless otherwise specified

(a) *Description:* A tasteless, reddish-brown, crystalline powder
(b) *Melting-point:* 183-188°C (dec.).
(c) *Spectroscopy data:* λ_{max} (in aqueous phosphate buffer, pH 7.38) 237 nm, A (1%, 1 cm) = 40; 255 nm, A(1%, 1 cm) = 39; 334 nm, A(1%, 1cm) = 33; 475 nm, A(1%, 1 cm) = 19. Infrared, nuclear magnetic resonance and mass spectral data have been tabulated (Gallo & Radaelli, 1976).
(d) *Optical rotation:* $[\alpha]_D^{25}$ = +10.6° (c = 5% in deuterated chloroform) (Gallo & Radaelli, 1976)
(e) *Solubility:* Practically insoluble in water; freely soluble in chloroform; soluble in ethyl acetate, methanol and dimethyl sulphoxide; slightly soluble in ethanol and acetone (Gallo & Radaelli, 1976)
(f) *Stability:* Stable as dry powder. Subject to oxidation and photodegradation at temperatures above 40°C

1.4 Technical products and impurities

Various national and international pharmacopoeias give specifications for the purity of rifampicin in pharmaceutical products. For example, it is available in the US as a USP grade containing not less than 90.0% rifampicin calculated on the dried basis. It is also available in 300 mg doses as capsules containing 90.0-130.0% of the stated amount of rifampicin (US Pharmacopeial Convention, Inc., 1975). Under US Food & Drug Administration (1978) regulations, all rifampicin must be batch certified and fulfill certain standards of identity, potency, quality and purity.

In the UK, rifampicin is available in 150 and 300 mg doses as capsules and in 450 and 600 mg doses as tablets. It is also available in a syrup containing 100 mg rifampicin in each 5 ml, and in combination tablets containing 150 mg rifampicin and 100 mg isonicotinic acid hydrazide (Wade, 1977).

In Japan, rifampicin is available in 450 mg doses as capsules.

The main impurities of rifampicin have been reported to be 3-formylrifamycin SV and rifampicin-quinone (Gallo & Radaelli, 1976).

2. Production, Use, Occurrence and Analysis

2.1 Production and use

(a) Production

Rifampicin is a semi-synthetic derivative of rifamycin antibiotics which are produced by the fermentation of *Streptomyces mediterranei*, a species which was first isolated in Italy in 1957 from a soil sample collected in France. The fermentation produces a complex mixture from which rifamycin B is isolated. Rifamycin B is transformed by a series of reactions into 3-formylrifamycin SV, which in turn is condensed with 1-amino-4-methylpiperazine in peroxide-free tetrahydrofuran to give rifampicin (Harvey, 1975; Gallo & Radaelli, 1976).

There is no evidence that rifampicin has ever been produced commercially in the US. US imports of rifampicin through principal US customs districts in recent years have shown a steady growth from a level of 321 kg in 1972 (US Tariff Commission, 1973) to 6190 kg in 1978 (US International Trade Commission, 1979).

One company in Switzerland has fermentation facilities to produce rifamycin B. Two manufacturers, one in Brazil and one in Argentina, produce rifampicin, but the basic fermentation step is carried out elsewhere. One company in Italy produces both rifamycin B and rifampicin.

No evidence was found that rifampicin has ever been commercially produced in Japan. Imports were 9000 kg in 1976, 10,000 kg in 1977 and 12,000 kg in 1978, principally from Italy, Switzerland and Thailand.

(b) Use

Rifampicin is a very broad spectrum, semi-synthetic antibiotic with bactericidal activity against most gram-positive and gram-negative bacteria at concentrations attainable *in vivo*. It acts by inhibiting DNA-dependent RNA polymerase, which leads to the suppression of RNA chain synthesis (Goodman & Gilman, 1975). Rifampicin is especially active against the following gram-positive bacteria: *Staphylococcus pyogenes, Streptococcus pyogenes, Strep. viridans,* and *Diplococcus pneumoniae*; and it is variably active against gram-negative organisms, especially *Hemophilus influenzae, meningococci* and *gonococci*. Both *Myocobacterium tuberculosis* and *M. leprae* are very susceptible to the drug (Harvey, 1975).

The main use of rifampicin is in the treatment of leprosy and tuberculosis, in association with other antimycobacterial drugs (WHO, 1977). The usual daily dose is 450 mg in patients weighing less than 50 kg and 600 mg in patients weighing more than 50 kg. The dosage for children is 10-20 mg/kg, maximum 600 mg daily. For intermittent regimens, 600 mg are given to adult patients twice a week (Harvey, 1975; Wade, 1977).

Rifampicin is also used in the chemoprophylactic treatment of asymptomatic carriers of *Neisseria meningitidis*, although it is not used for treatment of meningococcal infections (Goodman & Gilman, 1975; American Society of Hospital Pharmacists, 1979).

2.2 Occurrence

The rifamycins are a group of structurally similar antibiotics produced by *Streptomyces mediterranei*. Rifampicin does not occur in nature.

2.3 Analysis

Analytical methods for the determination of rifampicin in bulk products, pharmaceutical preparations and biological fluids based on spectrophotometric methods, fluorometric determination, complex formation, chromatographic methods and microbiological methods have been reviewed (Gallo & Radaelli, 1976). Typical methods for the analysis of rifampicin in various matrices are summarized in Table 1. Abbreviations used are: FL, fluorimetry; S, spectrometry; T, titration; TLC, thin-layer chromatography; DPA, diffusion plate assay; and HPLC/S, high-performance liquid chromatography with spectrometry.

Table 1. Analytical methods for rifampicin

Sample matrix	Sample preparation	Assay procedure	Limit of detection	Reference
Formulations	Transform into fluorescent product with hydrogen peroxide in aqueous carbonate-bicarbonate buffer	FL	not given	Finkel et al., 1971
	Dissolve in methanol; treat with aqueous solution of aluminium chloride	S	not given	Bârză, 1973a
	Dissolve in chloroform; develop with chloroform-methanol-water system	TLC	0.3 μg	Wilson et al., 1977
Capsules	Oxidize with excess ferric chloride	T	not given	Bârză, 1973b
	Dissolve in methanol; treat with aqueous solution of aluminium chloride	S	not given	Bârză, 1973a
Biological samples				
Bile	Extract with benzene	S	not given	Maggi et al., 1969
Serum	Extract with isoamyl alcohol	S	not given	Sunahara & Nakagawa, 1972
Plasma	Extract with chloroform in the presence of ascorbic acid and urea; dissolve in benzene and methanol; inject into chromotographic column; elute with ethyl acetate, piperidine and methanol	HPLC/S	not given	Murray et al., 1975

Table 1 (contd)

Sample matrix	Sample preparation	Assay procedure	Limit of detection	Reference
Biological samples (contd)				
Urine	Dissolve in methanol, treat with aqueous aluminium chloride	S	not given	Bârză, 1973a
	Extract with benzene	S	not given	Maggi et al., 1969
	Extract with isoamyl alcohol	S	not given	Sunahara & Nakagawa, 1972

RIFAMPICIN

3. Biological Data Relevant to the Evaluation of Carcinogenic Risk to Humans

3.1 Carcinogenicity studies in animals

(a) Oral administration

Mouse: Groups of 30-40 male and 36-44 female 8-week-old C3Hf mice received 0.0, 0.01, 0.03 or 0.06% rifampicin in the drinking-water with 0.05% sodium ascorbate for 60 weeks. An additional control group of 40 males and 40 females received only plain tap-water. Two males and 4 females died during treatment; 22-29 males and 23-28 females in the 5 groups were alive at 114 weeks of age, when the study was terminated. The combined incidences of benign and malignant liver-cell tumours in the 2 control groups and in the 3 treated groups were as follows: males, 16/40 (tap-water only), 18/30, 20/40, 21/40, 23/40; females, 9/39, 8/40, 16/40, 27/44 ($P<0.001$), 29/36 ($P<0.001$). There were no differences in the incidences of other types of tumour between treated and control groups of either sex (Della Porta *et al.*, 1978).

In a similar experiment, groups of 41-43 male and 36-38 female 8-week-old BALB/c mice received 0.0, 0.01, 0.03 or 0.06% rifampicin in drinking-water with 0.05% sodium ascorbate for 60 weeks. An additional control group received only plain tap-water. The experiment was terminated when the animals were 120 weeks of age. The median age at death was similar among animals of the same sex in all groups. The incidence of each tumour type was not significantly higher in treated than in control animals of either sex (Della Porta *et al.*, 1978).

Rat: Groups of 19-22 male and 19-20 female 6-week-old Wistar rats received 0.0, 0.03, or 0.06% rifampicin in drinking-water with 0.05% sodium ascorbate for 104 weeks. The experiment was terminated when the animals were 144 weeks of age. At the end of treatment, 33 males and 43 females, equally distributed among the different groups, were still alive. The incidence of each tumour type was not significantly different among animals of either sex in the three groups (Della Porta *et al.*, 1978).

(b) Subcutaneous and/or intramuscular administration

Mouse: A group of 30 male and 30 female young adult BALB/c mice were given 20 s.c. injections of 0.3 mg rifampicin in saline into the axilla over 2 months and kept under observation for 10 additional months; 2 similar groups were injected with saline or kept untreated. No malignant tumours were observed (Bichel, 1973). [Attention is drawn to the short duration of the experiment.]

3.2 Other relevant biological data

(a) Experimental systems

Toxic effects

The oral LD_{50}'s of rifampicin in rabbits, rats and mice are 2120, 1720 and in the range of 800-885 mg/kg bw, respectively. In mice, the i.v. LD_{50} is 260 mg/kg bw and the i.p. LD_{50} is in the range of 610-640 mg/kg bw; the i.p. LD_{50} in rats it is 550 mg/kg bw (Furesz, 1970; Goldberg et al., 1974).

In a 4-week toxicity study, rabbits that received 400 mg/kg bw per day orally showed considerable weight decrease and marked jaundice, together with fatty and hydropic degeneration of livers and kidneys. Liver and kidney degeneration was also observed in dogs that received 50 mg/kg bw per day in a 6-month chronic toxicity study; 2 dogs showed alterations in bone-marrow megakaryocytes (Furesz, 1970).

In rats, administration of 200 mg/kg bw per day rifampicin by gastric intubation for 8 days produced a transient decrease in body weight, especially in females; 400 mg/kg bw daily for 8 days produced a very pronounced decrease in body weight, early anorexia, apathy, ataxia and marked dorsal hair loss. It induced fatty liver and a significant increase in the total cholesterol in the livers of male and female rats and in total lipids and triglycerides in the livers of female rats (Piriou et al., 1979).

Prenatal toxicity

Oral administration of doses over 150 mg/kg bw rifampicin to mice, rats and rabbits during the active period of organogenesis produced spina bifida in offspring of rats and mice and cleft palates in mouse fetuses; no effects were observed on rabbit fetuses (Tuchmann-Duplessis & Mercier-Parot, 1969). An incidence of 59% cleft palate was observed in mouse fetuses exposed prenatally to doses of 500 mg/kg bw per day on days 9 and 10 of gestation (Jäger et al., 1974).

Absorption, distribution, excretion and metabolism

Absorption of orally administered doses of 1.25-10 mg/kg bw rifampicin was faster in mice and rats than in dogs: maximum blood levels were reached in approximately 90 minutes in mice and rats and in 5-6 hours in dogs (Furesz, 1970).

Rifampicin administered intravenously to albino mice undergoes rapid tissue distribution (Boman, 1975a). A high untake of ^{14}C-rifampicin was initially observed in the liver of rats and mice (Akimoto et al., 1970; Boman, 1975a); in mice, lung, myocardium, brown fat, salivary glands, gastrointestinal mucosa, pancreas and kidney all showed higher uptakes than the blood (Boman, 1975a).

Rifampicin accumulates in melanin-containing tissues and is transferred transplacentally (Boman, 1975b).

In male rats, following oral administration of 50 mg/kg bw ^{14}C-rifampicin, 21.3% and 40.6% of the dose was excreted in urine and faeces, respectively, by 48 hours (Akimoto et al., 1970). Elimination of the drug from plasma was rapid in rats and guinea-pigs, slower in mice and very slow in dogs (Furesz, 1970). Two metabolites were identified in liver, bile and faeces of rats: 25-deacetylrifampicin and N-demethylrifampicin (Akimoto et al., 1970). Deacetylation of rifampicin also occurs in dogs and guinea-pigs (Furesz, 1970).

Mutagenicity and other, related short-term tests

Rifampicin was not mutagenic in spot tests using reversion assays with *Salmonella typhimurium his*⁻ G46 and TA1532 or with *Escherichia coli trp*⁻ WP2, in forward mutations in *Escherichia coli* (to azetidine carboxylic acid-resistance) or in *Saccharomyces cerevisiae* (to canavanine-resistance), nor in gene conversion in *Saccharomyces cerevisiae*. There was no differential sensitivity of *E. coli* WP2 *uvr A*⁺ and *uvr A*⁻ strains, but with the *S. typhimurium uvr B+* (D 3052) and *uvr B*⁻ (TA1534) strains different growth inhibition was observed (Mitchell, 1974).

Feeding of *Drosophila melanogaster* males for 3 days with 0.5 mg/ml rifampicin did not result in increased recessive lethality among the progeny (Vogel & Obe, 1973). Kočišová & Šrám (1974) obtained the same result by injecting male flies with a 0.15% rifampicin solution.

In a dominant lethal assay, i.p. injection of 750 mg/kg rifampicin to male mice produced no significant increase in the number of early fetal deaths in the first mating week (Epstein et al., 1972).

No significant increase in chromosomal aberrations was found in metaphase I of meiosis when mice were treated intraperitoneally with 150 mg/kg bw rifampicin at the preleptotene stage of spermatocytes or at the spermatogonial stage (Šrám & Kočišová, 1975).

In human leucocytes treated *in vitro* with rifampicin, the chromosomes showed no evidence of a clastogenic effect (Vogel & Obe, 1973). However, an increase in chromatid breaks was seen when whole blood cell cultures were treated with rifampicin (Roman & Georgian, 1977). No significant effect on chromosome breakage in HeLa cells was observed after 30 passages of the cells in medium containing 150 µg/ml rifampicin (Klen et al., 1973). It has been reported (Srb et al., 1974) that treatment with rifampicin induces no chromosome aberrations in HEp-2 cells; however, the actual numbers of structural aberrations observed (16 in 1098 control chromosomes; 38 in 1094 chromosomes in treated cells) would seem to indicate a significant difference using the tables of Kastenbaum & Bowman (1970).

Rifampicin does not form a complex with isolated, double-stranded DNA (Neogy et al., 1974). It acts by inhibiting DNA-dependent RNA polymerase, which leads to the suppression of RNA chain synthesis (Goodman & Gilman, 1975).

(b) Humans

Toxic effects

There are numerous reports of acute renal failure due to rifampicin. A case report and a survey of the literature are given by Nessi et al. (1976).

Cutaneous reactions, consisting of flushing of the face and neck sometimes with itching or a rash; gastrointestinal reactions, consisting of loss of appetite, nausea, mild abdominal pain and, occasionally, vomiting and diarrhoea; hepatitis; and thrombocytopenic purpura can occur following rifampicin administration, irrespective of whether it is given daily or intermittently. Reactions such as the 'flu' syndrome - i.e., episodes of fever, chills, and sometimes headache, dizziness and bone pain starting 1-2 hours after each dose of rifampicin and lasting up to 8 hours - collapse and shock, shortness of breath, haemolytic anaemia and renal failure usually occur only if rifampicin is given intermittently, and in particular if given once or twice a week (Ferguson, 1971; Scheuer et al., 1974; Vaughan, 1977; Bedir et al., 1978; Girling & Hitze, 1979). Ocular toxicity has also been reported (Cayley & Majumdar, 1976).

After administration of 1200 mg rifampicin daily for 14 days to healthy volunteers, the half-life of thyroxine (T4) was decreased from 157 to 106 hours. A significant decrease in reverse triiodothyronine (rT_3) and an increase in triidothyronine (T_3) were also observed (Ohnhaus & Studer, 1980).

Prenatal toxicity

Warkany (1979) reviewed this subject and reported on 118 pregnancies of women exposed to rifampicin in whose offspring no increase in malformation rate was observed.

Steen & Stainton-Ellis (1977) reported on 229 pregnancies in which there was exposure to rifampicin. There were 202 live births, 22 abortions (17 induced) and 5 intrauterine deaths. Nine (4.5%) of the live-born children had malformations, including anencephaly (1), hydrocephaly (2), skeletal reduction anomalies (3), urinary anomalies (1) and a dislocated hip (unlikely to have been produced by rifampicin). In 10 a hemorrhagic tendency was observed. [Attention is drawn to the fact that this report did not specify the method of selecting the treated women.]

Absorption, distribution, excretion and metabolism

After oral administration of rifampicin on an empty stomach, the absorption is rapid and practically complete (Acocella, 1978).

Rifampicin induces drug-metabolizing enzymes in the liver (Zilly *et al.*, 1975). Its apparent half-life in serum decreases after repeated administration: the half-life of rifampicin after daily oral doses of 300 mg was 2.7 hours on day 1 and 1.5 hours on day 8 (Nitti *et al.*, 1972; Acocella, 1978; Emmerson *et al.*, 1978). With doses above 300-450 mg, the kinetics of elimination become non-linear, with more than proportional increases in serum concentration and slower elimination (Acocella, 1978).

Rifampicin is excreted unchanged in urine and bile (Acocella, 1978) and is also metabolized. The major metabolite of rifampicin is deacetylrifampicin (Maggi *et al.*, 1969), which is excreted principally in bile (Maggi *et al.*, 1969; Acocella, 1978). Other identified urinary metabolites are 3-formylrifampicin (Sunahara & Nakagawa, 1972; Acocella, 1978), rifampicinquinone, deacetylrifampicinquinone and 3-formyldeacetylrifampicin (Sunahara & Nakagawa, 1972).

Mutagenicity and other, related short-term tests

No differences were found in the frequency of chromosomal aberrations in leucocytes of tuberculous patients before treatment and during chemotherapy with either isoniazid/streptomycin/*para*-aminosalicylic acid, replaced by ethambutol after 3 months, or isoniazid/rifampicin/ethambutol (Obe *et al.*, 1976).

3.3 Case reports and epidemiological studies of carcinogenicity in humans

No data were available to the Working Group.

4. Summary of Data Reported and Evaluation

4.1 Experimental data

Rifampicin has been tested in two strains of mice and in rats by oral administration. It was also tested in mice by subcutaneous administration. After oral administration, it significantly increased the incidence of benign and malignant liver-cell tumours only in female mice of one strain; no evidence of carcinogenicity was observed in animals of the other strain. In rats, no increased tumour incidence was found. The experiment by subcutaneous administration was inadequate.

The available studies on mutagenicity indicated the absence of a mutagenic effect.

Rifampicin is teratogenic for mice and rats.

4.2 Human data

Rifampicin is a commonly used antimycobacterial drug. Its use in human medicine has increased recently.

No case reports or epidemiological studies were available to the Working Group.

In a preliminary report, nine malformations occurred among the children of 229 women exposed to the drug. (Three had defects of the central nervous system, and three had skeletal reduction defects.)

4.3 Evaluation

In view of the *limited evidence*[1] for the carcinogenicity of rifampicin in mice and the absence of epidemiological studies, no evaluation of the carcinogenicity of rifampicin to humans could be made.

---

[1] See preamble, p. 18.

5. References

Acocella, G. (1978) Clinical pharmacokinetics of rifampicin. *Clin. Pharmacokinet., 3,* 108-127

Akimoto, T., Ono, K. & Nanpo, T. (1970) Absorption, distribution, metabolism and excretion of rifampicin (RFP) in the rat (Jpn.). *Jpn. J. Antibiot., 23,* 250-256

American Society of Hospital Pharmacists (1979) *American Hospital Formulary Service,* Washington DC, Section 8:16

Bârză, P. (1973a) Contribution to the analytical study of rifampicin. V. A new spectrophotometric method for the determination of rifampicin (Rom.). *Farmacia (Bucharest), 21,* 435-439

Bârză, P. (1973b) Contributions to the analytical study of rifampicin. IV. Indirect iodometric determination of rifampicin (Rom.) *Farmacia (Bucharest), 21,* 121-126

Bedir, Ö., Yalcin, E. & Eskinasis, N. (1978) Rifampicin induced hepatitis in childhood (Ger.). *Monatsschr. Kinderheilkd., 126,* 337-339

Bichel, J. (1973) Rifampicin in a carcinogenic experiment. *Lancet, ii,* 1209

Boman, G. (1975a) Tissue distribution of ^{14}C-rifampicin. I. Whole body autoradiography of albino mice. *Acta pharmacol. toxicol., 36,* 257-266

Boman, G. (1975b) Tissue distribution of ^{14}C-rifampicin. II. Accumulation in melanin-containing structures. *Acta pharmacol. toxicol., 36,* 267-283

Cayley, F.E. & Majumdar, S. (1976) Ocular toxicity due to rifampicin. *Br. med. J., i,* 199-200

Della Porta, G., Cabral, J.R. & Rossi, L. (1978) Carcinogenicity study of rifampicin in mice and rats. *Toxicol. appl. Pharmacol., 43,* 293-302

Emmerson, A.M., Grüneberg, R.N. & Johnson, E.S. (1978) The pharmacokinetics in man of a combination of rifampicin and trimethoprim. *J. antimicrob. Chemother., 4,* 523-531

Epstein, S.S., Arnold, E., Andrea, J., Bass, W. & Bishop, Y. (1972) Detection of chemical mutagens by the dominant lethal assay in the mouse. *Toxicol. appl. Pharmacol., 23,* 288-325

Ferguson, G.C. (1971) Rifampicin and thrombocytopenia. *Br. med. J., ii,* 638

Finkel, J.M., Pittillo, R.F. & Mellett, L.B. (1971) Fluorometric and microbiological assays for rifampicin and the determination of serum levels in the dog. *Chemotherapy, 16,* 380-388

Furesz, S. (1970) Chemical and biological properties of rifampicin. *Antibiot. Chemother., 16,* 316-351

Gallo, G.G. & Radaelli, P. (1976) *Rifampin.* In: Florey, K., ed., *Analytical Profiles of Drug Substances,* Vol. 5, New York, Academic Press, pp. 467-513

Girling, D.J. & Hitze, K.L. (1979) Adverse reactions to rifampicin. *Bull. World Health Organ., 57,* 45-49

Goldberg, L.E., Stepanova, E.S., Muraveiskaya, V.S., Belova, I.P., Vertogradova, T.P. & Shepelevtseva, N.G. (1974) Toxicity and pharmacological properties of rifampicin (Russ.). *Antibiotiki (Moscow), 19,* 427-432

Goodman, L.S. & Gilman, A., eds (1975) *The Pharmacological Basis of Therapeutics,* 5th ed., New York, Macmillan, pp. 1208-1210

Harvey, S.C. (1975) *Antimicrobial drugs.* In: Osol, A., eds., *Remington's Pharmaceutical Sciences,* 15th ed., Easton, PA, Mack Publishing Co., p. 1124

Jäger, E., Merker, H.-J. & Bass, R. (1974) Investigations on the mode of teratogenic action of high doses of rifampicin (Abstract). *Teratology, 10,* 312

Kastenbaum, M.A. & Bowman, K.O. (1970) Tables for determining the statistical significance of mutation frequencies. *Mutat. Res., 9,* 527-549

Klen, R., Skalská, H., Srb, V. & Heger, J. (1973) The influence of rifampicin on the chromosomes of HeLa cells. *Folia biol. (Prague), 19,* 354-358

Kočišová, J. & Šrám, R.J. (1974) Effect of simultaneous administration of antibiotics and TEPA on the realization of potential chromosome breaks as translocations in *Drosophila melanogaster. Folia biol. (Prague), 20,* 325-332

Maggi, N., Furesz, S., Pallanza, R. & Pelizza, G. (1969) Rifampicin desacetylation in the human organism. *Arzneimittel-forsch., 19,* 651-654

Mitchell, I. de G. (1974) A comparison of the sensitivity and specificity of microbial systems for assessing genetic damage. *Agents Actions, 4,* 286-294

Murray, J.F., Jr, Gordon, G.R. & Peters, J.H. (1975) Determination of rifampin and desacetylrifampin in plasma (Abstract no. 497). *Pharmacologist, 17,* 266

Neogy, R.K., Chowdhury, K. & Kerr, I. (1974) Nitrocellulose filter retention method for studying drug-nucleic acid interactions. *Biochim. biophys. Acta, 374,* 96-107

Nessi, R., Bonoldi, G.L., Redaelli, B. & di Filippo, G. (1976) Acute renal failure after rifampicin: a case report and survey of the literature. *Nephron, 16,* 148-159

Nitti, V., Delli Veneri, F., Ninni, A. & Meola, G. (1972) Rifampicin blood serum levels and half-life during prolonged administration in tuberculous patients. *Chemotherapy, 17,* 121-129

Obe, G., Beek, B. & Slacik-Erben, R. (1976) The use of the human leukocyte test system for the evaluation of potential mutagens. *Proc. Eur. Soc. Toxicol., 17,* 118-127

Ohnhaus, E.E. & Studer, H. (1980) The effect of different doses of rifampicin on thyroid hormone metabolism. *Br. J. Pharmacol.* (in press)

Piriou, A., Warnet, J.-M., Jacqueson, A., Claude, J.-R. & Truhaut, R. (1979) Fatty liver induced by high doses of rifampicin in the rat: possible relation with an inhibition of RNA polymerases in eukariotic cells. *Arch. Toxicol., Suppl. 2,* 333-337

Roman, I.C. & Georgian, L. (1977) Cytogenetic effects of some anti-tuberculosis drugs *in vitro. Mutat. Res., 48,* 215-224

Scheuer, P.J., Summerfield, J.A., Lal, S. & Sherlock, S. (1974) Rifampicin hepatitis. A clinical and histological study. *Lancet, i,* 421-425

Šrám, R.J. & Kočišová, J. (1975) Effect of antibiotics on the mutagenic activity induced by chemicals. I. Chromosome aberrations during spermatogenesis in mice. *Folia biol. (Prague), 21,* 60-64

Srb, V., Puža, V., Spurná, V. & Keprtová, J. (1974) The action of rifampicin on stabilized cell lines HEp-2 and HeLa. *Experientia, 30,* 484-486

Steen, J.S.M. & Stainton-Ellis, D.M. (1977) Rifampicin in pregnancy. *Lancet, ii,* 604-605

Sunahara, S. & Nakagawa, K. (1972) Metabolic study and controlled clinical trials of rifampicin. *Chest, 61,* 526-532

Tuchmann-Duplessis, H. & Mercier-Parot, L. (1969) Influence of an antibiotic, rifampicin, on the prenatal development of rodents (Fr.). *C.R. Acad. Sci. (Paris), 269,* 2147-2149

US Food & Drug Administration (1978) Food and drugs. *US Code Fed. Regul.,* Title 21, parts 300-499, pp. 183, 711-712

US International Trade Commission (1979) *Imports of Benzenoid Chemicals and Products, 1978,* USITC Publication 990, Washington DC, US Government Printing Office, p. 81

US Pharmacopeial Convention, Inc. (1975) *The US Pharmacopeia,* 19th rev., Rockville, MD, pp. 442 and 673

US Tariff Commission (1973) *Imports of Benzenoid Chemicals and Products, 1972,* TC Publication 601, Washington DC, US Government Printing Office, p. 82

Vaughan, R.B. (1977) *Drugs used in tuberculosis and leprosy.* In: Dukes, M.N.G., ed., *Side Effects of Drugs Annual 1, A Worldwide Yearly Survey of New Data and Trends,* Amsterdam, Excerpta Medica, pp. 231-233

Vogel, E. & Obe, G. (1973) Testing of rifampicin on possible genetic effects on *Drosophila melanogaster* and human leukocyte chromosomes *in vitro. Experientia, 29,* 124-125

Wade, A., ed. (1977) *Martindale, The Extra Pharmacopoeia,* 27th ed., London, The Pharmaceutical Press, pp. 1596-1601

Warkany, J. (1979) Antituberculous drugs. *Teratology, 20,* 133-138

WHO (1977) WHO Expert Committee on leprosy. Fifth Report. *World Health Organ. Tech. Rep. Ser., 607,* 22

Wilson, W.L., Graham, K.C. & Lebelle, M.J. (1977) Thin-layer chromatographic identity and purity test for rifampin. *J. Chromatogr., 144,* 270-274

Windholz, M., ed. (1976) *The Merck Index,* 9th ed., Rahway, NJ, Merck & Co., p. 1068

Zilly, W., Breimer, D.D. & Richter, E. (1975) Induction of drug metabolism in man after rifampicin treatment measured by increased hexobarbital and tolbutamide clearance. *Eur. J. clin. Pharmacol., 9,* 219-227

SPIRONOLACTONE

1. Chemical and Physical Data

1.1 Synonyms and trade names

Chem. Abstr. Services Reg. No.: 52-01-7

Chem. Abstr. Name: Pregn-4-ene-21-carboxylic acid, 7-(acetylthio)-17-hydroxy-3-oxo-, γ-lactone, (7α, 17α)

IUPAC Systematic Name: 7α-Acetylthio-3-oxo-17α-pregn-4-ene-21,17β-carbolactone

Synonyms: β-(7α-Acetylthio-17β-hydroxy)-3-oxoandrost-4-en-17α-yl)propionic acid, lactone; 7α-acetylthio-17β-hydroxy-3-oxo-17α-pregn-4-ene-21-carboxylic acid γ-lactone; 7α-acetylthio-3-oxo-17β-pregn-4-ene-21, 17β-carbolactone; 17-hydroxy-7α-mercapto-3-oxo-17α-mercapto-3-oxo-17α-pregn-4-ene-21-carboxylic acid γ-lactone 7-acetate; 3-(3-keto-7α-acetylthio-17β-hydroxy-4-androsten-17α-yl) propionic acid lactone; 3-(3-oxo-7α-acetylthio-17β-hydroxy-4-androsten-17α-yl)propionic acid γ-lactone; 3'-(3-oxo-7α-acetylthio-17β-hydroxyandrost-4-en-17β-yl)propionic acid lactone; spiro[17H-cyclopenta(a)phenanthrene-17,2'(5'H)furan], pregn-4-ene-21-carboxylic acid deriv.; spirolactone; spirolakton; spironolactone A; S-ester with 17-hydroxy-7α-mercapto-3-oxo-17α-pregn-4-ene-21-carboxylic acid, γ-lactone

Trade names: Aldactazide; Aldactide; Aldactone; Aldactone A; Osiren; Osyrol; SC 9420; SC 15983; Spiresis; Spiridon; Spiroctanie; Spirolang; Spirone; Uractone; Verospiron; Verospirone

1.2 Structural and molecular formulae and molecular weight

$C_{24}H_{32}O_4S$ Mol. wt: 416.6

1.3 Chemical and physical properties of the pure substance

From Wade (1977) or Windholz (1976), unless otherwise specified

(a) *Description:* Buff-coloured, crystalline powder with a slightly bitter taste
(b) *Melting-point:* 201-205°C (melting and resolidification at lower temperatures, 134-135°C, is sometimes noted)
(c) *Spectroscopy data:* λ_{max} (in methanol) 238 nm, A(1% 1 cm) = 47. Infrared, nuclear magnetic resonance and mass spectral data have been tabulated (Sutter & Lau, 1975).
(d) *Optical rotation:* $[\alpha]_D^{20}$ −33.5° (1% in chloroform)
     $[\alpha]_D^{20}$ −50.0° (1% in dioxane)
(e) *Solubility:* Practically insoluble in water; freely soluble in benzene and chloroform (1 in 3); soluble in ethyl acetate, diethyl ether (1 in 100) and ethanol (1 in 80); slightly soluble in methanol and fixed oils
(f) *Stability:* Sensitive to oxidation and hydrolysis

1.4 Technical products and impurities

Various national and international pharmacopoeias give specifications for the purity of spironolactone in pharmaceutical products. For example, it is available in the US as a USP grade containing 97.0-101.5% active ingredient on a dried basis. It is also available in 25 mg doses as tablets containing 95.0-105% of the stated amount of spironolactone (US Pharmacopeial Convention, Inc., 1975). The *British Pharmacopoeia* (British Pharmacopoeia Commission, 1973) requires a minimum content of at least 96% and includes limit tests for a number of potential impurities, including mercapto compounds, sulphur and chromium (see IARC, 1980). Tablets containing 25 mg and 100 mg and combination products with a thiazide (usually hydroflumethiazide) are available (Wade, 1977). In Japan, spironolactone is available as powders and tablets.

SPIRONOLACTONE

2. Production, Use, Occurrence and Analysis

2.1 Production and use

(a) Production

Spironolactone was first synthesized in 1959 by the reaction of 3-(3-oxo-17β-hydroxy-4-androsten-17α-yl)propanoic acid γ-lactone with chloranil and *para*-toluenesulphonic acid in xylene to produce 3-(3-oxo-17β-hydroxy-4,6-androstandien-17α-yl)propanoic acid lactone, which was treated with thioacetic acid to give spironolactone (Cella & Tweit, 1959; Tweit *et al.*, 1962). It is not known whether this is the method used for commercial production.

Commercial production of spironolactone was first reported in the US in 1964 (US Tariff Commission, 1965). Only one US company is believed to produce spironolactone, and data on its production and sales are not published (see preamble, p. 21). Data on US imports and exports are not reported separately.

The drug is believed to be produced by one company in France, one company in The Netherlands, 2 companies in Italy and 3 companies in the Federal Republic of Germany. Spironolactone is not produced in Japan. Japanese imports amounted to 2.4 thousand kg in 1976, 2.9 thousand kg in 1977 and 3.3 thousand kg in 1978, all of which were imported from the US.

(b) Use

Spironolactone is an aldosterone antagonist used for the treatment of: essential hypertension; oedema associated with congestive heart failure; hepatic cirrhosis; the nephrotic syndrome and idiopathic oedema; and oedema associated with hyper-aldosteronism. It increases sodium excretion and reduces potassium excretion in the distal renal tubules (Goodman & Gilman, 1975; Swinyard, 1975; Wade, 1977).

In the treatment of essential hypertension, 50-100 mg of spironolactone are administered orally in divided doses daily, often in combination with a thiazide diuretic (Baker, 1979).

In the treatment of oedema, an initial dose of 100 mg is administered in divided doses continued for at least 5 days to determine the diuretic response. If a satisfactory response is obtained, dosage may be continued at the same or at a reduced level (American Society of Hospital Pharmacists, 1974). The average daily dosage of spironolactone for children is 1.5-3.0 mg/kg bw (Wade, 1977; Baker, 1979).

Spironolactone has also been used in the treatment of hypertension associated with hyperaldosteronism (Wade, 1977).

The US Food & Drug Administration (1979) has established regulations controlling the use of spironolactone in human medicine, because of its tumorigenic potential.

Spironolactone is reportedly used in veterinary medicine as an aldosterone antagonist (Windholz, 1976).

2.2 Occurrence

Spironolactone is not known to occur in nature.

2.3 Analysis

Analytical methods for the determination of spironolactone based on its partition coefficient, its phase solubility, and using ultra-violet spectrometry, colorimetry, fluorimetry and high-pressure liquid and thin-layer chromatography have been reviewed (Sutter & Lau, 1975).

Typical methods for the analysis of spironolactone in various matrices are summarized in Table 1. Abbreviations used are: FL, fluorimetry; UV, ultra-violet spectrometry; HPLC, high-performance liquid chromatography; BTA, blue tetrazolium assay; and TLC/FL, thin-layer chromatography with fluorimetry.

Table 1. Analytical methods for spironolactone

Sample matrix	Sample preparation	Assay procedure	Limit of detection	Reference
Formulations				
Bulk	Dissolve in methanol	UV	not given	US Pharmacopeial Convention, Inc., 1975
Tablets	Powder; triturate with hexane; extract with benzene; dissolve in methanol	UV	not given	US Pharmacopeial Convention, Inc., 1975
	Dilute in water or ethanol	HPLC	not given	Das Gupta & Ghanekar, 1978
	Dilute in ethanol	BTA	not given	Das Gupta & Ghanekar, 1978
Biological samples				
Serum	Add hydrochloric acid; extract with diethyl ether; add sodium hydroxide and reextract; evaporate; dissolve in chloroform; develop with carbon tetrachloride-ethyl acetate	TLC/FL	2 µg/l	Van der Merwe *et al.*, 1979
Plasma, bile, urine, gastric fluids	Dethioacetylate under mild acidic or alkaline conditions; measure fluorescence in 62% sulphuric acid	FL	10 µg/l	Sadée *et al.*, 1972a, 1973

3. Biological Data Relevant to the Evaluation of Carcinogenic Risk to Humans

3.1 Carcinogenicity studies in animals

Oral administration

Rat: Groups of 36 male and 36 female 7-week-old Sprague-Dawley rats received 50, 150 or 500 mg/kg bw per day spironolactone mixed in the diet for 78 weeks; a control group of 72 males and 72 females were kept untreated. In a second experiment, groups of 30 male and 30 female rats received 0, 10, 30 or 100 mg/kg bw per day spironolactone mixed in the diet for 104 weeks. Both studies were terminated at the end of treatment. In the 78-week study, an excess of thyroid adenomas in animals of both sexes and of interstitial-cell adenomas in the testis was observed with the mid- and high-dose levels. Of males of the control, low-, mid- and high-dose groups, 0/59, 4/33, 15/31 and 18/28, respectively, developed thyroid tumours; in females the incidences were 1/62, 1/31, 12/34 and 13/34, respectively. Testicular tumours occurred in 0/72, 0/36, 5/36 and 12/36 males, respectively (Lumb *et al.*, 1978). [Due to the incomplete reporting and to several inconsistencies in the observations, the Working Group considered that these results, although indicating an increased incidence of tumours at certain sites in the treated animals, were inadequate for an assessment of the overall carcinogenicity of spironolactone. The results generate sufficient concern to indicate the urgency for further testing of this chemical.]

3.2 Other relevant biological data

(a) Experimental systems

Toxic effects

The i.p. LD_{50} in rats, mice and rabbits was 790, 360 and 870 mg/kg bw, respectively, while the intragastric LD_{50} in all three species was more than 1000 mg/kg (Lumb *et al.*, 1978).

Pituitaries, adrenals and kidneys of rats, dogs and rhesus monkeys treated chronically with doses in excess of 100 times the recommended human dose were not altered histologically. In the rats, which received 100 and 500 mg/kg bw, the thyroid weight was increased in a dose-related manner, and uniformly small follicles were found; the liver was enlarged. No significant weight changes occurred in the rat testes, but maturational arrest was found. In male rhesus monkeys, mammary acinar tissue was increased. Seminal vesicles and prostates in the rats, dogs and monkeys were significantly reduced in weight (Lumb *et al.*, 1978).

Prenatal toxicity

No defects were produced in the offspring of rats and mice given i.p. doses of up to 80 mg/kg bw SC 14266 [potassium canrenoate, which is a metabolite of spironolactone in humans (Funder *et al.*, 1974; Sadée *et al.*, 1974)] during days 8-14 (rats) or 7-13 (mice) of pregnancy, although with 80 mg/kg bw some resorptions occurred in mice (Miyakubo *et al.*, 1977). Selye *et al.* (1971) reported increased resorptions in rats that received 100 mg/kg bw daily for various periods after the 6th day of pregnancy.

Absorption, distribution, excretion and metabolism

Spironolactone is well absorbed in dogs (Sadée *et al.*, 1972b), rats and rhesus monkeys (Karim *et al.*, 1976) after oral administration.

It is extensively metabolized, and there is considerable species variation both in the metabolic handling and elimination of spironolactone and its metabolites (Karim *et al.*, 1977). The plasma half-life in dogs is less than 10 minutes (Sadée *et al.*, 1972c). Biliary excretion is an important route of elimination; the total recovery in urine plus faeces together (with the amount in faeces given in parentheses) during 6 days following a single i.v. dose of 5 mg/kg bw was 97 (90), 88 (66) and 101 (55)% of the dose, respectively, in rats, dogs and rhesus monkeys (Karim *et al.*, 1976).

Metabolites of spironolactone may be divided into those in which the sulphur of spironolactone is removed and those in which the sulphur is retained. Canrenone (CAN) is the primary metabolite in the first class (Karim *et al.*, 1977) and is a biologically active metabolite (antimineralocorticoid) (Gochmann & Gantt, 1962; Sadée *et al.*, 1972a). It is further metabolized by three main pathways: (1) opening of the γ-lactone ring to canrenoic acid, which is excreted as canrenoate ester glucuronide; (2) hydroxylation to 15α-hydroxy-CAN, 15β-hydroxy-CAN and 21-hydroxy-CAN; and (3) reduction to 6,7-dihydro-CAN, 4,5β,6,7-tetrahydro-CAN, 4,5α,6,7-tetrahydro-CAN, 3β-hydroxy,4,5α-tetrahydro-CAN, 3β-hydroxy,4,5β,6,7-hexahydro-CAN and 3α-hydroxy,4,5β6,7-hexahydro-CAN. Metabolites in the second class are 7α-sulphoxide-spirolactones (two epimers), 7α-sulphone-spirolactone, 6β-hydroxy-thiomethyl analogue and 6β-hydroxy-sulphoxide. Canrenoate ester glucuronide, 21-hydroxy-CAN (excreted as a conjugate) and sulphur-containing metabolites are quantitatively important in monkeys, while the reduced metabolites are important in dogs (Karim *et al.*, 1977).

The first pathway that leads to the sulphur-containing metabolites is postulated to be the hydrolysis of the thioacetate group of spironolactone to 7α-thio-spirolactone, followed by S-methylation to 7α-thiomethyl-spirolactone (Karim et al., 1977). These two compounds have antimineralocorticoid activity in rats and dogs (Hofmann, 1974) and have also shown affinity for aldosterone-binding proteins in vitro (Funder et al., 1974). Their presence in biological fluids has not been established, but they would appear to be the precursors of the isolated metabolites.

6,7-Dihydro-CAN also possesses aldosterone antagonist activity (Kagawa et al., 1957).

Spironolactone induces a sex-dependent increase in hepatic microsomal enzyme activity in rats (Stripp et al., 1971). Pretreatment of female rats with spironolactone shortens the half-life of its main metabolite, canrenone (Solymoss et al., 1970), protects against the adrenal necrosis caused by injection of 7, 12-dimethylbenz[a]anthracene (DMBA) (Somogyi et al., 1971) and delays the development and decreases the incidence of DMBA-induced mammary tumours in rats (Kovacs & Somogyi, 1970).

Spironolactone inhibits the binding of dihydrotestosterone to its receptor in rat ventral prostate (Pita et al., 1975).

No data on mutagenic effects were available.

(b) Humans

Spironolactone is an aldosterone antagonist, which increases sodium excretion and reduces potassium excretion in the distal renal tubules (Goodman & Gilman, 1975; Wade, 1977).

Toxic effects

Gynaecomastia and impotence are recognized side-effects of the administration of spironolactone in men, especially at doses exceeding 100 mg daily but also at doses of 50 mg/day (Clark, 1965; Zarren & Black, 1975; Huffman et al., 1977).

Spironolactone treatment increased the dialysable fraction of testosterone in serum by 20% ($P<0.01$). Concentrations of canrenone similar to those found in serum after the daily oral administration of 400 mg spironolactone displaced testosterone from its serum-binding protein in vitro (Caminos-Torres et al., 1977).

Cytoplasmic bodies with a predominant phospholipid content were found in the cells of the adrenal glomerulosa at *post mortem* in 18 patients, all of whom had been treated with spironolactone, and not in the adrenals of 62 patients, many with similar diseases, who had not received spironolactone (Janigan, 1963).

Absorption, distribution, excretion and metabolism

Spironolactone is absorbed rapidly: after oral administration of +100 μCi ^{3}H-spironolactone, plasma radioactivity levels reached a maximum within 30-60 minutes. At that time, approximately 60% of the plasma radioactivity was due to unchanged spironolactone; this decreased with a half-life of some hours (Abshagen *et al*., 1976).

Spironolactone is extensively metabolized (Karim *et al*., 1975; Abshagen *et al*., 1976). Approximately 90% of a radio-labelled oral dose of 500 mg was recovered in urine (53%) and faeces (36%) within 6 days (Abshagen *et al*., 1976).

The major metabolite formed is canrenone, which reaches a rapid equilibrium with potassium canrenoate in the plasma (Sadée *et al*., 1974). The half-lives of the terminal log-linear phase of elimination of these two metabolites from plasma is about 17-22 hours Both compounds appear to only a small extent in urine and are predominantly eliminated by metabolism (Sadeé *et al*., 1973).

Other identifed urinary metabolites are: the 6β-hydroxy-sulphoxide, which is 3-(3-oxo-7α-methylsulphinyl-6β,17β-dihydroxy-4-androsten-17α-yl propionic acid γ-lactone; the 7α-sulphone-spirolactone, which is 17-hydroxy-7α-methyl-sulphonyl-3-oxo-17α-pregn-4-ene-21-carboxylic acid γ lactone; the 15α-hydroxy-canrenone, which is 15α,17-dihydroxy-3-oxo-17α-pregna-4,6-diene-21-carboxylic acid γ lactone; the 7α-sulphoxide-spirolactones (two epimers), which are 17-hydroxy-7α-methylsulphinyl-3-oxo-17α-pregn-4-ene-21-carboxylic acid γ lactones, and are unstable (Karim *et al*., 1975); and the 6β-hydroxy-7α-methylsulphonyl derivative which is the main excretion product during the first hours after dosing (Abshagen *et al*., 1976).

No data on mutagenic or teratogenic effects were available.

3.3 Case reports and epidemiological studies of carcinogenicity in humans

In a case report (Loube & Quirk, 1975), 5 women developed breast cancer after administration of 'Aldactazide' (a combination of 25 mg spironolactone plus 25 mg hydrochlorothiazide) for periods of 4-24 months.

From two of the earliest studies that investigated an association between reserpine and breast cancer (Armstrong et al., 1974; Boston Collaborative Drug Surveillance Program, 1974), data on spironolactone were subsequently reported (Jick & Armstrong, 1975). In one of the studies (Boston Collaborative Drug Surveillance Program, 1974), 1(0.7%) of 150 breast cancer patients was a user of a spironolactone-containing drug, while in the age-matched controls this frequency was 6 (1.0%) of 600. In the other study (Armstrong et al., 1974), the frequencies of spironolactone use were 1/708 (0.1%) in the breast cancer patients and 2/1430 (0.1%) in age-matched controls. The overall estimate of relative risk was 0.8, with an upper 95% one-sided confidence limit of 3.0.

Williams et al. (1978) conducted a case-control study of antihypertensive drugs and breast cancer, mainly to evaluate the previously reported association of reserpine with breast cancer (see also monograph on reserpine, p.211). From 80,000 women screened for breast cancer at several centres in the US, 2446 subjects were selected and questioned about their use of antihypertensive medication and about possible confounding factors related to breast cancer. Among the 88% who replied, there were 481 cases of breast cancer, 421 with a negative breast biopsy, and 1268 controls without breast lesions. Previous spironolactone use was reported by 13 cases (2.7%), by 9 with negative biopsies (2.1%) and by 26 controls (2.0%). Two cases (0.4%) and 7 controls (0.6%) had used spironolactone for 5 years or more. The relative risk of breast cancer for spironolactone versus no drug, adjusted for age, race and screening centre location, was 1.4 for use ever and 0.5 for therapy of 5 or more years' duration.

Data were also available from a hypothesis-seeking retrospective cohort study in which 95 commonly used drugs were tested for association with primary cancers at each main site (Friedman & Ury, 1980). As part of this study, 1475 persons who had received at least one dispensed prescription for spironolactone between 1969 and 1973 were followed up for cancer development through 1976. Expected cases were based on age- and sex-specific incidence rates for all the 143,574 subscribers to a medical care programme who had received prescriptions from the same pharmacy during the same period. Among spironolactone users, 9 cases of breast cancer were observed and 8.3 were expected. In these screening analyses, in which a number of nominally significant associations may have appeared by chance, statistically significant excesses among spironolactone users were noted only for pharyngeal cancer (2 observed and 0.1 expected, $P<0.01$) and for all cancers combined (84 observed and 63.1 expected, $P<0.05$). The excess of all cancers, 21 cases, was partly explained by an excess of 9 cases of prostatic cancer, most of which were diagnosed within 2 years of first mention of use of the drug. [This type of screening study does not include consideration of some important confounding variables, dose-response relationships, and other factors of interest in evaluating drug-cancer associations.]

4. Summary of Data Reported and Evaluation

4.1 Experimental data

Spironolactone was tested by oral administration in two experiments in rats. An increased incidence of thyroid and testicular tumours was reported in one experiment but not in another experiment of longer duration with lower doses.

Attention is drawn to the absence of studies on the teratogenicity and mutagenicity of this compound.

4.2 Human data

Spironolactone is an aldosterone antagonist commonly used as a potassium-sparing diuretic.

Five cases of breast cancer were reported in women who had used a drug containing spironolactone. Four analytical studies, however, showed no consistent evidence of an association.

4.3 Evaluation

The experimental studies, while providing *limited evidence*[1] of a carcinogenic effect, were difficult to interpret because of inadequacies and inconsistencies in reporting. Epidemiological studies have not confirmed the suspicion raised by case reports that spironolactone may cause breast cancer in humans. The data are insufficient, however, to permit confident exclusion of such an effect.

---

[1] See preamble, p. 18.

5. References

Abshagen, U., Rennekamp, H. & Luszpinski, G. (1976) Pharmacokinetics of spironolactone in man. *Naunyn-Schmiedeberg's Arch. Pharmacol., 296,* 37-45

American Society of Hospital Pharmacists (1974) *American Hospital Formulary Service,* Washington DC, p. 40:28

Armstrong, B., Stevens, N. & Doll, R. (1974) Retrospective study of the association between use of *Rauwolfia* derivatives and breast cancer in English women. *Lancet, ii,* 672-675

Baker, C.E., Jr, ed. (1979) *Physicians' Desk Reference,* Oradell, NJ, Medical Economics Co., pp. 1582-1585

Boston Collaborative Drug Surveillance Program (1974) Reserpine and breast cancer. *Lancet, ii,* 669-671

British Pharmacopoeia Commission (1973) *British Pharmacopoeia,* London, Her Majesty's Stationery Office, p. 442

Caminos-Torres, R., Ma, L. & Snyder, P.J. (1977) Gynecomastia and semen abnormalities induced by spironolactone in normal men. *J. clin. Endocrinol. Metab., 45,* 255-260

Cella, J.A. & Tweit, R.C. (1959) Steroidal aldosterone blockers. II. *J. org. Chem., 24,* 1109-1110

Clark, E. (1965) Spironolactone therapy and gynecomastia. *J. Am. med. Assoc., 193,* 157-158

Das Gupta, V. & Ghanekar, A.G. (1978) Stability-indicating methods for quantitative determination of spironolactone using high-pressure liquid chromatography and blue tetrazolium reaction. *J. pharm. Sci., 67,* 889-891

Friedman, G.D. & Ury, H.K. (1980) Initial screening for carcinogenicity of commonly used drugs. *J. natl Cancer Inst., 65* (in press)

Funder, J.W., Feldman, D., Highland, E. & Edelman, I.S. (1974) Molecular modifications of anti-aldosterone compounds: effects on affinity of spirolactones for renal aldosterone receptors. *Biochem. Pharmacol., 23,* 1493-1501

Gochman, N. & Gantt, C.L. (1962) A fluorimetric method for the determination of a major spironolactone (aldactone) metabolite in human plasma. *J. Pharmacol. exp. Ther., 135,* 312-316

Goodman, L.S. & Gilman, A., eds (1975) *The Pharmacological Basis of Therapeutics,* 5th ed., New York, Macmillan, pp. 837-838

Hofmann, L.M. (1974) *Aldosterone antagonists in laboratory animals.* In: Wesson, L.G. & Fanelli, G.M., eds, *Recent Advances in Renal Physiology and Pharmacology,* Baltimore, MD, University Park Press, pp. 305-316

Huffman, D.H., Azarnoff, D.L. & Kampmann, J. (1977) Spironolactone and gynecomastia: relationship with the metabolic clearance of androgens (Abstract). *Clin. Res., 25,* 271A

IARC (1980) *IARC Monographs on the Evaluation of the Carcinogenic Risk of Chemicals to Humans,* Vol. 23, *Some Metals and Metallic Compounds,* Lyon (in press)

Janigan, D.T. (1963) Cytoplasmic bodies in the adrenal cortex of patients treated with spirolactone. *Lancet, i,* 850-852

Jick, H. & Armstrong, B. (1975) Breast cancer and spironolactone. *Lancet, ii,* 368-369

Kagawa, C.M., Cella, J.A. & Van Arman, C.G. (1957) Action of new steroids in blocking effects of aldosterone and deoxycorticosterone on salt. *Science, 126,* 1015-1016

Karim, A., Hribar, J., Aksamit, W., Doherty, M. & Chinn, L.J. (1975) Spironolactone metabolism in man studied by gas chromatography-mass spectrometry. *Drug Metab. Disposition, 3,* 467-478

Karim, A., Kook, C., Zitzewitz, D.J., Zagarella, J., Doherty, M. & Campion, J. (1976) Species differences in the metabolism and disposition of spironolactone. *Drug. Metab. Disposition, 4,* 547-555

Karim, A., Hribar, J., Doherty, M., Aksamit, W., Chappelow, D., Brown, E., Markos, C., Chinn, L.J., Liang, D. & Zagarella, J. (1977) Spironolactone: diversity in metabolic pathways. *Xenobiotica, 7,* 585-600

Kovacs, K. & Somogyi, A. (1970) Suppression by spironolactone of 7,12-dimethylbenz[a]-anthracene-induced mammary tumors. *Eur. J. Cancer, 6,* 195-201

Loube, S.D. & Quirk, R.A. (1975) Breast cancer associated with administration of spironolactone. *Lancet, i,* 1428-1429

Lumb, G., Newberne, P., Rust, J.H. & Wagner, B. (1978) Effects in animals of chronic administration of spironolactone. A review. *J. environ. Pathol. Toxicol., 1,* 641-660

Miyakubo, H., Saito, S., Tokunaga, Y., Ando, H. & Nanba, H. (1977) SC-14266 was administered intraperitoneally to pregnant rats and mice for the examination of pre- and post-natal development in their offsprings (Jpn.). *Nichidai Igaku Zasshi, 36,* 261-282

Pita, J.C., Lippmann, M.E., Thompson, E.B. & Loriaux, D.L. (1975) Interaction of spironolactone and digitalis with the 5α-dihydrotestosterone (DHT) receptor of rat ventral prostate. *Endocrinology, 97,* 1521-1527

Sadée, W., Dagcioglu, M. & Riegelman, S. (1972a) Fluorometric microassay for spironolactone and its metabolites in biological fluids. *J. pharm. Sci., 61,* 1126-1129

Sadée, W., Riegelman, S. & Jones, S.C. (1972b) Disposition of tritium-labelled spironolactones in the dog. *J. pharm. Sci., 61,* 1132-1135

Sadée, W., Riegelman, S. & Jones, S.C. (1972c) Plasma levels of spironolactones in the dog. *J. pharm. Sci., 61,* 1129-1132

Sadée, W., Dagcioglu, M. & Schröder, R. (1973) Pharmacokinetics of spironolactone, canrenone and canrenoate-K in humans. *J. Pharmacol. exp. Ther., 185,* 686-695

Sadée, W., Schröder, R., Leitner, E.V. & Dagcioglu, M. (1974) Multiple dose kinetics of spironolactone and canrenoate-potassium in cardiac and hepatic failure. *Eur. J. clin. Pharmacol., 7,* 195-200

Selye, H., Taché, Y. & Szabo, S. (1971) Interruption of pregnancy by various steroids. *Fertil. Steril., 22,* 735-740

Solymoss, B., Toth, S., Varga, S. & Krajny, M. (1970) The influence of spironolactone on its own biotransformation. *Steroids, 16,* 263-275

Somogyi, A., Kovacs, K., Solymoss, B., Kuntzman, R. & Conney, A.H. (1971) Suppression of 7,12-dimethylbenz[a]anthracene-produced adrenal necrosis by steroids capable of inducing aryl hydrocarbon hydroxylase. *Life Sci., 10,* 1261-1271

Stripp, B., Hamrick, M.E., Zampaglione, N.G. & Gillette, J.R. (1971) The effect of spironolactone on drug metabolism by hepatic microsomes. *J. Pharmacol. exp. Ther., 176,* 766-771

Sutter, J.L. & Lau, E.P.K. (1975) *Spironolactone.* In: Florey, K., ed., *Analytical Profiles of Drug Substances,* Vol. 4, New York, Academic Press, pp. 431-451

Swinyard, E.A. (1975) *Diuretic drugs.* In: Osol, A., ed., *Remington's Pharmaceutical Sciences,* 15th ed., Easton, PA, Mack Publishing Co., pp. 867-868

Tweit, R.C., Colton, F.B., McNiven, N.L. & Klyne, W. (1962) Steroid aldosterone blockers. V. Stereochemistry of the addition of ethanethiolic acid to $\Delta^{4,6}$-3-oxosteroids. *J. org. Chem., 27,* 3325-3327

US Food & Drug Administration (1979) Spironolactone; drugs for human use; drug efficacy study implementaton; announcement. *Fed. Regist., 44,* No. 119, 35295-35296

US Pharmacopeial Convention, Inc. (1975) *The US Pharmacopeia,* 19th rev., Rockville, MD, pp. 469-470

US Tariff Commission (1965) *Synthetic Organic Chemicals, US Production and Sales, 1964,* TC Publication 167, Washington DC, US Government Printing Office, p. 137

Van der Merwe, P.J., Muller, D.G. & Clark, E.C. (1979) Quantitation of spironolactone and its metabolite, canrenone, in human serum by thin-layer spectrofluorimetry. *J. Chromatogr., 171,* 519-521

Wade, A., ed. (1977) *Martindale, The Extra Pharmacopoeia,* 27th ed., London, The Pharmaceutical Press, pp. 567-569

Williams, R.R., Feinleib, M., Connor, R.J. & Stegens, N.L. (1978) Case-control study of antihypertensive and diuretic use by women with malignant and benign breast lesions detected in a mammography screening program. *J. natl Cancer Inst., 61,* 327-335

Windholz, M., ed. (1976) *The Merck Index,* 9th ed., Rahway, NJ, Merck & Co., p. 1132

Zarren, H.S. & Black, P.M. (1975) Unilateral gynecomastia and impotence during low-dose spironolactone administration in men. *Mil. Med., 140,* 417-419

SULFAFURAZOLE (SULPHISOXAZOLE)

1. Chemical and Physical Data

1.1 Synonyms and trade names:

Chem. Abstr. Services Reg. No.: 127-69-5

Chem. Abstr. Name: Benzenesulfonamide, 4-amino-*N*-(3,4-dimethyl-5-isoxazolyl)-

IUPAC Systematic Name: *N'*-(3,4)Dimethylisoxazol-5-yl-sulphanilamide

Synonyms: 5-(*para*-Aminobenzenesulphonamide)-3,4-dimethylisoxazole; 4-amino-*N*-(3,4-dimethyl-5-isoxazolyl)benzenesulphonamide; 5-(4-aminophenylsulphonamido)-3,4-dimethylisoxazole; 3,4-dimethylisoxazole-5-sulphanilamide; N^1-(3,4-dimethyl-5-isoxazolyl)sulphanilamide; 3,4-dimethyl-5-sulphanilamidoisoxazole; 3,4-dimethyl-5-sulphonamidoisoxazole; sulphadimethylisoxazole; sulphafuraz; sulphafurazol; sulphafurazole; sulphafurazolum; sulphaisoxazole; 5-sulphanilamido-3,4-dimethylisoxazole; sulphisoxazol; sulphofurazole

Trade names: Accuzole; Alphazole; Amidoxal; Astrazolo; Azo Gantrisin; Azosulfizin; Bactesulf; Barazae; Chemouag; Dorsulfan; Entusil; Entusul; Ganda; Gantrisin; Gantrisine; Gantrisona; Gantrosan; Isoxamin; J-Sul; Koro-Sulf; Neazolin; Neoxazol; Norilgan-S; Novazolo; Novosaxazole; NU 445; Pancid; Renosulfan; Resoxol; Roxosul; Roxoxol; Saxosozine; Sodizole; Sosol; Soxamide; SK - Soxazole; Soxisol; Soxitabs; Soxo; Soxomide; Stansin; Sulbio; Sulfagan; Sulfagen; Sulfalar; Sulfapolar; Sulfasan; Sulfasol; Sulfazin; Sulfazole; Sulfisin; Sulfizin; Sulfizol; Sulfizole; Sulfoxol; Suloxsol; Sulsoxin; Thiasin; TL-azole; Unisulf; Urisoxin; Uritrisin; Urogan; U.S. - 67; Vagilia; V-Sul

1.2 Structural and molecular formulae and molecular weight

$C_{11}H_{13}N_3O_3S$　　　　　　　　　　Mol. wt: 267.3

1.3 Chemical and physical properties of the pure substance

From Wade (1977), unless otherwise specified

(a) Description: White, odourless, crystalline powder with a slightly bitter taste
(b) Melting-point: 195-198°C
(c) Spectroscopy data: λ_{max} (in phosphate buffer pH 7.5) 253 nm, A(1%, 1 cm) = 79. Infrared, nuclear magnetic resonance and mass spectral data have been tabulated (Rudy & Senkowski, 1973).
(d) Solubility: Practically insoluble in water; soluble in ethanol (1 in 50), chloroform (1 in 1000), diethyl ether (1 in 800), acetone, 5% aqueous sodium bicarbonate (1 in 30) and dilute hydrochloric acid
(e) Stability: Sensitive to oxidation and light

1.4 Technical products and impurities

Various national and international pharmacopoeias given specifications for the purity of sulfafurazole in pharmaceutical products. For example, it is available in the US as a USP grade containing 99.0-101.0% active ingredient calculated on the dried basis. Specifications are given for the melting-point range (194-199°C), the loss on drying (not to exceed 0.5%), and residue on ignition (limited to 0.1%). Selenium content should not exceed 0.003% and heavy metals should not exceed 0.002%. It is available in 500 mg doses as tablets containing 95.0-105.0% of the stated amount of sulfafurazole (US Pharmacopeial Convention, Inc., 1975).

In the *British Pharmacopoeia,* sulfafurazole contains not less than 99% and complies with a thin-layer chromatography test for related sulfonamide-based impurities (British Pharmacopoeia Commission, 1973). It is also available in the UK in 500 mg doses as tablets (Wade, 1977).

SULFAFURAZOLE (SULPHISOXAZOLE)

In Japan, sulfafurazole is available in tablets, powder, syrups and as 10 and 20% injections.

2. Production, Use, Occurrence and Analysis

2.1 Production and use

(a) Production

Sulfafurazole was first synthesized in 1947 by Wuest and Hoffer (Windholz, 1976). In one reported method for its manufacture, *para*-acetaminobenzene sulphonyl chloride is condensed with 3,4-dimethyl-5-amino-isoxazole in pyridine to give 5-acetaminobenzene-sulphonylamino-3,4-dimethylisoxazole. The acetyl group is then removed by treatment with 20% hydrochloric acid to give sulfafurazole. It is not known whether this is the method used for its commercial production.

Commercial production of sulfafurazole was first reported in the US in 1965 (US Tariff Commission, 1967). Only one US company currently manufactures an undisclosed amount (see preamble, p. 21) (US International Trade Commission, 1979a). US imports of sulfafurazole through the principal US customs districts amounted to 23.9 thousand kg in 1978 (US International Trade Commission, 1979b). Data on US exports of sulfafurazole are not available.

One company in Italy is believed to produce the compound.

Sulfafurazole has been produced in Japan since 1965. The production from the single manufacturer is estimated to have been 5 thousand kg in 1976, 18 thousand kg in 1977 and 10 thousand kg in 1978. There is no evidence of Japanese imports or exports in recent years.

(b) Use

Sulfafurazole is widely used in human medicine as a short acting, rapidly absorbed sulfonamide, particularly for the treatment of urinary tract infections caused by susceptible organisms (usually *Escherichia coli*, *Klebsiella aerobacter*, *Staphylococcus*, *Proteus mirabiles* and, less frequently, *Proteus vulgaris*). It is also used in the treatment of vaginitis and may be used in the prevention of meningitis. It may also be used alone or with various other drugs for the treatment of toxoplasmosis, trachoma, inclusion conjunctivitis, nocardiosis, chancroids, and chloroquinine-resistant malaria. It is usually administered orally as an initial dose of 4 g followed by 1-2 g every 4-6 hours. The dosage for children over 2 months of age is 75 mg/kg bw initially, then 150 mg/kg bw in divided doses every 4 hours (maximum, 6 g daily). As a treatment for vaginitis, a 10% cream is used in a 2.5-5.0 ml dose twice daily (Goodman & Gilman, 1975; Harvey, 1975; Wade, 1977).

Sulfafurazole is used as an intermediate in the manufacture of its diethanolamine salt (sulphisoxazole diolamine; Nu 445; Gantrisin diethanolamine; Suladrin; Sulfium) and its N^1-acetyl derivative (sulphisoxazole acetyl; Lipo Gantrisin), both of which are also used as antibacterial agents. It reportedly has been used as an antimicrobial agent in veterinary medicine (Windholz, 1976).

2.2 Occurrence

Sulfafurazole is not known to occur in nature.

2.3 Analysis

Analytical methods for the determination of sulfafurazole based on phase solubility, thin-layer chromatography, spectrometry, colorimetry, fluorimetry and titrimetric analysis have been reviewed (Rudy & Senkowski, 1973). Typical methods for the analysis of sulfafurazole in various matrices are summarized in Table 1. Abbreviations used are: T, titrimetric analysis; FL, fluorimetry; and HPLC/UV, high performance liquid chromatography with ultra-violet detection.

Table 1. Analytical methods for sulfafurazole

Sample matrix	Sample preparation	Assay procedure	Limit of detection	Reference
Formulation	Dissolve in dimethylformamide; add solution of thymol blue in dimethylformamide	T (sodium methoxide)	not given	US Pharmacopeial Convention, Inc., 1975
Plasma	Form derivative (such as dansylsulphonamide) or react with 4,5-methylene-dioxy-phthalaldehyde to form phthalimidine derivative	FL	0.3 mg/l or 6 mg/l, respectively	de Silva & D'Arconte, 1969
	Vortex-mix with acetonitrile and centrifuge	HPLC/UV	2.0 mg/l	Peng et al., 1977

3. Biological Data Relevant to the Evaluation of Carcinogenic Risk to Humans

3.1 Carcinogenicity studies in animals

(a) Oral administration

Mouse: Groups of 50 male and 50 female 7-week-old B6C3F mice received by gavage, 0, 500 or 2000 mg/kg bw sulfafurazole (USP grade) suspended in 0.5% aqueous carboxymethyl cellulose, 7 days per week for 103 weeks; an additional control group was kept untreated. The experiment was terminated when the animals were 111-113 weeks of age. The survival rate was similar in all groups. Although variations in tumour incidences were observed, no significant differences attributable to treatment were found for any tumour type (National Cancer Institute, 1979).

Rat: Groups of 50 male and 50 female 5-week-old Fischer 344 rats received by gavage 0, 100 or 400 mg/kg bw sulfafurazole (USP grade) suspended in 0.5% aqueous carboxymethyl cellulose, 7 days per week for 103 weeks; an additional control group was kept untreated. The experiment was terminated when the animals were 109-111 weeks of age. No significant differences attributable to treatment were found for any tumour type (National Cancer Institute, 1979).

3.2 Other relevant biological data

(a) Experimental systems

Toxic effects

The oral LD_{50} of sulfafurazole is more than 1.0 g/kg bw in rabbits (Schnitzer et al., 1955) and 6.8 g/kg bw in mice. The oral LD_{50} of sodium sulfafurazole in mice is 10 g/kg bw (Windholz, 1976).

Prenatal toxicity

When mice and rats were administered 1000 mg/kg bw sulfafurazole orally on days 7-12 and 9-14 of pregnancy, respectively, a significant increase in cleft palate and skeletal defects was found in offspring of both species; in addition, mandibular defects were present in the rat fetuses (Kato & Kitagawa, 1973).

Absorption, distribution, excretion and metabolism

An oral dose of 1g/kg bw was absorbed rapidly in mice, and peak plasma levels of approximately 2.0 mg/ml were achieved 1 hour after administration (Nishimura *et al.*, 1958). In dogs, 75-82 and 88-96% of oral (a 250 mg tablet) and i.v. (9 mg/kg bw) doses were recovered, respectively, in the urine within 24 hours (Osbaldiston & Walker, 1972).

Mutagenicity and other, related short-term tests

Sulfafurazole was not mutagenic in *Escherichia coli* Sd-4-73 when tested in the absence of a metabolic activation system (Szybalski, 1958).

(b) Humans

Toxic effects

Adverse reactions severe enough to require discontinuation of sulfafurazole administration occurred with an incidence of 3.1% in a series of 1002 treated patients. Skin rashes, eosinophilia and drug fever were the common manifestations (Koch-Weser *et al.*, 1971).

Prenatal toxicity

Sulfafurazole has been shown to transfer into the amniotic fluid during early fetal life (Blum *et al.*, 1975). Mellin (1964) found no increase in the defect rate when mothers were treated in the first trimester. Heinonen *et al.* (1977), who examined records of 796 offspring of mothers treated in the first 4 lunar months of pregnancy, also found no increase in malformation rate.

Absorption, distribution, excretion and metabolism

Absorption of sulfafurazole is rapid and essentially complete. In fasted subjects given oral doses of 4.0 g of the sodium salt in solution, peak plasma levels occurred within the first 30 minutes after dosing (Van Petten *et al.*, 1971). The half-life of sulfafurazole is approximately 6 hours (Nelson & O'Reilly, 1960; Kaplan *et al.*, 1972).

Urinary excretion of drug following a dose of 2.0 g (oral, i.v. or i.m.) is greater than 90% of the dose; 40-60% is excreted unchanged as sulfafurazole (Kaplan *et al.*, 1972). Identified urinary metabolites of sulfafurazole are acetylsulphisoxazole, sulphisoxazole-*N*-glucuronide, sulphisoxazole-*N*-sulphonate and sulphanilamide (Uno & Kono, 1960, 1962).

No data were available on the mutagenicity of sulfafurazole in humans.

3.3 Case reports and epidemiological studies of carcinogenicity in humans

In a hypothesis-seeking study involving determination of the incidence of all forms of cancer in relation to drug exposure in 143,574 members of a health plan, no significant excess of any cancer was observed in 11,659 subjects who had received sulfafurazole. Follow-up was for a minimum of 3 years (Friedman & Ury, 1980). [About 54,000 person-years of follow-up would have been accumulated by subjects given sulfafurazole. Data on the age and sex distributions of the exposed subjects and the doses and durations of use of the drug were not given.]

4. Summary of Data Reported and Evaluation

4.1 Experimental data

Sulfafurazole was tested in mice and rats by oral administration: no increases in tumour incidences were observed.

No adequate studies of mutagenicity were available.

It is teratogenic for mice and rats.

4.2 Human data

Sulfafurazole is one of the most commonly used sulfonamide drugs in the treatment of urinary tract infections. Its production has remained stable during recent years.

In one hypothesis-seeking epidemiological study, no association was observed between sulfafurazole use and any cancer.

In two large studies of women exposed during pregnancy, no increase in malformation rate was observed in the offspring.

4.3 Evaluation

The data from studies in experimental animals and in humans were not indicative of a carcinogenic effect but were not sufficient for an evaluation of the carcinogenicity of sulfafurazole to humans.

5. References

Blum, M., Elian, I. & Ben-Tovim, R. (1975) Transfer of antibiotics across the placenta in early pregnancy (Heb.). *Harefuah, 88,* 510-512

British Pharmacopoeia Commission (1973) *British Pharmacopoeia,* London, Her Majesty's Stationery Office, p. 450

Friedman, G.D. & Ury, H.K. (1980) Initial screening for carcinogenicity of commonly used drugs. *J. natl Cancer Inst., 65* (in press)

Goodman, L.S. & Gilman, A., eds (1975) *The Pharmacological Basis of Therapeutics,* 5th ed., New York, Macmillan, pp. 1009,1124-1127

Harvey, S.C. (1975) *Antimicrobial drugs.* In: Osol, A., ed., *Remington's Pharmaceutical Sciences,* 15th ed., Easton, PA, Mack Publishing Co., p. 1111

Heinonen, O.P., Slone, D. & Shapiro, S. (1977) *Birth Defects and Drugs in Pregnancy,* Littleton, MA, Publishing Sciences Group, Inc., p. 301

Kaplan, S.A., Weinfeld, R.E., Abruzzo, C.W. & Lewis, M. (1972) Pharmacokinetic profile of sulfisoxazole following intravenous, intramuscular, and oral administration to man. *J. pharm. Sci., 61,* 773-778

Kato, T. & Kitagawa, S. (1973) Production of congenital skeletal anomalies in the fetuses of pregnant rats and mice treated with various sulfonamides. *Congenital Anomalies, 13,* 17-23

Koch-Weser, J., Sidel, V.W., Dexter, M., Parish, C., Finer, D.C. & Kanarek, P. (1971) Adverse reactions to sulfisoxazole, sulfamethoxazole, and nitrofurantoin. Manifestations and specific reaction rates during 2,118 courses of therapy. *Arch. intern. Med., 128,* 399-404

Mellin, G.W. (1964) Drugs in the first trimester of pregnancy and the fetal life of *Homo sapiens. Am. J. Obstet. Gynecol., 90,* 1169-1180

National Cancer Institute (1979) *Bioassay of Sulfisoxazole for Possible Carcinogenicity (Tech. Rep. Ser. No. 138),* Department of Health, Education & Welfare Publications No. (NIH) 79-1393, Washington DC, US Government Printing Office

Nelson, E. & O'Reilly, I. (1960) Kinetics of sulfisoxazole acetylation and excretion in humans. *J. Pharmacol. exp. Ther., 129,* 368-372

Nishimura, H., Nakajima, K., Okamoto, S., Shimaoka, N. & Sasaki, K. (1958) Part II. Comparative evaluation of MS-53 and sulfisoxazole: therapeutic effectiveness, absorption, excretion, and tissue distribution. *Ann. Rep. Shionogi Res. Lab., 8,* 779-790

Osbaldiston, G.W. & Walker, W.S. (1972) Blood concentration and renal excretion of penicillin G. and sulfisoxazole in the dog. *Am. J. vet. Res., 33,* 1479-1483

Peng, G.W., Gadalla, M.A.F. & Chiou, W.L. (1977) High pressure liquid chromatographic determination of sulfisoxazole in plasma. *Res. Commun. chem. Pathol. Pharmacol., 18,* 233-246

Rudy, B.C. & Senkowski, B.Z. (1973) *Sulfisoxazole.* In: Florey, K., ed., *Analytical Profiles of Drug Substances,* Vol. 2, New York, Academic Press, pp. 487-506

Schnitzer, R.J., Grunberg, E., Marusich, W. & Engelberg, R. (1955) The toxicity of triple mixtures of sulfonamides under conditions of continous oral administration. *Antiobiot. Chemother., 5,* 281-288

de Silva, J.A.F. & D'Arconte, L. (1969) The use of spectrophotofluorometry in the analysis of drugs in biological materials. *Forensic Sci., 14,* 184-204

Szybalski, W. (1958) Special microbiological systems. II. Observations on chemical mutagenesis in micro-organisms. *Ann. N.Y. Acad. Sci., 76,* 475-489

Uno, T. & Kono, M. (1960) Studies on the metabolism of sulfisoxazole. I. On the excrements in the human urine after administration of sulfisoxazole (Jpn.). *J. pharm. Soc. Jpn., 80,* 201-204

Uno, T. & Kono, M. (1962) Studies on the metabolism of sulfisoxazole. VI. On the new metabolite of sulfisoxazole in human. *J. pharm. Soc. Jpn., 82,* 1660-1663

US International Trade Commission (1979a) *Synthetic Organic Chemicals, US Production and Sales, 1977,* USITC Publication 920, Washington DC, US Government Printing Office, p. 160

US International Trade Commission (1979b) *Imports of Benzenoid Chemicals and Products, 1978,* USITC Publication 990, Washington DC, US Government Printing Office, p. 88

US Pharmacopeial Convention, Inc. (1975) *The US Pharmacopeia,* 19th rev., Rockville, MD, pp. 480-481

US Tariff Commission (1967) *Synthetic Organic Chemicals, US Production and Sales, 1965,* TC Publication 206, Washington DC, US Government Printing Office, p. 118

Van Petten, G.R., Becking, G.C., Withey, R.J. & Lettau, H.F. (1971) Studies on the physiological availability and metabolism of sulfonamides. II. Sulfisoxazole. *J. clin. Pathol., 11,* 35-41

Wade, A., ed. (1977) *Martindale, The Extra Pharmacopoeia,* 27th ed., London, The Pharmaceutical Press, pp. 1480-1482

Windholz, M., ed. (1976) *The Merck Index,* 9th ed., Rahway, NJ, Merck & Co., p. 1160

SULFAMETHOXAZOLE

1. Chemical and Physical Data

1.1 Synonyms and trade names

Chem. Abstr. Services Reg. No.: 723-46-6

Chem. Abstr. Name: Benzenesulfonamide, 4-amino-*N*-(5-methyl-3-isoxazolyl)-

IUPAC Systematic Name: *N'*-(5-Methylisoxazol-3-yl)sulphanilamide

Synonyms: 3-*para*-Aminobenzenesulphonamido-5-methylisoxazole; 4-amino-*N*-(5-methyl-3-isoxazolyl)benzene sulphonamide; 3-(*para*-aminophenylsulphonamido)-5-methylisoxazole; N^1-(5-methyl-3-isoxazolyl)sulphanilamide; 5-methyl-3-sulphanilamidoisoxazole; sulphamethalazole; sulphamethoxazol; sulphamethoxazole; sulphamethoxizole; sulphamethylisoxazole; 3-sulphanilamido-5-methylisoxazole; sulphisomezole

Trade names: Azo-Gantanol; Bactrim; Co-trimoxazole; Eusaprim; Fectrim; Gantanol; Metoxal; MS 53; Radonil; Ro 4-2130; Septra; Septran; Septrin; Sinomin; Trib; Trimetoprim-Sulfa

1.2 Structural and molecular formuale and molecular weight

$C_{10}H_{11}N_3O_3S$ Mol. wt: 253.3

1.3 Chemical and physical properties of the pure substance

From Wade (1977), unless otherwise stated

(a) *Description:* White or yellowish-white, odourless, crystalline powder
(b) *Melting-point:* 169-172°C
(c) *Spectroscopy data:* λ_{max} (in phosphate buffer pH 7.5) 256-257 nm, A(1%, 1cm) = 68. Infrared, mass spectral and nuclear magnetic resonance data have been tabulated (Rudy & Senkowski, 1973).
(d) *Solubility:* Practically insoluble in water; soluble in ethanol (1 in 50), acetone (1 in 3) and aqueous alkaline hydroxides; practically insoluble in chloroform and diethyl ether
(e) *Stability:* Sensitive to oxidation and light

1.4 Technical products and impurities

Various national and international pharmacopoeias give specifications for the purity of sulfamethoxazole in pharmaceutical products. For example, it is available in the US as a NF grade containing 98.5-101.0% active ingredient on a dried basis. The loss on drying at 105°C for 4 hours should not exceed 0.5%; the residue on ignition should not exceed 0.1%; and the amount of selenium should not exceed 0.003%. A thin-layer chromatographic trace test is outlined for sulphanilamide and sulphanilic acid. Sulfamethoxazole is available as an oral suspension containing 500 mg active ingredient (95.0-110.0% of the stated amount) in 5 ml solution, and in tablets as 500 mg doses containing 95.0-105.0% of the stated amount (National Formulary Board, 1975).

In the *British Pharmacopoeia* (British Pharmacopoeia Commission, 1973), specifications require a purity of not less than 99%; it also includes a limit test for related substances based on thin-layer chromatography.

In the US, UK and most other western European countries, sulfamethoxazole is available in a combination with trimethoprim called Co-trimoxazole (5 parts sulfamethoxazole and 1 part trimethoprim); this formulation is available as tablets, injections and mixtures (Wade, 1977).

2. Production, Use, Occurrence and Analysis

2.1 Production and use

(a) Production

A method of preparing sulfamethoxazole was first reported in 1957 (Windholz, 1976). One method involves the condensation of *N*-acetyl-*para*-aminobenzenesulphonyl chloride with 5-methyl-3-aminoisoxazole in pyridine. The acetyl group is then cleaved to yield sulfamethoxazole (Sittig, 1979). It is not known whether this is the method used for its commercial production.

Sulfamethoxazole reportedly was introduced in the US in 1959 (Sittig, 1979), but commercial production was not reported until 1965 (US Tariff Commission, 1967). Only one US company currently manufactures an undisclosed amount (see preamble, p. 21) (US International Trade Commission, 1978). US imports of sulfamethoxazole through the principal US customs districts amounted to 7840 kg in 1978 (US International Trade Commission, 1979).

The drug is believed to be produced by 3 companies in Italy and 1 in the UK.

Sulfamethoxazole is produced by a single Japanese company; annual production was 60 thousand kg in 1976, 49 thousand kg in 1977, and 69 thousand kg in 1978. During those years, Japan imported an average of 3 thousand kg per year from Switzerland.

(b) Use

Sulfamethoxazole is an antibacterial agent used primarily in the treatment of urinary tract infections caused by susceptible organisms (usually *Escherichia coli*, *Klebsiella aerobacter*, *Staphylococcus*, *Proteus mirabilis*, and, less frequently, *Proteus vulgaris*). It may be used in the prevention of susceptible meningitis and may also be used alone or with various other drugs for the treatment of gonorrhoea, respiratory infections, toxoplasmosis, brucellosis, trachoma, inclusion conjunctivitis, nocardiosis, chancroids and acute otitis media. The drug is used in an initial dose of 2 g, followed by 1 g 2 or 3 times per day. A total daily dose of 3 g should not be exceeded. Children are given 50-60 mg per kg bw initially, followed by 25-30 mg/kg bw twice daily (Goodman & Gilman, 1975; Harvey, 1975; Wade, 1977; Baker, 1979).

Sulfamethoxazole in combination with trimethoprim is the sulfonamide most commonly used around the world. It is also used in combination with pyrimethamine in the treatment of chloroquine-resistant falciparum malaria (Harvey, 1975).

2.2 Occurrence

Sulfamethoxazole is not known to occur in nature.

2.3 Analysis

Analytical methods for the determination of sulfamethoxazole based on phase solubility, thin-layer chromatography, spectrophotometry, colorimetry, fluorimetry and titrimetric analysis have been reviewed (Rudy & Senkowski, 1973). Typical methods for the analysis of sulfamethoxazole in various matrices are summarized in Table 1. Abbreviations used are: T, titrimetric analysis; NMR, nuclear magnetic resonance; and HPLC/UV, high-performance liquid chromatography with ultra-violet detection.

Table 1. Analytical methods for sulfamethoxazole

Sample matrix	Sample preparation	Assay procedure	Limit of detection	Reference
Formulations	Dissolve in glacial acetic acid; add water and hydrochloric acid; titrate with sodium nitrate solution	T	not given	National Formulary Board, 1975
	Powder; dissolve in dimethyl sulphoxide-d_6; centrifuge	NMR	not given	Rodriguez et al., 1977
Biological samples				
Serum	Dilute with water; add perchloric acid; centrifuge	HPLC/UV	0.5 mg/l	Vree et al., 1978a
Urine	Add perchloric acid	HPLC/UV	10 mg/l	Vree et al., 1978a

SULFAMETHOXAZOLE

3. Biological Data Relevant to the Evaluation of Carcinogenic Risk to Humans

3.1 Carcinogenicity studies in animals

Oral administration

Rat: Groups of 25-26 male and 24-25 female Charles River CD rats received 25, 50, 150, 300 or 600 mg/kg bw/day sulfamethoxazole mixed with the diet for 60 weeks, at which time the animals were killed; two groups of 50 rats were kept untreated. At the end of the treatment, some of the animals were sacrificed and thyroid nodules or adenomas were observed in treated males and females combined as follows: 0/28, 7/30, 20/29, 19/27, 23/23. Lung metastases were observed in 4 rats of the three higher dose groups. No thyroid tumours were observed in the two control groups of 28 and 26 rats that were sacrificed (Swarm *et al.*, 1973). [Attention is drawn to the short duration of the study and the absence of information on tumours other than of the thyroid.]

3.2 Other relevant biological data

(a) Experimental systems

The administration of sulfamethoxazole to rats, mice and dogs produces thyroid hyperplasia, as a result of the release of the pituitary thyroid stimulating hormone. The goitrogenic effect of this sulfonamide does not occur in monkeys (Swarm *et al.*, 1973).

No data on prenatal effects were available.

Absorption, distribution, excretion and metabolism

An oral dose of 1.0 g/kg bw sulfamethoxazole is absorbed rapidly in mice, and peak plasma levels of approximately 1.0 mg/ml were achieved 1 hour after administration. The plasma elimination half-life is approximately 6 hours. Tissue distribution studies in rats showed high concentrations of sulfamethoxazole in kidney, lung, liver, spleen and brain. The rate of elimination of the drug from these tissues paralleled that from the blood (Nishimura *et al.*, 1958).

Mutagenicity and other, related short-term tests

No chromosome aberrations were observed in human lymphocytes treated with sulfamethoxazole *in vitro* (Stevenson *et al.*, 1973). Sulfamethoxazole in combination with trimethoprim also had no effect on chromatid breaks in human fibroblasts *in vitro* (Byarugaba *et al.*, 1975).

(b) Humans

Toxic effects

Adverse reactions severe enough to require discontinuation of sulfamethoxazole administration occurred with an incidence of 3.3% in a series of 359 treated patients. Skin rashes, eosinophilia and drug fever were the common manifestations. No adverse effects on the thyroid were observed (Koch-Weser *et al.*, 1971; Swarm *et al.*, 1973).

Prenatal toxicity

Sulfamethoxazole crosses the human placenta and reaches a peak at 10 hours. After a few gestational weeks, the concentration of sulfamethoxazole is lower in amniotic fluid and in the foetus than in maternal serum (Reid *et al.*, 1975). Williams *et al.* (1969) treated 120 pregnant women and found no increase in defects in their offspring; only 10 of the women were treated before the 16th week. Heinonen *et al.* (1977) reported no increase in malformation rates in the offsping from 46 pregnancies when treatment was given in the first 4 lunar months.

Absorption, distribution, excretion and metabolism

Absorption of an orally administered dose of 800 mg sulfamethoxazole in combination with 160 mg trimethoprim is virtually complete (Schwartz & Rieder, 1970), and peak plasma levels (40-60 µg/ml) are achieved between 2 and 4 hours after administration of solid dosage forms (Bach *et al.*, 1973; Nolte & Büttner, 1974).

The plasma half-life of sulfamethoxazole, whether administered alone or in combination with trimethoprim (Bactrim®, etc.), is about 9 hours (Schwartz & Rieder, 1970; Nolte & Büttner, 1974).

Elimination of sulfamethoxazole and its metabolites from the body takes place by urinary excretion and is practically complete within 96 hours (Schwartz & Rieder, 1970); it is not significantly affected by the subject's acetylation phenotype (Vree *et al.*, 1978b). N^4-Acetylsulfamathoxazole is the major metabolite (Nishimura *et al.*, 1958). Other identified urinary metabolites are sulfamethoxazole-N^1-glucuronide (Ueda & Kuribayashi, 1964), sulfamethoxazole-$N^{2'}$-glucuronide (Ueda *et al.*, 1967) and hydroxysulfamethoxazole (Ueda *et al.*, 1971).

SULFAMETHOXAZOLE

Mutagenicity and other, related short-term tests

Administration of sulfamethoxazole in combination with trimethoprim to patients (adults or children) in therapeutic doses (about 2 g per day) did not increase the frequency of chromosome aberrations in peripheral lymphocytes (Stevenson *et al.*, 1973; Gebhart, 1973, 1975a,b).

3.3 Case reports and epidemiological studies of carcinogenicity in humans

Data were available only from a hypothesis-seeking, retrospective cohort study in which 95 commonly used drugs were tested for association with primary cancers of each main site (Friedman & Ury, 1980). As part of this study, 1709 subjects received at least one prescription for sulfamethoxazole between 1969 and 1973 and were followed up for cancer development through 1976. Expected numbers of cancers were based on age- and sex-specific incidence rates for all 143,574 individuals who had received prescriptions from the same pharmacy during the same period. In the screening analyses, in which a number of nominally significant associations may have appeared by chance, statistically significant excesses among sulfamethoxazole users were noted for nasopharyngeal cancer (3 cases observed and 0.1 expected; $P<0.002$) and cervical cancer (7 cases observed and 2.2 expected; $P<0.05$). A possible explanation of the latter association is sexual activity, which is related to both cervical cancer and to urinary infection for which sulfamethoxazole is used. There was no associaton with all cancers combined (42 observed and 43.9 expected). [This type of screening study does not include consideration of some important confounding variables, dose-response relationships, and other factors important in evaluating drug-cancer associations.]

4. Summary of Data Reported and Evaluation

4.1 Experimental data

Sulfamethoxazole was tested in one experiment in rats by oral administration: it produced thyroid tumours.

No mutagenic effects were observed. Attention is drawn to the absence of studies on the teratogenicity of this compound.

4.2 Human data

Sulfamethoxazole is commonly used in the treatment of urinary-tract infections.

In one hypothesis-seeking epidemiological study, an association between sulfamethoxazole use and nasopharyngeal and cervical cancers was noted.

4.3 Evaluation

There is *limited evidence*[1] for the carcinogenicity of sulfamethoxazole in experimental animals. The epidemiological data were insufficient. No evaluation of the carcinogenicity of sulfamethoxazole to humans could be made.

---

[1] See preamble, p. 18.

5. References

Bach, M.C., Gold, O. & Finland, M. (1973) Absorption and urinary excretion of trimethoprim, sulfamethoxazole, and trimethoprim-sulfamethoxazole: results with single doses in normal young adults and preliminary observations during therapy with trimethoprim-sulfamethoxazole. *J. infect. Dis., 128* (Suppl.), S584-S599

Baker, C.E., Jr, ed. (1979) *Physicians' Desk Reference*, Oradell, NJ, Medical Economics Co., pp. 750-751, 1428-1430, 1436-1437

British Pharmacopoeia Commission (1973) *British Pharmacopoeia*, London, Her Majesty's Stationery Office, p. 451

Byarugaba, W., Rüdiger, H.W., Koske-Westphal, T., Wohler, W. & Passarge, E. (1975) Toxicity of antibiotics on cultured human skin fibroblasts. *Humangenetik, 28*, 263-267

Friedman, G.D. & Ury, H.K. (1980) Initial screening for carcinogenicity of commonly used drugs. *J. natl Cancer Inst., 65* (in press)

Gebhart, E. (1973) Chromosome examination after Bactrim® therapy (Ger.). *Med. Klin., 68*, 878-881

Gebhart, E. (1975a) Chromosomal studies in Bactrim® therapy (Abstract no. 54). *Mutat. Res., 29*, 280

Gebhart, E. (1975b) Chromosome studies in children treated with Bactrim® (Ger.). *Z. Kinderheilkd., 119*, 47-52

Goodman, L.S. & Gilman, A., eds (1975) *The Pharmacological Basis of Therapeutics*, 5th ed., New York, Macmillan, pp. 1009, 1058

Harvey, S.C. (1975) *Antimicrobial drugs*. In: Osol, A., ed., *Remington's Pharmaceutical Sciences*, 15th ed., Easton, PA, Mack Publishing Co., p. 1110

Heinonen, O.P., Slone, D. & Shapiro, S. (1977) *Birth Defects and Drugs in Pregnancy*, Littleton, MA, Publishing Sciences Group, Inc., pp. 298, 301

Koch-Weser, J., Sidel, V.W., Dexter, M., Parish, C., Finer, D.C. & Kanarek, P. (1971) Adverse reactions to sulfisoxazole, sulfamethoxazole, and nitrofurantoin. Manifestations and reaction rates during 2,118 courses of therapy. *Arch. intern. Med., 128*, 399-404

National Formulary Board (1975) *National Formulary,* 14th ed., Washington DC, American Pharmaceutical Association, pp. 665-667

Nishimura, H., Nakajima, K., Okamoto, S., Shimaoka, N. & Sasaki, K. (1958) Part II. Comparative evaluation of MS-53 and sulfisoxazole: therapeutic effectiveness, absorption, excretion and tissue distribution. *Ann. Rep. Shionogi Res. Lab., 8,* 779-790

Nolte, H. & Büttner, H. (1974) Investigations on plasma levels of sulfamethoxazole in man after single and chronic oral administration alone and in combination with trimethoprim. *Chemotherapy, 20,* 321-330

Reid, D.W.J., Caillé, G. & Kaufmann, N.R. (1975) Maternal and transplacental kinetics of trimethoprim and sulfamethoxazole, separately and in combination. *Can. med. Assoc. J., 112,* 67S-72S

Rodriguez, M.R., Pizzorno, M.T. & Albonico, S.M. (1977) NMR determination of trimethoprim and sulfamethoxazole in tablets and powders. *J. pharm. Sci., 66,* 121-123

Rudy, B.C. & Senkowski, B.Z. (1973) *Sulfamethoxazole.* In: Florey, K., ed., *Analytical Profiles of Drug Substances,* Vol. 2, New York, Academic Press, pp. 467-486

Schwartz, D.E. & Rieder, J. (1970) Pharmacokinetics of sulfamethoxazole + trimethoprim in man and their distribution in the rat. *Chemotherapy, 15,* 337-355

Sittig, M. (1979) *Pharmaceutical Manufacturing Encyclopedia,* Park Ridge, NJ, Noyes Data Corporation, pp. 579-580

Stevenson, A.C., Clarke, G., Patel, C.R. & Hughes, D.T.D. (1973) Chromosomal studies *in vivo* and *in vitro* of trimethoprim and sulphamethoxazole (Co-trimoxazole). *Mutat. Res., 17,* 255-260

Swarm, R.L., Roberts, G.K.S., Levy, A.C. & Hines, L.R. (1973) Observations on the thyroid gland in rats following the administration of sulfamethoxazole and trimethoprim. *Toxicol. appl. Pharmacol., 24,* 351-363

Ueda, M. & Kuribayashi, K. (1964) Studies on metabolism of drugs. V. On the new metabolite of sulfisomezole in human (Jpn.). *J. pharm. Soc. Jpn., 84,* 1104-1107

Ueda, M., Nakagawa, Y. & Murakami, N. (1967) Studies on metabolism of drugs. VI. On the new metabolite of sulfisomezole in human (2) (Jpn.). *J. pharm. Soc. Jpn., 87,* 451-454

Ueda, M., Takegoshi, I. & Koizumi, T. (1971) Studies on metabolism of drugs. X. New metabolite of sulfisomezole in man. *Chem. pharm. Bull., 19*, 2041-2045

US International Trade Commission (1978) *Synthetic Organic Chemicals, US Production and Sales, 1977*, USITC Publication 920, Washington DC, US Government Printing Office, p. 168

US International Trade Commission (1979) *Imports of Benzenoid Chemicals and Products, 1978*, USITC Publication 990, Washington DC, US Government Printing Office, p. 88

US Tariff Commission (1967) *Synthetic Organic Chemicals, US Production and Sales, 1965*, TC Publication 206, Washington DC, US Government Printing Office, p. 118

Vree, T.B., Hekster, Y.A., Baars, A.M., Damsma, J.E. & van der Kleijn, E. (1978a) Determination of trimethoprim and sulfamethoxazole (Co-trimoxazole) in body fluids of man by means of high-performance liquid chromatography. *J. Chromatogr., 146*, 103-112

Vree, T.B., Hekster, Y.A., Baars, A.M., Damsma, J.E. & van der Kleijn, E. (1978b) Pharmacokinetics of sulphamethoxazole in man; effects of urinary pH and urine flow on metabolism and renal excretion of sulphamethoxazole and its metabolite N_4-acetylsulphamethoxazole. *Clin. Pharmacokinet., 3*, 319-329

Wade, A., ed. (1977) *Martindale, The Extra Pharmacopoeia*, 27th ed., London, The Pharmaceutical Press, pp. 1484-1490

Williams, J.D., Brumfitt, W., Condie, A.P. & Reeves, D.S. (1969) The treatment of bacteriuria in pregnant women with sulphamethoxazole and trimethoprim. A microbiological, clinical and toxicological study. *Postgrad. med. J, Suppl. 45*, 71-76

Windholz, M., ed. (1976) *The Merck Index*, 9th ed., Rahway, NJ, Merck & Co., p. 1154

GENERAL CONSIDERATIONS ON N–NITROSATABLE DRUGS

Introduction

Many N-nitroso compounds (nitrosamines and nitrosamides) have been shown to be carcinogenic in experimental animals (IARC, 1978). The formation of N-nitroso compounds is theoretically possible with all compounds that contain amino groups. Secondary amines react directly; tertiary and, in some cases, primary amines may react by more complicated mechanisms. Since the endogenous formation of N-nitroso compounds from nitrosatable amine precursors and nitrosating agents, such as nitrite or nitrous gases, is not usually taken into account in carcinogenicity tests of the parent compound, additional investigations are necessary to evaluate this possible hazard.

The possibility that N-nitroso compounds are formed *in vivo* was first discussed by Druckrey & Preussmann (1962) and was first demonstrated in animal experiments by Sander & Bürkle (1969). Several detailed reviews on the subject are available (Mirvish, 1975; WHO, 1977; IARC, 1978; Olajos & Coulston, 1978; WHO, 1978).

Chemistry of N-nitrosation

The formation of nitrosamines from secondary amines and nitrite at acid pH can be described by the following equation:

$$\begin{array}{c} R_1 \\ \diagdown \\ NH + NaNO_2 \\ \diagup \\ R_2 \end{array} \xrightarrow{H^+} \begin{array}{c} R_1 \\ \diagdown \\ N - N{=}O \\ \diagup \\ R_2 \end{array} + Na^+ + OH^-$$

In reality, the chemistry of this reaction is much more complicated (Ridd, 1961; Challis & Butler, 1968; Fridman *et al.*, 1971). For amines, the effective nitrosating agent is N_2O_3, which is formed from nitrite in acidic aqueous media. Only the free, unprotonated amine, and not the amine salt, is available for nitrosation. As a result, the reaction rate is heavily dependent on pH: low pH favours formation of N_2O_3 from nitrite, but also favours protonation of the amine; at higher pH free amine is available, but N_2O_3 formation is reduced. It follows that the nitrosation of basic amines shows a pH optimum (usually pH 3.0-3.5) and is dependent on the basicity (pKa) of the amine.

The data in Table 1 demonstrate that less basic amines are much more easily nitrosated at the pH optimum than are strongly basic amines.

Table 1. Rate constants of nitrosation of amines with nitrite at optimal pH and 25°C[a]

Amine	pK_a	Optimal pH	Rate constant K_2 (mol^{-2} x sec^{-1})
Piperidine	11.2	3.0	0.00045
Dimethylamine	10.7	3.4	0.0017
N-Methylbenzylamine	9.5	3.0	0.013
Morpholine	8.7	3.4	0.42
Mononitrosopiperazine	6.8	3.0	6.7
Piperazine	5.6	3.0	83

[a] From Mirvish, 1975

The nitrosation of weakly basic secondary amides has in general no pH optimum: as the pH changes from 3 to 1, nitrosation increases by a factor of 10 per pH unit. The nitrosating agent is mainly the nitrosyl cation NO$^+$.

Contrary to some opinion, tertiary amines may also undergo nitrosation (Hein, 1963; Smith & Loeppky, 1967). The reaction rate, however, is usually appreciably lower than that of the nitrosation of secondary amines and is maximal at weakly acid pH (pH 3-6). The nitrosative cleavage of a C-N-bond probably leads to immonium intermediates, which either hydrolyse to form a secondary amine (Smith & Loeppky, 1967) or react directly with nitrite to form nitrite esters, which rearrange to form the nitrosamine (Lijinsky et al., 1972a).

Catalysis

Nitrosation reactions can be catalysed by a variety of chemicals. Chloride and thiocyanate ions are simple inorganic catalysts (Boyland et al., 1971; Fan & Tannenbaum, 1973), which probably act by forming highly reactive nitrosyl halides or analogous compounds, such as nitrosyl thiocyamates (Challis & Butler, 1968). Chloride is a normal component of the stomach fluid, and thiocyanate is present in saliva.

Aldehydes such as formaldehyde, chloral (Keefer & Roller, 1973), benzaldehyde and, especially, pyridoxal (vitamin B_6) (Archer et al., 1976) catalyse nitrosation reactions, probably by the formation of nitrite esters via methylene-immonium intermediates. The esters then rearrange to form nitrosamine and aldehyde. It is important to note that formaldehyde catalysis also leads to nitrosamine formation in neutral and even strongly alkaline media (Keefer & Roller, 1973).

Diphenols, such as 4-methylcatechol, are also effective catalysts (Challis & Bartlett, 1975; Davies et al., 1978; Pignatelli et al., 1980), as are micelle-forming surface-active compounds, such as lecithin (Okun & Archer, 1976). Bacteria have also been shown to catalyse nitrosation reactions (Archer et al., 1978).

Inhibition

Competition by inhibitors for the nitrosating agent may prevent nitrosamine formation or decrease reaction yields. Ascorbic acid is probably the most effective inhibitor (Mirvish et al., 1972); a reaction between ascorbic acid and the nitrosating agent forms NO from N_2O_3 and dehydroascorbic acid (Dahn et al., 1960). Another important nitrosation inhibitor is α-tocopherol (Mergens et al., 1978).

Examples of other compounds that compete with nitrosatable amines for available nitrite are amino acids, urea, amidosulphonic acid and primary amines. The simultaneous presence, for example, of primary and secondary amino groups in a nitrosation mixture often favours N-nitrosation over deamination (Paulsen & Mäckel, 1969; Mirvish, 1971).

N-Nitrosation *in vivo*

Many experiments in animals, and some observations in humans, have shown that nitrosation reactions can occur *in vivo*, mainly in the stomach. Their occurrence, however, depends on the relative concentrations of substrates, catalysts and inhibitors, and is influenced by the inhomogeneity of the stomach contents, by pH and by many other factors. Thus, quantitative prediction of nitrosation rates and yields *in vivo* is impossible.

One substrate, nitrite, is a normal constituent of human saliva. Its concentration depends largely on the nitrate intake in food and drinking-water. After reabsorption from the gut, dietary nitrate is partially secreted via the salivary glands into the mouth, where about 20% is reduced to nitrite by bacteria (Spiegelhalder et al., 1976; Tannenbaum et al., 1974, 1976). Recent investigations by Tannenbaum et al. (1978) have indicated that nitrite may also be formed in the gut by heterotrophic nitrification from ammonia. The practical relevance of this nitrite source is, however, uncertain.

The other class of substrate, amines, are present, with both catalysts and inhibitors, in food. Drugs may also contain nitrosatable amines.

Nitrosation of drugs

Lijinsky et al. (1972b,c) showed that amine-containing drugs may react with nitrite to form N-nitroso compounds. As would be expected, reactivity varies considerably within this group of chemicals. A selection of relevant data is given in Table 2.

Table 2. Some N-nitroso compounds formed from drugs

Drug	N-Nitroso compound formed	Reference
Piperazine	Mono- and dinitrosopiperazine	Mirvish (1975)
Phenmetrazine	N-Nitrosophenmetrazine	Greenblatt et al. (1972); Mirvish (1975)
Ephedrine	N-Nitrosoephedrine	Wogan et al. (1975); Eisenbrand et al. (1978); Kinawi & Schuster (1978)
Ethambutol	Dinitrosoethambutol	Montesano et al. (1974)
Chlordiazepoxide	N-Nitrosoderivative and rearrangement products	Walser et al. (1974); Mirvish (1975)
Phenacetin	N-Nitroso-2-nitro-4-ethoxyacet-anilide and other products	Eisenbrand & Preussmann (1975)
Aminophenazone	N-Nitrosodimethylamine	Lijinsky et al. (1972b)
Oxytetracycline	N-Nitrosodimethylamine	Lijinsky et al. (1972b); Lijinsky (1974)
Chlorpromazine	N-Nitrosodimethylamine	Lijinsky (1974); Mirvish (1975)
Dextropropoxyphene	N-Nitrosodimethylamine	Lijinsky (1974); Mirvish (1975)
Chlorpheniramine	N-Nitrosodimethylamine	Lijinsky (1974); Mirvish (1975)

Table 2 (contd)

Drug	N-Nitroso compound formed	Reference
Methadone	N-Nitrosodimethylamine	Lijinsky (1974); Mirvish (1975)
Methapyrilene	N-Nitrosodimethylamine	Lijinsky (1974); Mirvish (1975)
Quinacrine	N-Nitrosodiethylamine	Lijinsky (1974); Mirvish (1975)
Lucanthone	N-Nitrosodiethylamine	Lijinsky (1974); Mirvish (1975)
Tolazamide	N-Nitrosohexamethyleneimine	Lijinsky et al. (1972b); Lijinsky (1974)
Cyclizine	Dinitrosopiperazine	Lijinsky (1974); Mirvish (1975)
Tripelennamine	N-Nitrosodemethyltripelennamine	Rao & Krishna (1975)
Disulfiram	N-Nitrosodiethylamine and N-nitrosopiperidine	Lijinsky et al. (1972b)
Nikethamide	N-Nitrosodiethylamine and N-nitrosopiperidine	Lijinsky et al. (1972b)

It follows from these and similar data that most drugs that contain tertiary amino- or $N'N$-dialkylamido-groups react only very slowly under conditions of pH and temperature similar to those of the human stomach. Lijinsky (1974) investigated the nitrosatability of 12 drugs under defined conditions (in most cases: 5 mg of the drug per ml, 10 mg nitrite per ml, pH 3.4, 37°C, 4 hours' reaction time) and found that the yield of N-nitroso compounds was below 1% in almost all cases. Higher reactivity was seen with the oral antidiabetic drug tolazamide (3.4% yield of N-nitrosohexamethyleneimine, 3 hours' reaction time, pH 3.1), the antibiotic oxytetracycline (15% N-nitrosodimethylamine, 8 mg/ml drug, 16 mg/ml nitrite, pH 3) and the analgesic drug aminophenazone (amidopyrine, aminopyrine) (40% N-nitrosodimethylamine, 0.25 mg/ml drug, 0.25 mg/ml nitrite, 2 hours' reaction time, pH 3.2). Tripelennamine, under similar conditions, yielded 6% N-nitrosodemethyl compound (Rao & Krishna, 1975).

Drugs with secondary amino groups usually react more efficiently to form the corresponding N-nitrosated drug: piperazine gave a 62% yield (pH 3.0, 25°C, 10 minutes' reaction time) (Mirvish, 1975); phenmetrazine, up to 48 or 31% after 180 minutes in rat or rabbit stomach, respectively, with 0.8 or 4 mmol $NaNO_2$ (Greenblatt et al., 1972); ethambutol, 61% (pH 3.0, 37°C, 15 minutes) (Montesano et al., 1974); and ephedrine, 4% (pH 3.15, 37°C, 60 minutes) (Kinawi & Schuster, 1978).

Some drugs, such as chlordiazepoxide (Walser et al., 1974) and phenacetin (Eisenbrand & Preussmann, 1975), react via more complicated pathways, forming N-nitroso compounds at least as intermediates. The antihistamine drug methapyriline forms small quantities of N-nitrosodimethylamine together with several other N-nitroso compounds via fragmentation reactions (Mergens et al., 1979).

The induction of tumours in experimental animals by feeding a drug with nitrite (see below) is an expensive and relatively insensitive method of evaluating the hazard presented by nitrosation of drugs in vivo. Apart from the carcinogenicity of the N-nitroso compounds formed, the nitrosation rate in the gut is also of great importance. In most cases, unrealistically high doses of precursors have been used to obtain statistically significant results. One solution to this problem would be to measure the N-nitroso compounds formed at realistic levels of exposure. However, such an analysis must take into account the absorption rate from the stomach, and this is difficult to determine. Because the rate of metabolism is usually not known, the interpretation of measurements in blood or other body fluids is also difficult.

It may therefore be useful to study the nitrosation of drugs in vitro under standard conditions.

Nitrosation assay procedure (NAP test) (WHO, 1978)

If valid comparisons are to be made, the reactions must be carried out under standard conditions for set times, and the identity and yield of N-nitroso compounds established by mass spectrometry or other appropriate methods. The WHO Expert Group recommended a 'Nitrosation Assay Procedure' (NAP test) that must conform to the following criteria:

> Concentration of drug: 10 mmol/l
> Concentration of nitrite: 40 mmol/l
> Reaction temperature: 37°C
> pH: 3-4
> Reaction times: 1 hour and 4 hours

The relative concentrations of the reactants provide an adequate excess of nitrite to promote the reaction, and the absolute concentrations are appropriate to the sensitivity of available methods for measuring the resulting N-nitroso compounds. At 37°C there is little or no decomposition of nitrous acid; the pH range 3-4 is optimal for most nitrosation reactions and is also close to that prevailing in the stomach during digestion. Reaction times of 1 and 4 hours are set for rapidly and slowly reacting compounds, respectively, and ensure that complex reactions proceed to completion. If, however, some of the products are found to be unstable, the reaction time may need to be altered following a detailed examination of the chemical reactions.

In all cases, the substrates to be tested in the NAP test should be in the purest state obtainable, and particular care should be taken to eliminate preformed nitrosamines (Spiegelhalder et al., 1978; Eisenbrand et al., 1979), insofar as this is possible.

The assessment of combination products, containing more than one amino group, may present special problems. Similarly, if the compound is readily metabolized to other nitrosatable products, these must be considered separately and individually. While accelerators and inhibitors of N-nitrosation reactions may have a significant effect on yields, they are not selective in their action, and their use cannot, therefore, affect the relative positions of nitrosatable drugs on a scale such as that given in Table 3.

Table 3. The relative N-nitrosation of selected drugs: percent nitrosamine yield in a defined nitrosation assay procedure (NAP test)[a]

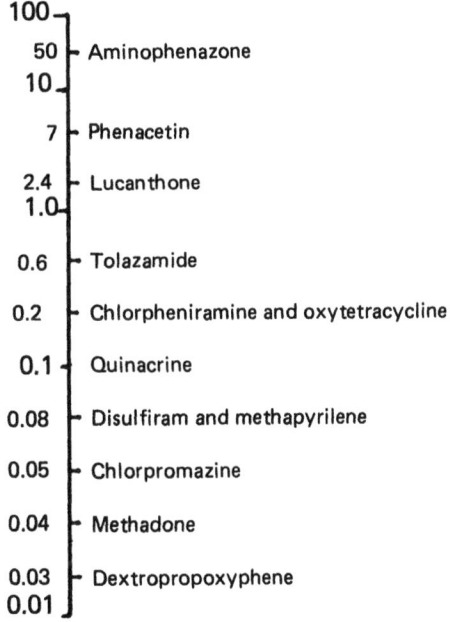

[a] From WHO (1978)

Experimental evidence of carcinogenic and other relevant biological effects of N-nitrosatable drugs

No review of such evidence will be attempted; however, references to the relevant studies are summarized in Tables 4, 5, 6 and 7.

Table 4. References to carcinogenicity tests on N-nitrosatable drugs administered in conjunction with sodium nitrite[a]

Drug	Mice	Rats
Aminophenazone	Alexandrov & Napalkov (1979) (prenatal exposure)	Lijinsky et al. (1973); Taylor & Lijinsky (1975); Chan & Fong (1977); Scheunig et al. (1979)
		Alexandrov & Napalkov (1979) (prenatal exposure)
Chlordiazepoxide		Lijinsky & Taylor (1977a,b)
Disulfiram		Lijinsky & Reuber (1980)
Ephedrine hydrochloride		Schneider et al. (1977)
Ethambutol	Biancifiori et al. (1975)	
Lucanthone hydrochloride		Lijinsky & Taylor (1977a,b)
Methapyrilene		Lijinsky & Taylor (1977a,b)
Methapyrilene hydrochloride		Frederick Cancer Research Center (1979)
Oxytetracycline hydrochloride		Taylor & Lijinsky (1975)
Piperazine	Greenblatt et al. (1971); Greenblatt & Mirvish (1972)	Garcia & Lijinsky (1973); Schneider et al. (1977) Schneider et al. (1977) (prenatal exposure)
Propylhexedrine hydrochloride		Schneider et al. (1977)

[a] Test compounds were administered by the oral route, unless otherwise specified.

Table 5. References to carcinogenicity tests on nitrosation products of N-nitrosatable drugs

Nitrosation product	Mice	Rats
N-Nitrosoephedrine	Wogan et al. (1975) (i.p. injections)	Eisenbrand et al. (1978)
N-Nitrosopiperazine	Greenblatt & Mirvish (1972)	Garcia et al. (1970); Love et al. (1977)
N,N'-Dinitrosopiperazine	Zabezhinsky (1969); Greenblatt et al. (1971); Schmähl & Thomas (1965); Zabezhinsky (1969) (s.c. administration)	Druckrey et al. (1967); Druckrey et al. (1964, 1967) (s.c. administration); Weisburger et al. (1966); Hadidian et al. (1968); Garcia & Lijinsky (1972); Lijinsky & Taylor (1975)
N-Nitrosophenmetrazine		Lijinsky & Taylor (1976)
N-Nitrosophenidate		Lijinsky & Taylor (1976)

Table 6. References to mutagenicity and other, related short-term tests on N-nitrosatable drugs

Compound	Mutagenicity	Chromosomal aberrations
Aminophenazone		
+ sodium nitrite	Arisawa et al. (1978) (S. typhimurium)	Newton & Lilly (1977) (rat lymphocytes)
+ nitrite	Blijleven (1979) (Drosophila)	
+ sodium nitrite	Inui et al. (1978) (hamster embryo cells)	

Table 7. References to mutagenicity and other, related short-term tests on nitrosation products of N-nitrosatable drugs

Compound	Mutagenicity	Gene conversion
N-Nitrosochlor-diazepoxide		Krafft & Onken, 1976 (*S. cerevisiae*)
N,N'-Dinitroso-ethambutol	Bartsch et al. (1980) (*S. typhimurium*)	
N-Nitrosopiperazine	Zeiger et al. (1972); Braun et al. (1977); Rao et al. (1978) (*S. typhimurium*)	
N,N'-Dinitroso-piperazine	Zeiger et al. (1972); Braun et al. (1977); Andrews et al. (1978); Rao et al. (1978) (*S. typhimurium*)	
N,N'-Dinitroso-piperazine	Trams & Künkel (1965); Elespuru & Lijinsky (1976) (*E. coli*)	

References

Alexandrov, V.A. & Napalkov, N.P. (1979) Transplacental carcinogenic effect as a result of a combined injection of amidopyrine and nitrite in mice (Russ.). *Vopr. Onkol., 25,* 48-52

Andrews, A.W., Thibault, L.H. & Lijinsky, W. (1978) The relationship between mutagenicity and carcinogenicity of some nitrosamines. *Mutat. Res., 51,* 319-326

Archer, M.C., Tannenbaum, S.R. & Wishnok, J.S. (1976) *Nitrosamine formation in the presence of carbonyl compounds.* In: Walker, E.A., Bogovski, P. & Griciute, L., eds, *Environmental* N-*Nitroso Compounds: Analysis and Formation (IARC Scientific Publications No. 14),* Lyon, International Agency for Research on Cancer, pp. 141-145

Archer, M.C., Yang, H.S. & Okun, J.D. (1978) *Acceleration of nitrosamine formation at pH 3.5 by microorganisms.* In: Walker, E.A., Castegnaro, M., Griciute, L. & Lyle, R.E., eds, *Environmental Aspects of* N-*Nitroso Compounds (IARC Scientific Publications No. 19),* Lyon, International Agency for Research on Cancer, pp. 239-246

Arisawa, M., Fujiu, M., Suhara, Y. & Maruyama, H.B. (1978) Differential mutagenicity of reaction products of various pyrazolones with nitrite. *Mutat. Res., 57,* 287-296

Bartsch, H., Malaveille, C., Camus, A.-M., Martel-Planche, G., Brun, G., Hautefeuille, A., Sabadie, N., Barbin, A., Kuroki, T., Drevon, C., Piccoli, C. & Montesano, R. (1980) Validation and comparative studies on 180 chemicals with *S. typhimurium* strains and V79 Chinese hamster cells in the presence of various metabolizing systems. *Mutat. Res., 76,* 1-50

Biancifiori, C., Montesano, R. & Bolis, G.B. (1975) Investigation on the carcinogenicity of sodium nitrite and/or ethambutol in BALB/c/Cb/Se mice (Ital.). *Lav. Anat. Patol. Perugia, 35,* 45-56

Blijleven, W.G.H. (1979) Mutagenicity testing of amines and amides combined with nitrite in *Drosophila melanogaster* (Abstract no. 43). *Mutat. Res., 64,* 128

Boyland, E., Nice, E. & Williams, K. (1971) The catalysis of nitrosation by thiocyanate from saliva. *Food Cosmet. Toxicol., 9,* 639-643

Braun, R., Schöneich, J. & Ziebarth, D. (1977) *In vivo* formation of N-nitroso compounds and detection of their mutagenic activity in the host-mediated assay. *Cancer Res., 37,* 4572-4579

Challis, B.C. & Bartlett, C.D. (1975) Possible cocarcinogenic effects of coffee constituents. *Nature, 254*, 532-533

Challis, B.C. & Butler, A.R. (1968) *Substitution at an amino nitrogen*. In: Patai, S., ed., *The Chemistry of the Amino Group*, Vol. 1, New York, Interscience, pp. 305-320

Chan, W.C. & Fong, Y.Y. (1977) Ascorbic acid prevents liver tumour production by aminopyrine and nitrite in the rat. *Int. J. Cancer, 20*, 268-270

Dahn, H., Loewe, L. & Bunton, C.A. (1960) Oxidation of ascorbic acid by nitrous acid. VI. Review and discussion of the results (Ger.). *Helv. chim. Acta, 43*, 320-333

Davies, R., Dennis, M.J., Massey, R.C. & McWeeny, D.J. (1978) *Some effects of phenol- and thiol-nitrosation reactions on N-nitrosamine formation*. In: Walker, E.A., Castegnaro, M., Griciute, L. & Lyle, R.E., eds, *Environmental Aspects of N-Nitroso Compounds (IARC Scientific Publications No. 19)*, Lyon, International Agency for Research on Cancer, pp. 183-197

Druckrey, H. & Preussmann, R. (1962) Formation of carcinogenic nitrosamines in tobacco smoke (Ger.). *Naturwissenschafften, 49*, 498-499

Druckrey, H., Ivankovic, S., Mennel, H.D. & Preussmann, R. (1964) Selective production of carcinomas of the nasal cavity in rats with N,N-dinitrosopiperazine, nitrosopiperidine, nitrosomorpholine, methylallyl-, dimethyl- and methylvinylnitrosamines (Ger.). *Z. Krebsforsch., 66*, 138-150

Druckrey, H., Preussmann, R., Ivankovic, S. & Schmähl, D. (1967) Organotropic carcinogenic action of 65 different *N*-nitroso compounds in BD rats (Ger.). *Z. Krebsforsch., 69*, 103-201

Eisenbrand, G. & Preussmann, R. (1975) Nitrosation of phenacetin. Formation of *N*-nitroso-2-nitro-4-ethoxyacetanilide as an unstable product of the nitrosation in dilute aqueous-acidic solution. *Arzneimittel.-forsch., 25*, 1472-1475

Eisenbrand, G., Preussmann, R. & Schmähl, D. (1978) Carcinogenicity of *N*-nitrosoephedrine in rats. *Cancer Lett., 5*, 103-106

Eisenbrand, G., Spiegelhalder, B., Kann, J., Klein, R. & Preussmann, R. (1979) Carcinogenic *N*-nitrosodimethylamine as a contamination in drugs containing 4-dimethylamino-2,3-dimethyl-1-phenyl-3-pyrazolin-5-one (amidopyrine, aminophenazone). *Arzneimittel.-forsch., 29*, 867-869

Elespuru, R.K. & Lijinsky, W. (1976) Mutagenicity of cyclic nitrosamines in *Escherichia coli* following activation with rat liver microsomes. *Cancer Res., 36*, 4099-4101

Fan, T.-Y. & Tannenbaum, S.R. (1973) Factors influencing the rate of formation of nitrosomorpholine from morpholine and nitrite: acceleration by thiocyanate and other anions. *J. Agric. Food Chem., 21*, 237-240

Frederick Cancer Research Center (1979) *Interim Report of the Subchronic Bioassay of Methapyrilene in Rats and the Chronic Toxicity Study with Methapyrilene and Sodium Nitrite in Rats as of April 30, 1979*, Frederick, MD

Fridman, A.L., Mukhametshin, F.M. & Novikov, S.S. (1971) Advances in the chemistry of aliphatic *N*-nitrosamines. *Russ. chem. Rev., 40*, 34-50

Garcia, H. & Lijinsky, W. (1972) Tumorigenicity of five cyclic nitrosamines in MRC rats. *Z. Krebsforsch., 77*, 257-261

Garcia, H. & Lijinsky, W. (1973) Studies of the tumorigenic effect in feeding of nitrosamino acids and of low doses of amines and nitrite to rats. *Z. Krebsforsch., 79*, 141-144

Garcia, H., Keefer, L., Lijinsky, W. & Wenyon, C.E.M. (1970) Carcinogenicity of nitrosothiomorpholine and 1-nitrosopiperazine in rats. *Z. Krebsforsch., 74*, 179-184

Greenblatt, M. & Mirvish, S. (1972) Dose-response studies with concurrent administration of piperazine and sodium nitrite to strain A mice. *J. natl Cancer Inst., 49*, 119-124

Greenblatt, M., Mirvish, S. & So, B.T. (1971) Nitrosamine studies: induction of lung adenomas by concurrent administration of sodium nitrite and secondary amines in Swiss mice. *J. natl Cancer Inst., 46*, 1029-1034

Greenblatt, J.M., Kommineni, V., Conrad, E., Wallcave, L. & Lijinsky, W. (1972) In vivo conversion of phenmetrazine into its *N*-nitroso derivative. *Nature (New Biol.), 236*, 25-26

Hadidian, Z., Fredrickson, T.N., Weisburger, E.K., Weisburger, J.H., Glass, R.M. & Mantel, N. (1968) Tests for chemical carcinogens. Report on the activity of derivatives of aromatic amines, nitrosamines, quinolines, nitroalkanes, amides, epoxides, aziridines, and purine antimetabolites. *J. natl Cancer Inst., 41*, 985-1036

Hein, G.E. (1963) The reaction of tertiary amines with nitrous acid. *J. chem. Educ., 40*, 181-184

IARC (1978) *IARC Monographs on the Evaluation of the Carcinogenic Risk of Chemicals to Humans* Vol. 17, *Some N-Nitroso Compounds*, Lyon

Inui, N., Nishi, Y., Taketomi, M. & Mori, I. (1978) Somatic mutation on hamster embryonic cells by concurrent transplacental administrations of sodium nitrite and aminopyrine (Abstract). *Proc. Jpn. Cancer Assoc., 11*, 11

Keefer, L.K. & Roller, P.P. (1973) *N*-Nitrosation by nitrite ion in neutral and basic medium. *Science, 181*, 1245-1247

Kinawi, A. & Schuster, T. (1978) Reaction kinetic studies on the formation of *N*-nitrosoephedrine *in vitro* and *in vivo* (Ger.). *Arzneimittel.-forsch., 28*, 219-225

Krafft, S. & Onken, A. (1976) Induction of mitotic gene conversion in *Saccharomyces cerevisiae* with chlordiazepoxide and its *N*-nitroso derivative in a host-mediated assay. *Mutat. Res., 34*, 333-336

Lijinsky, W. (1974) Reaction of drugs with nitrous acid as a source of carcinogenic nitrosamines. *Cancer Res., 34*, 255-258

Lijinsky, W. & Reuber, M.D. (1980) Tumours induced in Fischer 344 rats by the feeding of disulfiram together with sodium nitrite. *Food Cosmet. Toxicol., 18*, 85-87

Lijinsky, W. & Taylor, H.W. (1975) Carcinogenicity of methylated dinitrosopiperazines in rats. *Cancer Res., 35*, 1270-1273

Lijinsky, W. & Taylor, H.W. (1976) Carcinogenicity tests of *N*-nitroso derivatives of two drugs, phenmetrazine and methylphenidate. *Cancer Lett., 1*, 359-363

Lijinsky, W. & Taylor, H.W. (1977a) Feeding tests in rats on mixtures of nitrite with secondary and tertiary amines of environmental importance. *Food Cosmet. Toxicol., 15*, 269-274

Lijinsky, W. & Taylor, H.W. (1977b) *Nitrosamines and their precursors in food*. In: Hiatt, H.H., Watson, J.D. & Winsten, J.H. eds, *Origins of Human Cancer*, Vol. 4, Book C, Cold Spring Harbor, NY, Cold Spring Harbor Laboratory, pp. 1579-1590

Lijinsky, W., Keefer, L., Conrad, E. & Van de Bogart, R. (1972a) Nitrosation of tertiary amines and some biologic implications. *J. natl Cancer Inst., 49*, 1239-1249

Lijinsky, W., Conrad, E. & Van de Bogart, R. (1972b) Carcinogenic nitrosamines formed by drug/nitrite interactions. *Nature, 239*, 165-167

Lijinsky, W., Conrad, E. & Van de Bogart, R. (1972c) *Formation of carcinogenic nitrosamines by interaction of drugs with nitrite*. In: Bogovski, P., Preussmann, R. & Walker, E.A., eds, N-*Nitroso Compounds: Analysis and Formation (IARC Scientific Publications No. 3)*, Lyon, International Agency for Research on Cancer, pp. 130-133

Lijinsky, W., Taylor, H.W., Snyder, C. & Nettesheim, P. (1973) Malignant tumours of the liver and lung in rats fed aminopyrine or heptamethyleneimine together with nitrite. *Nature, 244*, 176-178

Love, L.A., Lijinsky, W., Keefer, L.K. & Garcia, H. (1977) Chronic oral administration of 1-nitrosopiperazine at high doses to MRC rats. *Z. Krebsforsch., 89*, 69-73

Mergens, W.J., Kamm, J.J., Newmark, H.L., Fiddler, W. & Pensabene, J. (1978) *Alphatocopherol: uses in preventing nitrosamine formation*. In: Walker, E.A., Castegnaro, M., Griciute, L. & Lyle, R.E., eds, *Environmental Aspects of* N-*Nitroso Compounds (IARC Scientific Publications No. 19)*, Lyon, International Agency for Research on Cancer, pp. 199-212

Mergens, W.J., Vane, F.M., Tannenbaum, S.R., Green, L. & Skipper, P.L. (1979) *In vitro* nitrosation of methapyrilene. *J. pharm. Sci., 68*, 827-832

Mirvish, S.S. (1971) Kinetics of nitrosamide formation from alkylureas, *N*-alkylurethans and alkylguanidines: possible implications for the etiology of human gastric cancer. *J. natl Cancer Inst., 46*, 1183-1193

Mirvish, S.S. (1975) Formation of *N*-nitroso compounds: chemistry, kinetics and *in vivo* occurrence. *Toxicol. appl. Pharmacol., 31*, 325-351

Mirvish, S.S., Wallcave, L., Eagen, M. & Shubik, P. (1972) Ascorbate-nitrite reaction: possible means of blocking the formation of carcinogenic *N*-nitroso compounds. *Science, 177*, 65-68

Montesano, R., Bartsch, H. & Brésil, H. (1974) Nitrosation of d-*N,N'*-bis-(1-hydroxymethylpropyl)ethylenediamine, an antitubercular drug. *J. natl Cancer Inst., 52*, 907-910

Newton, M.F. & Lilly, L.J. (1977) *Further assessment of a test for determining the mutagenicity of compounds metabolized* in vivo *in the rat*. In: Scott, D., Bridges, B.A. & Sobels, F.H., eds, *Progress in Genetic Toxicology*, Amsterdam, Elsevier/North Holland Biomedical Press, pp. 301-306

Okun, J.D. & Archer, M.C. (1976) *Micellar catalysis of nitrosamine formation*. In: Walker, E.A., Bogovski, P. & Griciute, L., eds, *Environmental N-Nitroso Compounds: Analysis and Formation (IARC Scientific Publications No. 14)*, Lyon, International Agency for Research on Cancer, pp. 147-151

Olajos, E.J. & Coulston, F. (1978) Comparative toxicology of *N*-nitroso compounds and their carcinogenic potential to man. *Ecotoxicol. environ. Saf., 2*, 317-367

Paulsen, H. & Mäckel, E. (1969) Monosaccharides with ring containing nitrogen. XXIV. Competition between nitrosation of neighbouring primary and secondary amino groups. Synthesis of nitrosamino sugars (Ger.). *Chem. Ber., 102*, 3844-3853

Pignatelli, B., Friesen, M. & Walker, E.A. (1980) *The role of phenols in catalysis of nitrosamine formation*. In: Walker, E.A., Castegnaro, M., Griciute, L. & Börzsönyi, M., eds, *N-Nitroso Compounds: Analysis, Formation and Occurrence (IARC Scientific Publications No. 31)*, Lyon, International Agency for Research on Cancer (in press)

Rao, G.S. & Krishna, G. (1975) Drug-nitrite interactions: formation of *N*-nitroso, *C*-nitroso, and nitro compounds from sodium nitrite and various drugs under physiological conditions. *J. pharm. Sci., 64*, 1579-1581

Rao, T.K., Young, J.A., Lijinsky, W. & Epler, J.L. (1978) Mutagenicity of *N*-nitrosopiperazine derivatives in *Salmonella typhimurium*. *Mutat. Res., 57*, 127-134

Ridd, J.H. (1961) Nitrosation, diazotisation, and deamination. *Q. Rev. chem. Soc. (Lond.), 15*, 418-441

Sander, J. & Bürkle, G. (1969) Induction of malignant tumours in rats by simultaneous feeding of nitrite and secondary amines (Ger.). *Z. Krebsforsch., 73*, 54-66

Scheunig, G., Horn, K.-H. & Mehnert, W.-H. (1979) Induction of tumours in Wistar rats after oral administration of aminophenazone and nitrite (Ger.). *Arch. Geschwulstforsch., 49*, 220-228

Schmähl, D. & Thomas, C. (1965) Production of lung and liver tumours in mice with *N,N'*-dinitrosopiperazine (Ger.). *Z. Krebsforsch., 67*, 11-15

Schneider, J., Warzok, R. & Schwarz, H. (1977) Endogenous formation of carcinogenic *N*-nitroso compounds in rats after application of drugs and nitrite (Ger.). *Exp. Pathol. 13*, 32-43

Smith, P.A.S. & Loeppky, R.N. (1967) Nitrosative cleavage of tertiary amines. *J. Am. chem. Soc., 89*, 1147-1157

Spiegelhalder, B., Eisenbrand, G. & Preussmann, R. (1976) Influence of dietary nitrate on nitrite content of human saliva: possible relevance to *in vivo* formation of *N*-nitroso compounds. *Food Cosmet. Toxicol., 14*, 545-548

Spiegelhalder, B., Eisenbrand, G. & Preussmann, R. (1978) *N*-Nitrosamine contamination of amines (Ger.). *Angew. Chem., 90*, 379-380

Tannenbaum, S.R., Sinskey, A.J., Weisman, M. & Bishop, W. (1974) Nitrite in human saliva. Its possible relationship to nitrosamine formation. *J. natl Cancer Inst., 53*, 79-84

Tannenbaum, S.R., Weisman, M. & Fett, D. (1976) The effect of nitrate intake on nitrite formation in human saliva. *Food Cosmet. Toxicol., 14*, 549-552

Tannenbaum, S.R., Fett, D., Young, V.R., Land, P.D. & Bruce, W.R. (1978) Nitrite and nitrate are formed by endogenous synthesis in the human intestine. *Science, 200*, 1487-1489

Taylor, H.W. & Lijinsky, W. (1975) Tumor induction in rats by feeding aminopyrine or oxytetracycline with nitrite. *Int. J. Cancer, 16*, 211-215

Trams, A. & Künkel, H.A. (1965) No mutation produced by *N*-nitrosopiperidine and *N,N*-dinitrosopiperazine in *Escherichia coli* (Ger.). *Naturwissenschaften, 52*, 650-651

Walser, A., Fryer, R.I., Sternbach, L.H. & Archer, M. (1974) Quinazolines and 1,4-benzodiazepines. LXV (1). Some transformations of chlordiazepoxide. *J. Heterocycl. Chem., 11*, 619-621

Weisburger, J.H., Weisburger, E.K., Mantel, N., Hadidian, Z. & Fredrickson, T. (1966) New carcinogenic nitrosamines in rats. *Naturwissenschaften, 53*, 508

WHO (1977) *Environmental Health Criteria*, Vol. 5, *Nitrates, Nitrites and N-Nitroso Compounds*, Geneva

WHO (1978) *Informal Consultation on the Potential Carcinogenicity of Nitrosatable Drugs (Report of a WHO Meeting, Geneva, June 12-16)*, Geneva

Wogan, G.N., Paglialunga, S., Archer, M.C. & Tannenbaum, S.R. (1975) Carcinogenicity of nitrosation products of ephedrine, sarcosine, folic acid, and creatinine. *Cancer Res., 35*, 1981-1984

Zabezhinsky, M.A. (1969) On carcinogenic effect of *N,N'*-dinitrosopiperazine on mice (Russ.). *Vopr. Onkol., 15*, 104-106

Zeiger, E., Legator, M.S. & Lijinsky, W. (1972) Mutagenicity of *N*-nitrosopiperazines for *Salmonella typhimurium* in the host-mediated assay. *Cancer Res., 32*, 1598-1599

SUPPLEMENTARY CORRIGENDA TO VOLUMES 1–23

Volume 23

Cumulative index, p. 422　*replace*　Cadmium cyclamate
　　　　　　　　　　　　by　　　Calcium cyclamate

CUMULATIVE INDEX TO IARC MONOGRAPHS ON THE EVALUATION

OF THE CARCINOGENIC RISK OF CHEMICALS TO HUMANS

Numbers in bold indicate volume, and other numbers indicate page. References to corrigenda are given in parentheses. Compounds marked with an asterisk (*) were considered by the Working Groups, but monographs were not prepared because adequate data on their carcinogenicity were not available.

A

Acetamide	**7**, 197	
Acetylsalicyclic acid*		
Acridine orange	**16**, 145	
Acriflavinium chloride	**13**, 31	
Acrolein	**19**, 479	
Acrylic acid	**19**, 47	
Acrylic fibres	**19**, 86	
Acrylonitrile	**19**, 73	
Acrylonitrile-butadiene-styrene copolymers	**19**, 91	
Actinomycins	**10**, 29	
Adipic acid*		
Adriamycin	**10**, 43	
Aflatoxins	**1**, 145	(corr. **7**,319)
		(corr. **8**,349)
	10, 51	
Aldrin	**5**, 25	
Amaranth	**8**, 41	
5-Aminoacenaphthene	**16**, 243	
para-Aminoazobenzene	**8**, 53	
ortho-Aminoazotoluene	**8**, 61	(corr. **11**,295)
para-Aminobenzoic acid	**16**, 249	
4-Aminobiphenyl	**1**, 74	(corr. **10**,343)
2-Amino-5-(5-nitro-2-furyl)-1,3,4-thiadiazole	**7**, 143	
4-Amino-2-nitrophenol	**16**, 43	

2-Amino-4-nitrophenol*
2-Amino-5-nitrophenol*
Amitrole   7,   31
Amobarbital sodium*
Anaesthetics, volatile   11, 285
Aniline   4,   27   (corr. **7,320**)
Anthranilic acid   16, 265
Apholate   9,   31
Aramite®   5,   39
Arsenic and arsenic compounds   1,   41
                                        2,   48
                                       23,   39

    Arsanilic acid
    Arsenic pentoxide
    Arsenic sulphide
    Arsenic trioxide
    Arsine
    Calcium arsenate
    Dimethylarsinic acid
    Lead arsenate
    Methanearsonic acid, disodium salt
    Methanearsonic acid, monosodium salt
    Potassium arsenate
    Potassium arsenite
    Sodium arsenate
    Sodium arsenite
    Sodium cacodylate

Asbestos   2,   17   (corr. **7,319**)
                                       14   (corr. **15,341**)
                                                   (corr. **17,351**)

    Actinolite
    Amosite
    Anthophyllite
    Chrysotile
    Crocidolite
    Tremolite

Auramine   1,   69   (corr. **7,319**)
Aurothioglucose   13,   39
Azaserine   10,   73   (corr. **12,271**)

Azathioprine*		
Aziridine	**9,** 37	
2-(1-Aziridinyl)ethanol	**9,** 47	
Aziridyl benzoquinone	**9,** 51	
Azobenzene	**8,** 75	

B

Benz[c]acridine	**3,** 241	
Benz[a]anthracene	**3,** 45	
Benzene	**7,** 203	(corr. **11,**295)
Benzidine	**1,** 80	
Benzo[b]fluoranthene	**3,** 69	
Benzo[j]fluoranthene	**3,** 82	
Benzo[a]pyrene	**3,** 91	
Benzo[e]pyrene	**3,** 137	
Benzyl chloride	**11,** 217	(corr. **13,**243)
Benzyl violet 4B	**16,** 153	
Beryllium and beryllium compounds	**1,** 17	
	23, 143	

    Bertrandite
    Beryllium acetate
    Beryllium acetate, basic
    Beryllium-aluminium alloy
    Beryllium carbonate
    Beryllium chloride
    Beryllium-copper alloy
    Beryllium-copper-cobalt alloy
    Beryllium fluoride
    Beryllium hydroxide
    Beryllium-nickel alloy
    Beryllium oxide
    Beryllium phosphate
    Beryllium silicate
    Beryllium sulphate and its tetrahydrate
    Beryl ore
    Zinc beryllium silicate

Bis(1-aziridinyl)morpholinophosphine sulphide	**9,** 55	
Bis(2-chloroethyl)ether	**9,** 117	

N,N-Bis(2-chloroethyl)-2-naphthylamine	4, 119	
Bischloroethyl nitrosourea*		
Bis(2-chloroisopropyl)ether*		
1,2-Bis(chloromethoxy)ethane	15, 31	
1,4-Bis(chloromethoxymethyl)benzene	15, 37	
Bis(chloromethyl)ether	4, 231	(corr. 13,243)
Blue VRS	16, 163	
Brilliant blue FCF diammonium and disodium salts	16, 171	
1,4-Butanediol dimethanesulphonate (Myleran)	4, 247	
Butyl-*cis*-9,10-epoxystearate*		
β-Butyrolactone	11, 225	
γ-Butyrolactone	11, 231	

C

Cadmium and cadmium compounds	2, 74	
	11, 39	
Cadmium acetate		
Cadmium carbonate		
Cadmium chloride		
Cadmium oxide		
Cadmium sulphate		
Cadmium sulphide		
Calcium cyclamate	22, 58	
Calcium saccharin	22, 120	
Cantharidin	10, 79	
Caprolactam	19, 115	
Carbaryl	12, 37	
Carbon tetrachloride	1, 53	
	20, 371	
Carmoisine	8, 83	
Catechol	15, 155	
Chlorambucil	9, 125	
Chloramphenicol	10, 85	
Chlordane	20, 45	
Chlordecone (Kepone)	20, 67	

Chlorinated dibenzodioxins	**15,**	41
Chlormadinone acetate	**6,**	149
	21,	365
Chlorobenzilate	**5,**	75
Chloroform	**1,**	61
	20,	401
Chloromethyl methyl ether	**4,**	239
Chloroprene	**19,**	131
Chloropropham	**12,**	55
Chloroquine	**13,**	47
para-Chloro-ortho-toluidine and its hydrochloride	**16,**	277
5-Chloro-ortho-toluidine*		
Chlorotrianisene	**21,**	139
Chlorpromazine*		
Cholesterol	**10,**	99
Chromium and chromium compounds	**2,**	100
	23,	205

    Barium chromate
    Basic chromic sulphate
    Calcium chromate
    Chromic acetate
    Chromic chloride
    Chromic oxide
    Chromic phosphate
    Chromite ore
    Chromium carbonyl
    Chromium potassium sulphate
    Chromium sulphate
    Chromium trioxide
    Cobalt-chromium alloy
    Ferrochromium
    Lead chromate
    Lead chromate oxide
    Potassium chromate
    Potassium dichromate
    Sodium chromate
    Sodium dichromate
    Strontium chromate
    Zinc chromate
    Zinc chromate hydroxide

Zinc potassium chromate
Zinc yellow

Chrysene	3, 159	
Chrysoidine	8, 91	
C.I. Disperse Yellow 3	8, 97	
Cinnamyl anthranilate	16, 287	
Citrus Red No. 2	8, 101	(corr. **19**,495)
Clofibrate	**24**, 39	
Clomiphene and its citrate	21, 551	
Conjugated oestrogens	21, 147	
Copper 8-hydroxyquinoline	15, 103	
Coumarin	10, 113	
Cycasin	1, 157	(corr. **7**,319)
	10, 121	
Cyclamic acid	22, 55	
Cyclochlorotine	10, 139	
Cyclohexylamine	22, 59	
Cyclophosphamide	9, 135	

D

2,4-D and esters	15, 111	
D & C Red No. 9	8, 107	
Dapsone	**24**, 59	
Daunomycin	10, 145	
DDT and associated substances	5, 83	(corr. **7**,320)
DDD (TDE)		
DDE		
Diacetylaminoazotoluene	8, 113	
N,N'-Diacetylbenzidine	16, 293	
Diallate	12, 69	
2,4-Diaminoanisole and its sulphate	16, 51	
2,5-Diaminoanisole*		
4,4'-Diaminodiphenyl ether	16, 301	
1,2-Diamino-4-nitrobenzene	16, 63	

1,4-Diamino-2-nitrobenzene	16, 73	
2,6-Diamino-3-(phenylazo)pyridine and its hydrochloride	8, 117	
2,4-Diaminotoluene	16, 83	
2,5-Diaminotoluene and its sulphate	16, 97	
Diazepam	13, 57	
Diazomethane	7, 223	
Dibenz[a,h]acridine	3, 247	
Dibenz[a,j]acridine	3, 254	
Dibenz[a,h]anthracene	3, 178	
7H-Dibenzo[c,g]carbazole	3, 260	
Dibenzo[h,rst]pentaphene	3, 197	
Dibenzo[a,e]pyrene	3, 201	
Dibenzo[a,h]pyrene	3, 207	
Dibenzo[a,i]pyrene	3, 215	
Dibenzo[a,l]pyrene	3, 224	
1,2-Dibromo-3-chloropropane	15, 139	
	20, 83	
ortho-Dichlorobenzene	7, 231	
para-Dichlorobenzene	7, 231	
3,3'-Dichlorobenzidine	4, 49	
trans-1,4-Dichlorobutene	15, 149	
3,3'-Dichloro-4,4'-diaminodiphenyl ether	16, 309	
1,2-Dichloroethane	20, 429	
Dichloromethane	20, 449	
Dichlorvos	20, 97	
Dicyclohexylamine	22, 60	
Dieldrin	5, 125	
Dienoestrol	21, 161	
Diepoxybutane	11, 115	(corr. 12,271)
1,2-Diethylhydrazine	4, 153	
Diethylstilboestrol	6, 55	
	21, 173	(corr. 23,417)
Diethylstilboestrol dipropionate	21, 175	
Diethyl sulphate	4, 277	

Diglycidyl resorcinol ether	11, 125	
Dihydrosafrole	1, 170	
	10, 233	
Dihydroxybenzenes	15, 155	
Dihydroxymethylfuratrizine	24, 77	
Dimethisterone	6, 167	
	21, 377	
Dimethoate*		
Dimethoxane	15, 177	
3,3'-Dimethoxybenzidine (o-Dianisidine)	4, 41	
para-Dimethylaminoazobenzene	8, 125	
para-Dimethylaminobenzenediazo sodium sulphonate	8, 147	
trans-2[(Dimethylamino)methylimino]-5-[2-(5-nitro-2-furyl)vinyl]-1,3,4-oxadiazole	7, 147	
3,3'-Dimethylbenzidine (o-Tolidine)	1, 87	
Dimethylcarbamoyl chloride	12, 77	
1,1-Dimethylhydrazine	4, 137	
1,2-Dimethylhydrazine	4, 145	(corr. 7,320)
Dimethyl sulphate	4, 271	
Dimethylterephthalate*		
Dinitrosopentamethylenetetramine	11, 241	
1,4-Dioxane	11, 247	
2,4'-Diphenyldiamine	16, 313	
Diphenylthiohydantoin*		
Disulfiram	12, 85	
Dithranol	13, 75	
Dulcin	12, 97	

E

Endrin	5, 157	
Eosin and its disodium salt	15, 183	
Epichlorohydrin	11, 131	(corr. 18,125)
1-Epoxyethyl-3,4-epoxycyclohexane	11, 141	
3,4-Epoxy-6-methylcyclohexylmethyl-3,4-epoxy-6-methylcyclohexane carboxylate	11, 147	

cis-9,10-Epoxystearic acid	11,	153
Ethinyloestradiol	6,	77
	21,	233
Ethionamide	13,	83
Ethyl acrylate	19,	57
Ethylene	19,	157
Ethylene dibromide	15,	195
Ethylene oxide	11,	157
Ethylene sulphide	11,	257
Ethylenethiourea	7,	45
Ethyl methanesulphonate	7,	245
Ethyl selenac	12,	107
Ethyl tellurac	12,	115
Ethynodiol diacetate	6,	173
	21,	387
Evans blue	8,	151

F

Fast green FCF	16,	187	
Ferbam	12,	121	(corr. 13,243)
Fluorescein and its disodium salt*			
2-(2-Formylhydrazino)-4-(5-nitro-2-furyl)thiazole	7,	151	(corr. 11,295)
Fusarenon-X	11,	169	

G

Glycidaldehyde	11,	175
Glycidyl oleate	11,	183
Glycidyl stearate	11,	187
Griseofulvin	10,	153
Guinea green B	16,	199

H

Haematite	1,	29
Haematoxylin*		
Heptachlor and its epoxide	5,	173
	20,	129
Hexachlorobenzene	20,	155
Hexachlorobutadiene	20,	179
Hexachlorocyclohexane (α-, β-, δ-, ϵ-, technical HCH and lindane)	5,	47
	20,	195
Hexachloroethane	20,	467
Hexachlorophene	20,	241
Hexamethylenediamine*		
Hexamethylphosphoramide	15,	211
Hycanthone and its mesylate	13,	91
Hydralazine and its hydrochloride	24,	85
Hydrazine	4,	127
Hydroquinone	15,	155
4-Hydroxyazobenzene	8,	157
17α-Hydroxyprogesterone caproate	21,	399
8-Hydroxyquinoline	13,	101
Hydroxysenkirkine	10,	265

I

Indeno[1,2,3-cd] pyrene	3,	229	
Iron-dextran complex	2,	161	
Iron-dextrin complex	2,	161	(corr. 7,319)
Iron oxide	1,	29	
Iron sorbitol-citric acid complex	2,	161	
Isatidine	10,	269	
Isonicotinic acid hydrazide	4,	159	
Isoprene*			
Isopropyl alcohol	15,	223	
Isopropyl oils	15,	223	
Isosafrole	1,	169	
	10,	232	

J

Jacobine   10, 275

L

Lasiocarpine   10, 281
Lead and lead compounds   1, 40   (corr. 7,319)
                                                 2, 52   (corr. 8,349)
                                                 2, 150
                                                 23, 325

    Lead acetate and its trihydrate
    Lead arsenate
    Lead carbonate
    Lead chloride
    Lead naphthenate
    Lead nitrate
    Lead oxide
    Lead phosphate
    Lead subacetate
    Lead tetroxide
    Tetraethyllead
    Tetramethyllead

Ledate   12, 131
Light green SF   16, 209
Lindane   5, 47
                                                 20, 195
Luteoskyrin   10, 163
Lynoestrenol   21, 407
Lysergide*

M

Magenta   4, 57   (corr. 7,320)
Maleic hydrazide   4, 173   (corr. 18,125)
Maneb   12, 137
Mannomustine and its dihydrochloride   9, 157
Medphalan   9, 168

Medroxyprogesterone acetate	6,	157
	21,	417
Megestrol acetate	21,	431
Melphalan	9,	167
Merphalan	9,	169
Mestranol	6,	87
	21,	257
Methacrylic acid*		
Methallenoestril*		
Methoxsalen	24,	101
Methoxychlor	5,	193
	20,	259
Methyl acrylate	19,	52
2-Methylaziridine	9,	61
Methylazoxymethanol	10,	121
Methylazoxymethanol acetate	1,	164
	10,	131
Methyl bromide*		
Methyl carbamate	12,	151
N-Methyl-N,4-dinitrosoaniline	1,	141
4,4'-Methylene bis(2-chloroaniline)	4,	65 (corr. 7,320)
4,4'-Methylene bis(2-methylaniline)	4,	73
4,4'-Methylenedianiline	4,	79 (corr. 7,320)
4,4'-Methylenediphenyl diisocyanate	19,	314
Methyl iodide	15,	245
Methyl methacrylate	19,	187
Methyl methanesulphonate	7,	253
N-Methyl-N'-nitro-N-nitrosoguanidine	4,	183
Methyl red	8,	161
Methyl selenac	12,	161
Methylthiouracil	7,	53
Metronidazole	13,	113
Mirex	5,	203
	20,	283
Mitomycin C	10,	171

Modacrylic fibres	19, 86	
Monocrotaline	10, 291	
Monuron	12, 167	
5-(Morpholinomethyl)-3-[(5-nitrofurfurylidene)-amino]-2-oxazolidinone	7, 161	
Mustard gas	9, 181	(corr. 13,243)

N

Nafenopin	24, 125	
1,5-Naphthalene diisocyanate	19, 311	
1-Naphthylamine	4, 87	(corr. 8,349)
		(corr. 22,187)
2-Naphthylamine	4, 97	
Native carrageenans	10, 181	(corr. 11,295)
Nickel and nickel compounds	2, 126	(corr. 7,319)
	11, 75	
Nickel acetate and its tetrahydrate		
Nickel ammonium sulphate		
Nickel carbonate		
Nickel carbonyl		
Nickel chloride		
Nickel-gallium alloy		
Nickel hydroxide		
Nickelocene		
Nickel oxide		
Nickel subsulphide		
Nickel sulphate		
Niridazole	13, 123	
5-Nitroacenaphthene	16, 319	
4-Nitrobiphenyl	4, 113	
5-Nitro-2-furaldehyde semicarbazone	7, 171	
1[(5-Nitrofurfurylidene)amino]-2-imidazolidinone	7, 181	
N-[4-(5-Nitro-2-furyl)-2-thiazolyl]acetamide	1, 181	
	7, 185	
Nitrogen mustard and its hydrochloride	9, 193	
Nitrogen mustard N-oxide and its hydrochloride	9, 209	
Nitrosatable drugs	24, 297	

N-Nitrosodi-n-butylamine	4, 197	
	17, 51	
N-Nitrosodiethanolamine	17, 77	
N-Nitrosodiethylamine	1, 107	(corr. 11,295)
	17, 83	(corr. 23,419)
N-Nitrosodimethylamine	1, 95	
	17, 125	
N-Nitrosodi-n-propylamine	17, 177	
N-Nitroso-N-ethylurea	1, 135	
	17, 191	
N-Nitrosofolic acid	17, 217	
N-Nitrosohydroxyproline	17, 303	
N-Nitrosomethylethylamine	17, 221	
N-Nitroso-N-methylurea	1, 125	
	17, 227	
N-Nitroso-N-methylurethane	4, 211	
N-Nitrosomethylvinylamine	17, 257	
N-Nitrosomorpholine	17, 263	
N'-Nitrosonornicotine	17, 281	
N-Nitrosopiperidine	17, 287	
N-Nitrosoproline	17, 303	
N-Nitrosopyrrolidine	17, 313	
N-Nitrososarcosine	17, 327	
Nitroxoline*		
Nivalenol*		
Norethisterone and its acetate	6, 179	
	21, 441	
Norethynodrel	6, 191	
	21, 461	
Norgestrel	6, 201	
	21, 479	
Nylon 6	19, 120	
Nylon 6/6*		

O

Ochratoxin A	10, 191
Oestradiol-17β	6, 99
	21, 279
Oestradiol 3-benzoate	21, 281
Oestradiol dipropionate	21, 283
Oestradiol mustard	9, 217
Oestradiol-17β-valerate	21, 284
Oestriol	6, 117
	21, 327
Oestrone	6, 123
	21, 343
Oestrone benzoate	21, 345
Oil Orange SS	8, 165
Orange I	8, 173
Orange G	8, 181
Oxazepam	13, 58
Oxymetholone	13, 131
Oxyphenbutazone	13, 185

P

Parasorbic acid	10, 199	(corr. 12,271)
Patulin	10, 205	
Penicillic acid	10, 211	
Pentachlorophenol	20, 303	
Pentobarbital sodium*		
Phenacetin	13, 141	
	24, 135	
Phenazopyridine and its hydrochloride	24, 163	
Phenelzine and its sulphate	24, 175	
Phenicarbazide	12, 177	
Phenobarbital and its sodium salt	13, 157	
Phenoxybenzamine and its hydrochloride	9, 223	
	24, 185	

Phenylbutazone	13,	183
ortho-Phenylenediamine*		
meta-Phenylenediamine and its hydrochloride	16,	111
para-Phenylenediamine and its hydrochloride	16,	125
N-Phenyl-2-naphthylamine	16,	325
N-Phenyl-para-phenylenediamine*		
Phenytoin and its sodium salt	13,	201
Piperazine oestrone sulphate	21,	148
Polyacrylic acid	19,	62
Polybrominated biphenyls	18,	107
Polychlorinated biphenyls	7,	261
	18,	43
Polychloroprene	19,	141
Polyethylene (low-density and high-density)	19,	164
Polyethylene terephthalate*		
Polyisoprene*		
Polymethylene polyphenyl isocyanate	19,	314
Polymethyl methacrylate	19,	195
Polyoestradiol phosphate	21,	286
Polypropylene	19,	218
Polystyrene	19,	245
Polytetrafluoroethylene	19,	288
Polyurethane foams (flexible and rigid)	19,	320
Polyvinyl acetate	19,	346
Polyvinyl alcohol	19,	351
Polyvinyl chloride	7,	306
	19,	402
Polyvinylidene fluoride*		
Polyvinyl pyrrolidone	19,	463
Ponceau MX	8,	189
Ponceau 3R	8,	199
Ponceau SX	8,	207
Potassium bis(2-hydroxyethyl)dithiocarbamate	12,	183
Prednisone*		

Proflavine and its salts	**24,** 195	
Progesterone	**6,** 135	
	21, 491	
Pronetalol hydrochloride	**13,** 227	(corr. **16,387**)
1,3-Propane sultone	**4,** 253	(corr. **13,243**)
		(corr. **20,591**)
Propham	**12,** 189	
β-Propiolactone	**4,** 259	(corr. **15,341**)
n-Propyl carbamate	**12,** 201	
Propylene	**19,** 213	
Propylene oxide	**11,** 191	
Propylthiouracil	**7,** 67	
Pyrazinamide*		
Pyrimethamine	**13,** 233	
Pyrrolizidine alkaloids	**10,** 333	

Q

Quinoestradol*		
Quinoestrol*		
para-Quinone	**15,** 255	
Quintozene (Pentachloronitrobenzene)	**5,** 211	

R

Reserpine	**10,** 217	
	24, 211	
Resorcinol	**15,** 155	
Retrorsine	**10,** 303	
Rhodamine B	**16,** 221	
Rhodamine 6G	**16,** 233	
Riddelliine	**10,** 313	
Rifampicin	**24,** 243	

S

Saccharated iron oxide	2, 161	
Saccharin	22, 111	
Safrole	1, 169	
	10, 231	
Scarlet red	8, 217	
Selenium and selenium compounds	9, 245	(corr. 12,271)
Semicarbazide and its hydrochloride	12, 209	(corr. 16,387)
Seneciphylline	10, 319	
Senkirkine	10, 327	
Sodium cyclamate	22, 56	
Sodium diethyldithiocarbamate	12, 217	
Sodium equilin sulphate	21, 148	
Sodium oestrone sulphate	21, 147	
Sodium saccharin	22, 113	
Soot, tars and shale oils	3, 22	
Spironolactone	24, 259	
Sterigmatocystin	1, 175	
	10, 245	
Streptozotocin	4, 221	
	17, 337	
Styrene	19, 231	
Styrene-acrylonitrile copolymers	19, 97	
Styrene-butadiene copolymers	19, 252	
Styrene oxide	11, 201	
	19, 275	
Succinic anhydride	15, 265	
Sudan I	8, 225	
Sudan II	8, 233	
Sudan III	8, 241	
Sudan brown RR	8, 249	
Sudan red 7B	8, 253	
Sulfafurazole (sulphisoxazole)	24, 275	
Sulfamethoxazole	24, 285	

Sunset yellow FCF	8, 257	

T

2,4,5-T and esters	15, 273	
Tannic acid	10, 253	(corr. 16,387)
Tannins	10, 254	
Terephthalic acid*		
Terpene polychlorinates (Strobane®)	5, 219	
Testosterone	6, 209	
	21, 519	
Testosterone oenanthate	21, 521	
Testosterone propionate	21, 522	
1,1,2,2-Tetrachloroethane	20, 477	
Tetrachloroethylene	20, 491	
Tetrafluoroethylene	19, 285	
Thioacetamide	7, 77	
4,4'-Thiodianiline	16, 343	
Thiouracil	7, 85	
Thiourea	7, 95	
Thiram	12, 225	
2,4-Toluene diisocyanate	19, 303	
2,6-Toluene diisocyanate	19, 303	
ortho-Toluenesulphonamide	22, 121	
ortho-Toluidine and its hydrochloride	16, 349	
Toxaphene (polychlorinated camphenes)	20, 327	
1,1,1-Trichloroethane	20, 515	
1,1,2-Trichloroethane	20, 533	
Trichloroethylene	11, 263	
	20, 545	
2,4,5- and 2,4,6-Trichlorophenols	20, 349	
Trichlorotriethylamine hydrochloride	9, 229	
Trichlorphon*		
Triethylene glycol diglycidyl ether	11, 209	

Tris(aziridinyl)-*para*-benzoquinone (Triaziquone)	9,	67
Tris(1-aziridinyl)phosphine oxide	9,	75
Tris(1-aziridinyl)phosphine sulphide (Thiotepa)	9,	85
2,4,6-Tris(1-aziridinyl)-*s*-triazine	9,	95
1,2,3-Tris(chloromethoxy)propane	15,	301
Tris(2,3-dibromopropyl) phosphate	20,	575
Tris(2-methyl-1-aziridinyl)phosphine oxide	9,	107
Trypan blue	8,	267

U

Uracil mustard	9,	235
Urethane	7,	111

V

Vinyl acetate	19,	341
Vinyl bromide	19,	367
Vinyl chloride	7,	291
	19,	377
Vinyl chloride-vinyl acetate copolymers	7,	311
	19,	412
4-Vinylcyclohexene	11,	277
Vinylidene chloride	19,	439
Vinylidene chloride-vinyl chloride copolymers	19,	448
Vinylidene fluoride*		
N-Vinyl-2-pyrrolidone	19,	461

X

2,4-Xylidine and its hydrochloride	16,	367
2,5-Xylidine and its hydrochloride	16,	377
2,6-Xylidine*		

Y

Yellow AB **8**, 279
Yellow OB **8**, 287

Z

Zectran **12**, 237
Zineb **12**, 245
Ziram **12**, 259

www.ingramcontent.com/pod-product-compliance
Ingram Content Group UK Ltd.
Pitfield, Milton Keynes, MK11 3LW, UK
UKHW051258180426
11947UKWH00020B/1786